Discovering Tuberculosis

Discovering Tuberculosis

A Global History, 1900 to the Present

Christian W. McMillen

Yale

UNIVERSITY PRESS

NEW HAVEN AND LONDON

Published with assistance from the Kingsley Trust Association Publication Fund established by the Scroll and Key Society of Yale College.

Yale University Press books may be purchased in quantity for educational, business, or promotional use. For information, please e-mail sales.press@yale.edu (U.S. office) or sales@yaleup.co.uk (U.K. office).

Set in Fournier MT type by IDS Infotech, Ltd.
Printed in the United States of America.

Library of Congress Cataloging-in-Publication Data
McMillen, Christian W., 1969–, author.
Discovering tuberculosis: a global history, 1900 to the present / Christian W. McMillen.

p. ; cm.
Includes bibliographical references and index.
ISBN 978-0-300-19029-8 (cloth: alk. paper)
I. Title.
[DNLM: 1. Tuberculosis, Pulmonary—history. 2. History, 20th Century. 3. History, 21st Century. 4. Tuberculosis Vaccines—history. 5. Tuberculosis, Pulmonary—prevention & control. WF 11.1]
RA644.T7
616.99′5—dc23

2014035013

A catalogue record for this book is available from the British Library.

This paper meets the requirements of ANSI/NISO Z39.48–1992 (Permanence of Paper).
10 9 8 7 6 5 4 3 2 1

For Stephanie, Maya, and Olin

Contents

Acknowledgments

The amount of help I received when researching and writing this book has been humbling—humbling because I needed so much of it and because I was reminded repeatedly how much in awe I am of the people working every day on tuberculosis and HIV. This project was a departure for me. Because of that I relied on friends, family, colleagues, and institutions to help me learn as much as I could about something I initially knew so little about.

I received financial support from the National Endowment for the Humanities, the Mellon Foundation (via a New Directions Fellowship), the Wellcome Trust, and the College of Arts and Sciences at the University of Virginia. Funding from UVA's Center for Global Health was instrumental in getting this book off the ground.

The research was far flung and in sources with which I was previously unfamiliar. I needed help. I did archival research in many places, and in each one accommodating archivists assisted me. Several deserve special mention, for without them much of the research would never have gotten done: Upasana Young at the UNICEF archives in New York; Marie Villemin and Reynald Erard at the World Health Organization in Geneva; and Guy Hall at the National Archives Atlanta Branch. Each of them went above and beyond the call of duty to help me navigate sources that were very hard to access. I have also benefited from outstanding research assistance. Chris Loomis gathered some materials from the National Archives, and Thomas Grillot did the same in Paris at the archives of the International Union Against Tuberculosis and Lung Disease. Richard Ambani's help was absolutely essential to working my way through the Kenya National Archives both while I was in Nairobi and from afar. Neeti Nair, a historian of modern India and my colleague in the history department at UVA, was a big help. I am grateful for all this help. The staff at UVA's Interlibrary Services, especially Lew Purifoy, also deserve special mention. They tirelessly tracked down what must have seemed like a stream of endless requests.

Many colleagues have read parts of the book, talked with me about TB and global health, and offered much useful advice over the years. Randall Packard's work was a source of inspiration. I've since come to know Randy and have benefited from our discussions—and his letters of recommendation! Sanjoy Bhattacharya, too, welcomed a neophyte into the history of global health and has been unflagging in his support. Erez Manela and I bounced ideas off each other and talked about sources on many occasions as we embarked on our respective histories of global health. Niels Brimnes's counsel and criticism have been priceless. For some years now Niels and I have been working in parallel on the history of TB in the twentieth century. When we realized that our research on and interests in India had converged, we decided to write an article together—it's been one of the highlights of my career. Our collective work is most evident in chapter 6. Niels has read most of the book, and his insights have been invaluable, as has his own work on the BCG vaccine. I am so pleased to have met Salmaan Keshavjee toward the end of writing the book. Salmaan read portions and offered very helpful comments. Rebecca Dillingham, now the director of UVA's Center for Global Health, has been a supporter of my work—and a good friend—for years. Two anonymous reviewers took extraordinary care with the manuscript. I am grateful for their comments and suggestions; I hope they recognize some of their work in the published book. Mel Leffler has been a friend and mentor since I arrived at UVA. I value his friendship and counsel immensely. Brian Owensby and Paul Halliday—good friends and colleagues in the history department—deserve thanks as well. And so too does Bruce Holsinger: he's listened to me talk about this book for years; he's read parts of it, and they're better as a result. Duane Osheim was chair of the history department during an especially trying time for my family. I am deeply grateful for his generosity, kindness, and understanding. I have now worked with Chris Rogers at Yale University Press on two books—thanks, Chris.

I made two trips to South Africa to learn about TB control in the era of HV/AIDS. I spent time with Tony Moll and others at the Church of Scotland Hospital in Tugela Ferry, KwaZulu-Natal, and with Gavin Churchyard and others at the Aurum Institute in Johannesburg. My aim was to see how those fighting the TB/HIV coepidemic work on a daily basis. It would be naive of me to say I have anything remotely like a complete understanding of the day-to-day challenges of controlling TB. I don't. But my two visits were immeasurably helpful in gleaning even a little insight. My observations, conversations, and encounters shaped much of the tenor and focus of the book. I imposed on many, many people. For their help with organizing my visits, for making me feel welcome when in South Africa, and for opening up their work to me, and in some cases their homes, I would like to thank Sheila Bamber, Stephan Lawn, Keren Middelkoop, Sheela Shennoi, Tania Thomas, Scott Heysell, Gerald Friedland, Tony Moll, Gavin Churchyard, Richard Chaisson, Jonathan Golub, Marianne Felix, and Amanda Miya. In this regard, I am also grateful to the Mellon Foundation. My New Directions Fellowship made it possible for me to take courses at Johns Hopkins in the epidemiology of TB and AIDS and funded my two trips to South Africa. The fellowship allowed me to learn about TB and HIV in a way I would never have been able to with conventional historical research funding. It provided me with an opportunity that changed the course of my research. For this I am grateful.

Finally, my friends and family. Brian, Paul, Bruce and Anna, Liz and John, Dodie and Allison, Risa and Rich, Sophie, Tico, Mel and Phyllis—these friendships sustain me. The unconditional support of my mother, Mary Ellen, my brother, Matt (who read and commented on the entire manuscript), and his partner, Clara, and my sister, Frances, means the world to me. My parents-in-law, David and Edie Tatel, too, have over many years now always taken a great interest in my work. But more important has been their love and support of my family. It's to my wife, Stephanie, and my children, Maya and Olin, that I owe my deepest gratitude. The years spent writing this book were tough ones for us all—and not least of all because of the book. Thank you.

Portions of chapters 1 and 2 were previously published in much different form: Christian W. McMillen, "'The Red Man and the White Plague': Rethinking Race, Tuberculosis, and American Indians, ca. 1890–1950," *Bulletin of the History of Medicine* 82, no. 3 (2008): 608–645, published by Johns Hopkins University Press, copyright 2009 by Johns Hopkins University Press, reprinted with permission. Portions of chapter 6 were previously published: Christian W. McMillen and Niels Brimnes, "Medical Modernization and Medical Nationalism: Resistance to Mass Tuberculosis

Vaccination in Postcolonial India, 1948–1955," *Comparative Studies in Society and History* 52, no. 1 (2010): 180–209, published by Cambridge University Press, copyright 2010 by Society for the Comparative Study of Society and History, reprinted with permission. I thank the two presses for allowing me to use portions of this previously published work.

Discovering Tuberculosis

Introduction

In the first two decades of the twenty-first century one billion people will become infected with tuberculosis. Two hundred million of them will live with active disease. By 2020, some estimate that thirty-five million of those will die; others think that it will be seventy million. History's most deadly disease remains so in the present and very likely will remain so in the future (see figure 1).[1]

Why? There's been plenty of time to learn TB's secrets and plot its demise. It's been a well-known human disease for millennia and has been well understood since the end of the nineteenth century. Its microscopic cause—*Mycobacterium tuberculosis*—was revealed by Robert Koch in 1882. A vaccine has been in use for almost a century. And antibiotics—drugs that actually kill the disease and cure the patient—have been around for more than six decades. They work.[2] Yet 1.5 to 2 million people, most of whom are in the developing world and many of whom also have HIV/AIDS, die of the disease each year. Like malaria, with which it shares its intractability and ability to prey upon poor people, TB has been and is again (finally!) the focus of attention. The World Health Organization's Stop TB Strategy addresses long-ignored problems like TB's synergistic relationship with HIV as well the ever-growing drug-resistant-TB crisis.[3] The Gates Foundation, too, devotes considerable time to the disease. And there's now even an international organization, the Global Fund to Fight AIDS, Malaria, and TB, that gives the disease a top spot in the pantheon of contemporary killers.

But in the developing world, especially sub-Saharan Africa, TB has never been under control (see figure 2). If you harbor the notion that at one

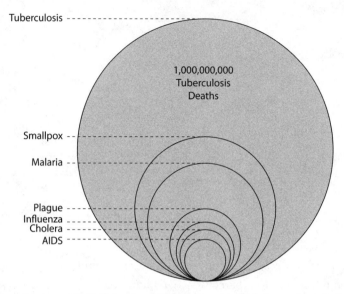

Tuberculosis

1,000,000,000
Tuberculosis
Deaths

Smallpox

Malaria

Plague
Influenza
Cholera
AIDS

Figure 1. Deaths worldwide from tuberculosis compared to deaths from other infectious diseases in the past 200 years. (From Tom Paulson, "Epidemiology: A Mortal Foe," *Nature* 502 [10 October 2013]: S2–S3, copyright 2013, adapted by permission from Macmillan Publishers Ltd.)

time TB was diminishing in force, abandon that notion now. We did not harness the disease and then let go of the reins; we've never even been able to hold on. One reads time and time again that TB is a treatable disease, that the drugs exist to cure it. With profound indignation people ask why, then, it remains such a scourge. It's true: the drugs do exist; they can work. They cure TB. All the outrage over the existence of a curable disease that nonetheless still kills millions is understandable, even expected. These theoretically avoidable deaths smack of a striking failure of political will and an almost deliberate disregard for the millions and millions of people at risk. It's sometimes hard to see things otherwise.

This book asks one question: why can't we control TB? It's mostly a historical book, and it looks to the past for the answer. Unfortunately, it's mostly about failures. By writing about TB control as a failure, I have not jettisoned alternative ways of telling the tale; there aren't any. To be sure, there is no TB epidemic in places such as well-off Western Europe, the United States, Japan, and Australia. And, miraculously, given the 1994 genocide and its aftermath—increased rates of TB, HIV, infant mortality, cholera—Rwanda has proved something of an African outlier. TB has been

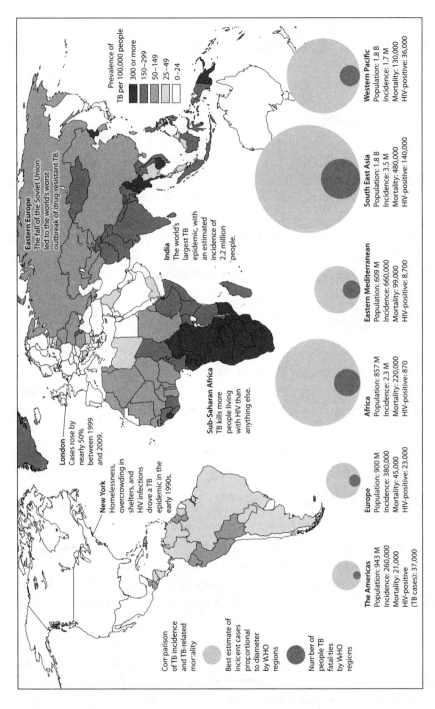

Figure 2. Tuberculosis around the world, circa 2012. (For source see figure 1.)

declining thanks to a government, donors, and groups like Partners in Health all committed to health equity.[4] But in much of the rest of the world not enough is being done, nor has enough ever been done, to control what is arguably the most intractable disease humans have ever known. For the better part of a century massive amounts of money and human energy, ingenuity, and dedication have been expended on this disease, with far fewer results than one would expect.

There is outrage and sadness in the world of TB control. In a relatively recent article in the *Bulletin of the World Health Association*, provocatively titled "Apocalypse or Redemption: Responding to Extensively Drug-Resistant Tuberculosis," the authors are refreshingly frank in their assessment of where we stand. "Drug-resistant TB, particularly the emergence of XDR-TB [extensively drug-resistant TB], is evidence of a new form of regression: we have taken the curable and made it nearly uncurable. The tendency has been to blame the most vulnerable and powerless—the patients who were unable, for a multitude of reasons, to follow treatment through to completion. It is time to recognize that we collectively bear responsibility for this. . . . If we cannot manage a disease as well known as TB, we have little justification to be stewards of the significant amount of resources given to health care globally."[5] In the biomedical literature such an admission is rare. It's a comment, of course, that a historian would find naturally appealing, for it reflects the way we think: human behavior, collectively and individually, is responsible for the predicament we find ourselves in. Which is this: We have had effective treatment for TB for more than half a century, and yet TB kills more people now than it ever has in the history of world.

The book unfolds in three discrete parts, each linked by a common concern: explaining why the decades-long effort to control TB has failed. The places, people, ideas, and developments I have chosen to write about—race and TB in East Africa, South Africa, and American Indian country from the turn of the twentieth century through the 1930s and into the 1940s; American Indian reservations, Kenya, and India in the years just before and the three decades after World War II; and the response of the World Health Organization, and others, to HIV/TB from the 1980s to the present—all have a particular place in the history of TB control and help to explain the disease's staying power. In the first part of the book I take up the question of race and biology and TB; this question was most vigorously debated using North American

Indians and Africans as subjects. When exploring methods of control, in part 2, it was on Indian reservations, and then in India and Kenya, where the pioneering work on the BCG (Bacillus Calmette-Guérin) vaccine and antibiotics was done. And Kenya is where one can track the emergence of drug resistant TB. Finally, in the last section, I examine the failure to get a handle on the HIV/TB coepidemic despite it being a well-known problem from the beginning of the AIDS pandemic. To look closely at the choices made regarding control strategies one must scrutinize the World Health Organization. And, again, as with antibiotics in the 1950s, 60s, and 70s, the pioneering research on methods of TB control done in the 1980s and 1990s—to the extent that there was any—was done in Africa.

This is a book in part on origin points, moments when things began. In this case, moments in the history of TB control when persistent problems emerged. But these are not problems of the past; they are not even past. As a historian I am of course inclined toward such moments. Historians like to figure out from where contemporary problems originate. My interest in doing so, however, does not spring solely from a historian's natural curiosity to discover something about the past. That impulse does certainly animate me. But much more than that I want to show how and when, and maybe even why, inertia and inaction set in, for example. To explain, very simply put, how we got where we are today. To do so I explore missed opportunities and show the tragic origins of contemporary problems as well as their at times profound impact on and place in the present.[6]

Discovering and rediscovering tuberculosis has been a feature of the twentieth-century history of medicine. The frank and brave assessment offered above of the multidrug-resistance problem and its human cause, this loud and clear admonishment from 2009, is not a new sentiment. Not at all. One only need look, as we will, to Kenya in the 1950s and 60s to see that it's a decades-old critique. Rediscovery is best illustrated by my chapters on drug resistance and the HIV/TB coepidemic. Drug-resistant TB is not, despite what one might see in the news, a new phenomenon. It's been around for decades. It was ineradicable by the mid-1970s. Problems like drug resistance and compliance on the part of patients, doctors, and others involved in drug delivery have been around since the beginning. And they've not been minor problems peeking in occasionally from the fringes. Drug resistance and compliance have been major international concerns since the 1950s. It is especially important to note that it was during the era of the greatest breakthroughs in TB treatment, a time characterized as an age of hubris and overconfidence, that drug resistance emerged as a problem almost impossible to control. HIV/TB is a newer problem. But it was a well-recognized one by the mid-1980s. TB is not newly out of control; it's never been under control.[7]

In thinking about repetition and rediscovery, about how there seems to be no historical consciousness in the world of TB control, I'm reminded of a scene Helen Epstein recounts in her book on AIDS in Africa, *The Invisible Cure*. Around 2005 Epstein found herself in Uganda at a conference organized by the Uganda AIDS Commission. After listening to one turgid presentation after another a USAID official at the meeting turned to Epstein and complained that no one knew how to do anything when it came to AIDS control. The official worried that all the money flowing in to Uganda would go to waste; she hoped to bring in some consultants from Brazil to show the Ugandans what to do. Epstein listened patiently. She then asked, "Why don't you speak to some of the Ugandans who worked on the AIDS program here in the 1980s?" After all, their approach has been universally recognized as innovative and effective. The official admitted she had not thought of *that*. Anyway, according to the official, "that all happened a long time ago."[8] It was history.

I have reached a point where I have been thinking about TB long enough now that I tend to forget that others haven't. It's front and center in my mind, and I assume the same is the case for everyone else. So it's always surprising to me—though of course it really shouldn't be—that when I tell people I am writing a book on TB common responses range from "Oh, I hear that's coming back!" to "TB? I didn't know *that* was still around." And I've yet to meet a soul who is anything but surprised by the synergistic relationship between HIV and TB. None of this is to say that these people are ill-informed, head-in-the-sand types. The opposite is often the case. When I explain things, they're generally shocked by both the magnitude of the problem and the fact that they knew nothing about it. Why?

Occasionally when talking with a friend or neighbor about what I'm working on someone will ask about polio—isn't *it* the true scourge of the developing world? "I heard that NPR series on it, and it sounds awful!" someone will say. It's true: polio is a terrible disease. Any reasonably compassionate person would wish it gone from the earth. In 2013, there were 406 reported cases.[9] Yet nearly twice as many children die before the age of one each year in Virginia, where I live; persistently high infant mortality in some counties is responsible for more death than polio in the entire world. The catalog of ailments that have a greater impact on mortality than polio is enormous. Yet the amount spent on polio eradication is staggering—well into the billions. The point here is not to argue for or against polio eradication—many besides me are already having that debate—or simply to point out that we live in a world of often confounding priorities, true as that might be. Rather, it is to ponder why TB gets so little attention and something like polio receives so much.

In other words: why on earth doesn't NPR do a story on TB?

TB has rarely been front-page news, certainty not in the developed world. It pops up occasionally. There was a great deal of noise about it in the early 1990s when drug-resistant TB threatened New York City. In 2005, when an American traveler returned from abroad and was discovered to have XDR-TB, the media was again briefly aflame. But otherwise TB gets virtually no attention. Commentators have lamented this for decades. "Tuberculosis is not a showy, 'tropical disease,'" noted the director of medical services in the Gold Coast in 1935, "and for this reason may fail to receive the public attention it merits. It is capable of killing throughout the length and breadth of the Gold Coast, and from a health standpoint is the most important problem for the future."[10] S. Lyle Cummins—of whom we will hear much more—lamented in 1939 that despite Burma having a tremendous amount of TB, most people in the country had no idea this was the case. It lay low because "no disease is more likely to escape public notice than pulmonary tuberculosis, because no disease is more insidious or better able to conceal itself behind an appearance of relatively good health."[11] Hugh Stott, a medical official in Kenya, acidly made the point in 1956, writing that "tuberculosis is not a 'headline' disease such as poliomyelitis, small pox or plague because of its insidious nature and chronicity; but there can be little doubt of the alarm which would be caused if 400 cases of any of these diseases, with a 33 per cent mortality, occurred annually in Nairobi."[12] TB was, and is, a deadly disease, but it kills slowly, with none of the drama of plague or cholera or the hideous disfigurement, so often seen in children, that polio wreaks on its victims. Different diseases elicit different responses, varying levels of panic and concern or indifference and neglect. These reactions often have nothing whatsoever to do with the actual threat a given disease might pose.[13] TB killed far more people in the nineteenth century than did cholera, but it elicited none of the same fears or attempts at control.

Interest in TB, as we will see, has peaked and plummeted, come and gone and come again. For decades—until about World War II—there was a great deal of attention paid to the question of race and TB among so-called primitive populations. But little was done to combat it. After the war, until the mid-1970s, TB was attacked like never before. The BCG vaccine, after being shown to be remarkably effective on American Indian reservations, captured the attention of UNICEF and the World Health Organization. Hundreds of millions of people were eventually vaccinated. The BCG vaccination program was the pioneer in the inchoate world of global health and led the way for other mass campaigns, like those against malaria and smallpox. Within a decade of the war antibiotics had been discovered and TB was attacked on two fronts: prevention and cure. But interest waned as priorities shifted, and by the end of the 1970s TB had become a neglected disease. Then came AIDS. And everything changed, again.

Tuberculosis is a resilient, powerful, protean bacterial infection. It can worm its way into any part of the body. It can be found in the blood and in the brain and in the bones. But what people talk about when they talk about TB is the pulmonary form of the disease. Being infected with TB is not the same as having active disease. TB can lie dormant; the bacilli can be, so to speak, at rest. It is this way in the vast majority of the billions of bodies around the planet that harbor the infection—an infection which was acquired at some point in their lives but which was not especially powerful or was fought off by a healthy immune system. Active disease occurs when the dormant infection is awakened or when someone catches TB from someone else with active disease. For example, a person with a latent infection who then tests positive for HIV, which subsequently develops into AIDS, is at great risk—the person's dormant disease is now likely to be woken up. That person, now with active, infectious TB, could cough near someone with no infection at all—and that bystander could become infected with active disease. These are the two ways people acquire active TB: someone's dormant infection is reactivated or someone is newly infected by a case of active TB. When infectious, TB can be highly so: singing, laughing, and of course coughing can spread the disease from person to person. (See figure 3.)

When TB wakes up and gets into the lungs, it eats them from the inside out, slowly diminishing their capacity, causing the chest to fill up with blood and the liquidy remains of the lungs. A wet, hacking cough is evocative of

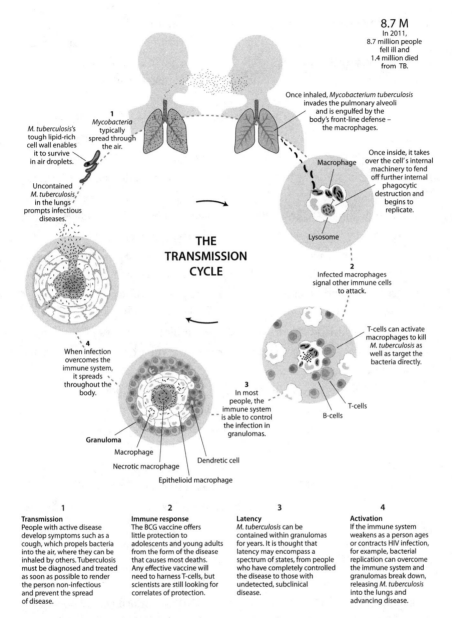

8.7 M
In 2011,
8.7 million people
fell ill and
1.4 million died
from TB.

Once inhaled, *Mycobacterium tuberculosis*
invades the pulmonary alveoli
and is engulfed by the
body's front-line defense –
the macrophages.

1
Mycobacteria
typically
spread through
the air.

M. tuberculosis's
tough lipid-rich
cell wall enables
it to survive
in air droplets.

Uncontained
M. tuberculosis
in the lungs
prompts infectious
diseases.

Once inside, it takes
over the cell's internal
machinery to fend
off further internal
phagocytic
destruction and
begins to
replicate.

Macrophage

Lysosome

**THE
TRANSMISSION
CYCLE**

2
Infected macrophages
signal other immune cells
to attack.

T-cells can activate
macrophages to kill
M. tuberculosis as
well as target the
bacteria directly.

4
When infection
overcomes the
immune system,
it spreads
throughout the
body.

3
In most
people, the
immune system
is able to control
the infection in
granulomas.

T-cells

B-cells

Granuloma

Macrophage

Necrotic macrophage

Dendretic cell

Epithelioid macrophage

1	2	3	4
Transmission	**Immune response**	**Latency**	**Activation**
People with active disease develop symptoms such as a cough, which propels bacteria into the air, where they can be inhaled by others. Tuberculosis must be diagnosed and treated as soon as possible to render the person non-infectious and prevent the spread of disease.	The BCG vaccine offers little protection to adolescents and young adults from the form of the disease that causes most deaths. Any effective vaccine will need to harness T-cells, but scientists are still looking for correlates of protection.	*M. tuberculosis* can be contained within granulomas for years. It is thought that latency may encompass a spectrum of states, from people who have completely controlled the disease to those with undetected, subclinical disease.	If the immune system weakens as a person ages or contracts HIV infection, for example, bacterial replication can overcome the immune system and granulomas break down, releasing *M. tuberculosis* into the lungs and advancing disease.

Figure 3. How tuberculosis is transmitted. (For source see figure 1.)

TB. The lungs now in liquid form are sloshing around in the chest. Cough that up—even in microscopic, impossible to see droplets—near other people, and they have a very good chance of getting TB too. Eventually, liquid replaces the lungs, the suffering patients cannot get enough oxygen, and respiratory failure occurs; they can no longer breathe and they drown. It's painful; it's drawn out. It's an awful way to die. But before any of this happens the disease weakens you, diminishes your capacity for work, and puts your family and friends—and anyone else you come into contact with—at risk. Individual death is only part of the problem.

TB is an ancient disease. Evidence of its antiquity comes from many parts of the world—it's been found in mummified remains in Egypt, grave sites in Europe, and in skeletons in the New World. It almost certainly originated in Africa, probably in the east, and left there when humans did seventy thousand years ago. It then further expanded its reach across the world, again as humans did, during what's known, rather aridly, as the Neolithic Demographic Transition—that period of extraordinary human population growth, settlement, and early agriculture.[14] It's possible that it's been evolving for three hundred million years. Though not exclusively found in humans—there are bovine and other forms of the disease—it is quite possibly the oldest of human diseases. Age, intractability, and prevalence—these are some of the essential characteristics of the disease.[15] It's a disease, too, as Helen Bynum has recently shown in her superb history of TB, that has been debated and pondered for as long as people have been writing.

Much of this history is fascinating. But what is most important for our story is what comes after the transition from what was known as consumption—by modern standards a vague term connoting a wasting, phlegmatic condition, rendering one's body weak, consumed by the disease—to tuberculosis—the single, infectious disease identified by the presence of the tubercle bacilli and only recognized as such in 1882. The transition did not happen immediately. When Robert Koch identified the source of the disease, previous notions of it did not all disappear overnight. Yet by the time our story really begins at the turn of the twentieth century the transition was well on its way toward completion. Ever since that transition occurred TB has been known as an infectious disease caused by the presence of the tubercle bacilli and passed from human to human. This modern way of seeing the disease has never, in any profound way, changed. Attacking the TB bacillus once it has arrived in the body or preventing it from getting there in the first place has been the focus of TB control ever since.

Many have written over the years about TB and offered explanations for why the disease has declined in some places and not in others.[16] As a historian I would consider it common sense that explaining the decline in TB in a given place must be done by considering many factors: a greater standard of living, especially adequate food and shelter; access to medical breakthroughs, especially antibiotics; and health and social policies that favor the improvement of the lives of those most vulnerable to diseases like TB.[17] All of these result in a decreasing risk of infection, and that in turn leads to less TB. It's become or remained a problem, conversely, in those places that foster it: places where access to drugs is limited and where risk factors like poor housing, malnutrition, and other health problems, such as HIV/AIDS, are abundant. The disease is complex, and thus it's no surprise that a variety of explanations help to explain why it's declined in some places and not in others. The general conditions that give rise to TB are not in dispute here. In addition, I am not arguing, naively, that biomedical approaches don't work or that poor countries, and thus poor people, should have access only to "appropriate technology," that somehow they are not up to the task of taking advantage of life-saving medical breakthroughs. Ideas about "primitive" peoples with regard to TB, or patients' inability to comply with medical regimens, as we will see, have done enough harm. I don't think waiting for the eradication of poverty is an adequate strategy for tackling tuberculosis. No one in the world of TB control, including the historical actors in this book, would dispute that stripping the world of inequality would drastically reduce the burden of TB. But that is not imminent, and so advances in biotechnology—a new, effective vaccine; a shorter, less toxic, antibiotic regimen; faster and more accurate diagnostic tools—should be, and are, sought, lauded, and supported. They are urgently needed.

This book, then, is not arguing against technological solutions to TB, nor is it suggesting that we wait for a radical change in social conditions for the decline of the disease. What the book offers are words of caution about persistent problems in the world of TB work, problems that date back to the earliest days. Ideas about who patients are, for one, are important. Race-based theories about who is and is not susceptible to TB have done, and still can do, great harm and have not been shown to do much good. Likewise, notions that patient compliance is at the heart of drug resistance are misguided and simplistic. So, too, is the notion that drug resistance itself is something new. On the contrary, its essential features have been known for more than half a century. Calculating cost effectiveness has the appearance of rationality and objectivity, but it can be, and has been, transformed into a rigid adherence to the single, cheapest solution at the expense of more nuanced and effective ones. Faith in a therapy or an approach can blind one to its flaws and prohibit the search for alternatives. Discovering what is old and calling it new is at a minimum inefficient and at worst regressive.

After all, what's at stake, of course, are the lives of millions and millions of people.

PART ONE
Discovery, 1900–1945

1. The Rise of Race

Where does TB come from? Who gets it and why? These questions have confounded researchers for decades. Over time, the answer has varied. In the past, researchers wondered if TB was native to Africa or the Americas, or among other populations alleged to have been cut off from civilization. Had people in such places had time to build up immunity—or was there really such a thing as immunity to TB? Then, as now, researchers thought that learning something about where TB came from, and how long it had been in a given area, might help them to understand its present profile. Wrapped up in the question of origins was, and is, the question of immunity. Immunity still captures the attention of TB researchers, especially as we begin to know more and more about genetics and interactions between genes and environment. But understanding immunity has eluded TB researchers for decades; its complexities plagued researchers in the past and still bedevil them in the present. And surely the most perplexing question has long been why TB lives latently in so many people—about two billion by current estimates—but only 10 percent of those develop active disease. Why is it that 90 percent of people infected with *Mycobacterium tuberculosis* never experience a single symptom? The majority of human beings appear to be "naturally resistant to tuberculosis." Why?[1]

The people who first mapped out the contours of the disease, debated its natural history, and explored its effects on different populations were in a position not altogether different from the one we find ourselves in today. As in the past, our knowledge of TB is undergoing change. Confronted by a disease old in nature but rapidly evolving, rapidly affecting populations for whom the disease was, if not absent, not common and certainly not well understood, TB workers throughout much of the twentieth century, just like their counterparts today, faced a lot of unanswered questions. For one, it's only been in the past decade, thanks to both the mapping of the TB genome and insights gleaned from molecular biology, that the evolutionary history of TB has come to be understood with a modicum of certainty. We now know that the differences between TB's various strains have important implications for disease virulence; genetic variation might even render some anti-TB drugs ineffective.[2] Also, it's now clear that the long-held view that humans acquired TB from cattle is in fact not true.[3] Just as TB forced those confronting the disease in decades past to devise new ways of thinking, so too are scientists, policy makers, and others now working hard to figure out how to control this still devastatingly deadly disease.

In one form or another the question has always boiled down to a debate over the influence of genes and environment. Is one more important than the other? Humans are of course products both of their environment and of their genetic heritage—and of course a person's or a population's genetic pedigree is in part determined by the environment.[4] In contemporary times there are those like Erwin Schurr, an expert on host resistance at McGill University in Montreal, who tend to favor genetics over environment. To be sure, when thinking about the disease, he attunes his analysis to the possibility that TB susceptibility is made possible by both genetics and environment—he notes that a person's exposure history might have an effect on that individual's genetic susceptibility in "extreme epidemiological settings." But genetics inches ahead. Schurr writes, "Tuberculosis is likely a fleeting target that depends on the specific exposure history of a population or a person. As shown, there are strong risk factors that can only be revealed in the context of gene-environment interactions, and possibly there will be instances when the environment overrides any existing genetic boundaries."[5]

To a historian, this last point seems obvious—of course the environment can determine one's risk of developing TB. Take two people with a similar genetic predisposition to TB (if such a genetic state exists); place one in an environment conducive to the disease, say urban sub-Saharan Africa, where the rate of infection and risk of exposure are high; place the other in a setting not especially conducive to TB, say an economically thriving, mid-sized college town in the United States, where the infection rate and the risk of exposure are low. Now, make one individual economically well off and the other not. Have one live in a single-family home; have the other living with ten others in a one-room apartment. One is well fed; the other is not. Now, keeping in mind that they are both genetically susceptible to the disease—but also keeping in mind that the person in sub-Saharan Africa more than likely is already infected with the bacillus and the person in the United States is not—increase the differences in their lives so that one moves ever closer to a low risk of TB and the other toward a high risk. Eventually, genetics will take a secondary role and the TB-friendly environment will take over in one case and the TB-hostile environment in the other. A genetic predisposition to TB will result in active disease only when triggered by the environment. It simply cannot be the case that the high rates of TB in India, China, and much of sub-Saharan Africa can be explained by genetics.

Looking to genetics to explain TB susceptibility is a wise idea, especially considering that vaccines could theoretically be directed at specific genes. And there have been such remarkable successes—as well as many setbacks—in treating some cancers at the molecular level that it only makes sense to do so with tuberculosis. We now know that the differences between TB's various strains have important implications for disease virulence and that genetic variation among strains might even render some anti-TB drugs ineffective.[6] It's possible, too, that researchers might find specific genetic reasons why a given ethnic group is more susceptible or less susceptible to TB; finding such a thing would aid in treatment.[7] What's more, whether or not human evolution worked that rapidly in conferring resistance to TB is open to debate, but at least some contemporary researchers argue that genetics alone could not have accounted for the decrease in incidence of TB in Europe—there simply was not enough time.[8] What many researchers argue now is that there are genetic associations that are ethnic specific, which might determine susceptibility or resistance to TB and thus might help with prevention and treatment. That is, there is the *possibility* that the genetics of a group has some bearing on its relationship with TB.[9]

But this is very difficult work. Adrian Hill, a prominent Oxford geneticist, noted when discussing predisposition to infectious disease generally that "analysis of the genetic basis of susceptibility to major infectious diseases is potentially the most complex area in the genetics of complex disease." Others agree: what makes some individuals, but not others, predisposed to TB is largely unknown. HIV researchers confront the same problem: because the immunology of the disease is not completely understood researchers are hard pressed to explain why some people appear to have natural resistance to HIV while others do not; developing a vaccine is also very difficult.[10]

But it is in explaining TB, perhaps more than any other disease, that we are most burdened by history. Those working on immunity to TB in the twenty-first century may be using new tools, but they are asking old questions. For more than a hundred years TB researchers have maintained a sustained interest in trying to determine just why some populations and not others succumb to tuberculosis. And that effort has left its mark on the history of TB control. No other disease before HIV/AIDS has so heavily relied on an interrogation of peoples' behavior and their bodies' ability to ward off infection to explain its prevalence and hold on humanity. As long ago as 1949, A. J. Walker, who was then a young medical officer confronting an uptick in TB in Kenya and who would become the director of medical services and a pioneer in TB control, wrote, "The mechanism of individual resistance has been studied perhaps to a greater degree in this disease [TB] than in any other."[11] Of course, explanations for its persistence are not solely couched in this way—whether a person or a "race" has resistance to it or not. Poverty and all it entails—overcrowding and malnutrition, most powerfully—explains a lot. Lack of access to good health care, too, fuels the disease's transmission. And exposure to the disease is of course more likely under these conditions. No one disputes these things; it's not hard to see why it's South Africa and not the United States that has a staggeringly high rate of TB. Yet, unlike with other diseases, malaria for instance, explaining TB's ability to become and remain one of the world's greatest killers has depended also on explaining its host, us. None of this is to say that understanding human biology and behavior is unimportant when looking at malaria or river blindness or cholera or measles. Of course it is. How could we explain cancer without resorting to human biology and in some cases behavior? Or develop vaccines? We could not. But that's not really the point. The point is that understanding TB's grip on some populations and not others has at times depended more on explaining them and less so on explaining the disease. *Those* people must have had the disease for *some* reason. What was it? Were some more resistant than others? If so, why? These questions animated TB researchers for decades, from roughly the turn of the twentieth century until World War II.

Before the era of antibiotics began in the late 1940s and early 1950s, initial work on TB in the developing world—and among indigenous populations in places like the United States and Canada—came in two waves. The first arrived in the early decades of the twentieth century (with data from the late nineteenth also trickling in) when conclusions about the disease were reached by speculation, anecdotal observation, limited clinical research, and the common wisdom of the times. Lyle Cummins—who did more than perhaps anyone to promote the notion of race-based resistance—might have been correct when he wrote in 1920 that "no disease has been more intensively studied than tuberculosis."[12] But when it came to the developing world and indigenous people, almost nothing was known; early assessments of TB among these populations were mostly guesswork.

Take a look at American Indians—a people who were the target of rampant speculation backed with very little data. From the time TB was identified as a major health problem among them—roughly the 1870s—race played a major role in explaining the TB epidemic. When Indians began dying and TB started to emerge as a regular feature of agents' and physicians' reports, racial, or hereditary, susceptibility was a common explanation. It was thought that susceptibility to the disease was built into their bodies, and more than one physician claimed, like the doctor among the Winnebagoes, that the "prevailing disease is tuberculosis, which is slowly, but surely, solving the Indian problem." And more often than not, when compelled to explain why, race was the reason. The physician at Yakama, William Coe, declared in 1887 that "their powers of resisting disease are inferior to any race of whom I have any knowledge."[13] Other explanations existed, to be sure, but that a belief in inherent susceptibility was the position of most Indian reservation physicians was made clear in 1904. After receiving and reviewing responses from reservation agents and doctors to a circular regarding health, the commissioner of Indian Affairs concluded that "the bulk of the evidence indicates that the Indian is more susceptible to this malady than the white man under like conditions." Children were especially prone. "A predisposition to tuberculosis unquestionably exists in the majority of young Indians, and the change from the freedom of the camp life to the crowded schoolroom and dormitory . . . acts as spark to tinder."[14] Woods Hutchinson, in 1907, summed up what many thought: "Resistance to or immunity from tuberculosis is a fixed characteristic of many races." Indians, especially, lacked resistance.[15] The following year, J. A. Carroll, the superintendent at the Mescalero Reservation, was blunt in his interpretation of what this meant: "An excessive mortality rate [from TB] is rapidly settling the Indian question at Mescalero. The causes of this deplorable state are varied . . . [but] the Indian's susceptibility to tuberculosis is well known."[16] Francis Leupp, the commissioner of Indian Affairs, thought that because they have "little immunity" Indians "like most uncivilized people [are] very susceptible to the diseases of the white man, especially tuberculosis."[17] That Indians were uniquely susceptible to TB was still a common belief into the 1920s. The tuberculosis committee of the National Research Council of Canada, in 1926, could confidently write that "it has long been known that Indians are far more susceptible to tuberculosis than are the White races of mankind."[18]

Like many ideas about American Indians these pronouncements arrived with little to back them up and represent more often than not a shared belief in the idea of the vanishing Indian—a well-known trope deployed ad nauseam in the late nineteenth century and well into the twentieth that suggested Indians were a dying race.[19] And while not everyone agreed—other early observers challenged what they perceived to be dubious racial explanations for the high incidence of TB—these were voices of dissent, decrying the common wisdom. In 1906, James Walker, the Pine Ridge physician, rejected race out of hand. TB in Indians was exactly the same disease as it was among whites. What's more, he wrote, "there is no inherent peculiarity of the Indian which renders him more liable to infection with tuberculosis than is a white man under like circumstances."[20] In 1910, Charles Laffer, the Warm Springs Agency physician, cast off easy racial explanations when he wrote that "tuberculosis has the reputation of being the most important factor [in the high death rate]. I no longer believe that the Indian 'is more susceptible' or has 'less resisting power' to tuberculosis than the white man. On the contrary, I am convinced that whites, living under similar conditions, would have a higher mortality and morbidity rate."[21] In 1923, the National Tuberculosis Association came to largely the same conclusion. The Bureau of Indian Affairs (BIA) had commissioned the association to do a nationwide survey of TB among Indians. Among its other findings—largely that TB was indeed a major killer and little was being done to combat it—was the following: "Those who believe that tuberculosis attacks without any racial preferences, but that the ravages of the disease are greatly influenced by unfavorable surroundings and economic conditions, and that the advent of the white man created a struggle for existence and subsistence which favored the development of the disease and that the red man, like the white or black races, responds to improved environments, will find in the following pages considerable evidence in support of this opinion."[22] It's true that any reader of the report would find evidence to support the notion that race-based explanations were at a minimum suspect.

Still, they prevailed. During the first wave of explaining TB's prevalence, common and conventional views on race colored most people's ability to explain who was struck by TB and why. The first wave was an era characterized by such things as an increased European presence in Africa and elsewhere, profound changes in American Indian life brought on by the wholesale movement to reservations and loss of resource base, and increased urbanization and migration across the developing world—all things that had an effect on rising rates of TB. In the first few decades of the century TB started to appear in places it had never been seen or where people had never looked for it. An explanation was necessary. Yet so little was known—in Kenya the best that could be said was that the "menace of tuberculosis remains vague but formidable"—that coming to any sort of definitive conclusion was all but impossible.[23] Yet, this did not stop many from making definitive claims. All the data most needed was the readily evident fact that TB *did* strike some people more powerfully than others. But to reason from effects to cause is of course going about things in the opposite direction.

It was not until the 1930s that a second wave of work on TB, characterized by thorough, systematic surveys, began. No fixed date separates one wave from the other, and thus there is some overlap between the two—some TB researchers, like the East African specialist Charles Wilcocks, produced work in both. But the differences are more important than the similarities. During the second wave sustained, systematic research carried out under the auspices, generally, of governments replaced forever a hallmark of the first wave—the lone investigator armed with scanty data making suspicions claims.

Despite the paucity of data, ideas born in the first wave wielded an enormous influence over those working in the world of TB for decades. Ideas from the first wave were not entirely washed away by the second. A few voices dominated the conversation, and their ideas were hard to overcome. Travelers' reports, histories, arcane medical texts, an old medical officer saying there had been little TB in the past and now there was a lot, very small-scale surveys, and autopsies—these were the sources for assessing TB before the 1930s. For decades, questions raised, but never adequately answered, in the first wave influenced TB research. One such question was whether or not

TB was, if not an entirely new disease, then at least one that had not yet wrought ravages akin to those in Europe. Wilcocks, who began looking into TB in Tanganyika in the 1920s, and who pioneered large-scale investigations in the 1930s, initially thought TB was a new disease. Based on reports that claimed 88 percent of Europeans and only 2–15 percent of Africans reacted positively to the tuberculin test (which demonstrates the presence of the bacillus but does not mean one has active disease), he surmised that TB was a recent arrival.[24] Others thought TB an older scourge. When the League of Nations published its report on TB and sleeping sickness in Africa, in 1923, the authors relied on the French researcher M. Kerandel, who had written the previous year that TB was not new in Africa. It was not a product of European colonization. It had been in Africa, particularly in the Sudan, for centuries and was spread by the caravan trade.[25] S. Lyle Cummins—of whom we will hear much more—surveyed a variety of "primitive populations" around the world in 1912 and surmised that TB had been present among some before contact with Europeans, but had never become endemic, much less epidemic. It took contact with Europeans for the disease to flourish. Using data gathered from several small surveys that employed an earlier form of testing for TB—the Von Pirquet cutaneous method—Cummins concluded, like Wilcocks, that low numbers of positives meant little exposure to TB.

Why was this an important question? There were those few who wanted to absolve Europeans of any responsibility for introducing the disease—if there was TB in the precontact population, then its presence was not the fault of civilization. Stephen Maher's 1929 inquiry into the origins of TB among American Indians set out to prove this very point and put to rest the "false doctrine" that the "white race" had passed TB on to the rest of the world. In Ontario, a Dr. D. A. Volume sent his paper "Tuberculosis and the Indians" to the Department of Indian Affairs, from where it was forwarded to R. G. Ferguson for his consideration as Canada's leading expert on Indians and TB. Dr. Volume's conclusion was the same as Maher's: TB was not introduced by whites; it had been in North America and prevalent among American Indians for centuries. Both Maher and Volume dug deep into historical sources for evidence of consumption or scrofula and found them everywhere. Volume's research in the seventeenth-century Jesuit Relations revealed, to him, a people plagued by TB.[26]

But most researchers, rather than trying to prove TB's ancient pedigree, thought that in its evolutionary history there might be clues to TB's virulence and thus to its control. A 1928 study of Mauritius came to the conclusion that the island's inhabitants—Indian, Chinese, and those of African descent—all possessed roughly the same amounts of chronic TB—or the "adult type" as it was then called. That acute TB, or the "child type," was rare led the author to conclude that each population had built up adequate resistance—the Chinese and Indian populations because of their history in tuberculous countries and the Creoles because of their roughly one hundred to two hundred years of contact with the disease. The Creole resistance was the takeaway point: a population, heretofore unexposed to TB, had built up resistance in historical time.[27] This conclusion, if correct and despite being based on a paucity of data modern researchers would likely consider insufficient, had important implications and speaks to what was really at the heart of most research into the evolutionary history of TB in the first wave: susceptibility. In the first large-scale examination of TB in an African country—Peter Allan's 1924 survey of South Africa—four factors were considered most important in the epidemiology of TB: the susceptibility of the different races and individuals to the disease; chances of infection and degrees of infection; resistance of infected persons to the disease; and economic conditions.[28] Allan, like others who followed, considered questions of immunity and susceptibility to be the most pressing. By trying to determine if TB was native to Africa or the Americas, for example, one might be able to gain clues to a population's immunity.

Had people in such places had time to build up immunity—or was there really such a thing as immunity to TB? Researchers in the 1930s finally began to get some useful numbers. What they found surprised them.

From the beginning of the twentieth century and continuing into the 1950s (it's of course impossible to date precisely the demise of an idea, but mid-century is pretty close) the notion that "primitive peoples" lacked immunity to tuberculosis—and other infectious diseases—was near universal. Not everyone everywhere thought it was true, but finding a population that was not, at one time or another, thought to be "virgin soil" is tough. And even if one did not subscribe to the theory, its prevalence in the first half of the twentieth century and its commonsense appeal were impossible to escape. In theory, "virgin soil" was a simple matter: if a population had not been exposed to a given disease then it was virgin soil for the disease to sprout in. In today's terms, the population was immunologically naive. But, like many theories, virgin soil too often ran into reality for it to remain so simple.

It's an idea that sounds reasonable (there's also, as discussed below, some truth embedded in its most basic principles). Imagine yourself, say in 1880, working for the Bureau of Indian Affairs and wondering why TB seemed to be so deadly. TB was still of course a major problem for the general population too, but Indians seemed especially vulnerable. Noticing this, and perhaps given to speculation on medical matters, you might have thought any number of things: Indian living conditions somehow differed, or, at a time before germ theory was commonly known or accepted, when diseases were thought to be "in the air," you might have thought they lived in a tuberculosis-laden climate. Or you might have thought there was something unique about Indians themselves. Given what you would likely have known about Indians (be it true or not)—that they had recently moved from the unrestricted life of the chase to the confines of the reservation and had rarely lived in what you would have considered civilized circumstances—you might have thought that they had previously lived relatively disease-free lives. Perhaps, like Washington Matthews, a prominent doctor and amateur anthropologist, who wrote in 1886, "'Idiosyncracy of race' and a score more theories, trivial and profound, might be advanced and shaken at the first question," you would have been skeptical of all explanations.[29] But if you wondered at all about the alarmingly high rate of TB among American Indians in the late nineteenth century—when the disease really latched on—there were a limited number of options available to you. And an explanation more obvious or appealing than virgin soil would be hard to come by.

Now, expand your horizon beyond North America to the rest of the world, a world in which you would have found many people in situations similar to those of American Indians. Think, as Cummins did, about all the populations who might fit a similar profile: high rates of TB combined with a presumed lack of experience with the disease, and, crucially, racial purity. Once you had surveyed the field it's entirely likely you would have come to the same conclusions as Cummins. He wrote in 1912 what he considered to be an epidemiological law: "That man, living under primitive conditions, is practically free from tuberculosis, and that man, when brought from a state of primitive existence and placed in contact with civilization, shews a very much greater liability to tuberculosis than does civilised man himself." Cummins went on to ask the question that would haunt TB research for the next forty or so years: "Whether the second of these propositions is a result of the first; whether, in short, primitive man owes his liability to the disease to the fact that, having no previous contact with the tubercle bacillus, he is, as it were, virgin soil for that organism."[30]

Virgin soil: it's evocative and simple; it makes sense. The term appeared in print as early as 1903 and caught on after Cummins first used it in 1912.[31] It quickly became a part of medicine's lingua franca. It's never disappeared. It jumped from medicine to other disciplines after Alfred Crosby published his seminal article "Virgin Soil Epidemics" in 1976. It's been a staple of American Indian history ever since. More recently, Jared Diamond's best-selling, Pulitzer Prize–winning *Guns, Germs, and Steel* gave the concept, if not the term, its most widespread exposure yet. Diamond made the central feature of virgin soil epidemics—a population's previous lack of exposure to a disease renders the population unable to resist it, and catastrophe ensues—a central feature of human history. The idea that populations, and not just individuals, are susceptible to disease became common wisdom. It works in some instances: there are populations—isolated, semi-closed-off, genetically homogenous—that have experienced virgin soil epidemics. Generally speaking these have been epidemics of such diseases as measles, whooping cough, and smallpox, diseases that have short incubation periods and that can kill quite rapidly—and that no population on the planet has developed resistance to.[32]

But when it comes to TB, virgin soil makes sense only when understood in the simplest of terms. What's more, when the term first gained ground in the early decades of the twentieth century it did so at a time when little was known about the disease. And just as important, the population most associated with the phenomenon—North American Indians—were far from virgin soil. That is: one of the most potent ideas regarding TB and "primitive" populations came into wide circulation when virtually nothing was known of the disease among those populations declared to be virgin soil. Men like Lyle Cummins, R. H. Ferguson, and George Bushnell dominated the thinking on TB among the "native races" during the first wave. And Cummins, whose influence is hard to underestimate, did his most influential work in the absence of much data. He formed his most influential opinions in the 1910s and 20s without the benefit of significant epidemiological research. We might wonder whether Cummins could really make the following claim in 1912: "It will be seen that there is reason to believe that the healthy adult who has grown up in civilised surroundings has, in ninety or more per cent. of cases, a demonstrable but isolated and harmless tubercular focus somewhere in his body, the African, under the natural conditions of his own country, is demonstrably free from such foci in 80 or 90 per cent. of cases."[33] Cummins seems to have had adequate data to support his claim for Europe; enough autopsies and Von Pirquet tests had been done to show that a large number of Europeans were infected with the tubercle bacillus. But did he have the data to make the opposite claim for Africa—that 80 to 90 percent of the population of the continent was virgin soil for TB? He cited a few papers, like one from French Guinea with a sample size of one hundred, and gave examples from his own explorations, but not research, in Sudan and Egypt. Such work—work based on scanty data—continued long after Cummins published his articles. In 1929, based on autopsy work that revealed healed tubercular lesions in only a small percentage of cases, another researcher claimed that the ability of Africans to resist TB was significantly less than that of Europeans. His sample size was small, too. Out of 176 autopsies, sixteen victims were found to have died from TB; among that number "healed lesions were rarely met with."[34] From a sample of sixteen a conclusion was reached. These small surveys do not add up to much—except a plausible-sounding idea.

Were Africans or other "primitive" populations virgin soil? Perhaps. But not until decades later was the research there to make the case one way or the other; a more accurate tuberculin test and the widespread use of x-rays in particular would call into question Cummins's assumptions, but they had not yet been invented. Cummins knew virgin soil was just a theory and might or might not be correct. But it caught on.

There is no doubt that virgin soil populations—ones untouched by a given disease and thus uniquely susceptible to it—have existed in historical and modern times. But the real question is why it is that these populations appear to not only catch diseases but also so quickly succumb to them. Cummins wondered this too. He wrote: "It is not to be denied, however, that uncivilised man usually makes a change for the worse in regard to his surroundings when he comes to or is reached by civilisation, but while this might explain his being as liable to tuberculosis as the civilised people with whom he mingled, it cannot account for his being much more so."[35] In other words, what was it about "primitives" that left them so vulnerable? Cummins and others acknowledged that Anglos, too, had suffered from TB, catching it in great numbers. They applied the same evolutionary logic to their forebears that they would come to apply to "primitives": susceptible individuals succumbed, and over time the "race" built up a collective immunity. Cummins was thus not necessarily arguing from a position of racial superiority; he acknowledged that at one time Anglos had had no defenses against the disease—and, in fact, some places, like parts of rural Wales, were still virgin soil for TB in the 1920s.[36] Over time, however, certain races had become "tubercularized." They acquired immunity. Cummins argued that races, not individuals, built up immunity. What this meant, among other things, was that Cummins and others considered some populations to be discrete enough that they could be considered a separate people, a separate race.

Cummins's notion of virgin soil was evolution at work in its baldest form. In the discussion of Cummins's 1912 article, "Primitive Tribes and Tuberculosis," Dr. W. A. Chapple, member of Parliament and prominent doctor, wrote what was perhaps the most Darwinian description of virgin soil. He did not think Cummins was looking hard enough at the level of population. "We must look at this," he wrote, "from a biological point of view, and consider the racial rather than the individual history. During generations of contact between the white races and tuberculosis there has been a dying off, in the early years of life, of those most susceptible to the disease. Being highly susceptible, originally they contracted the disease early in life and died off, leaving no progeny. Those less susceptible lived longer and left progeny, and these became the inheritors of a gradually increasing invulnerability." According to Chapple, primitive peoples' Darwinian inheritance was to live through "centuries of martyrdom" while their biology adapted. Removing the environmental triggers of TB—improving housing, cleaning up "bad air"—is well and good, but "you cannot remove that phylogenetic susceptibility" that primitive people possess.[37]

Chapple boiled down Darwin's central idea and applied it to TB. But Chapple did not base his conclusion on any research; it was based, rather, on casual observation. Again, this was all too common: reasoning from effect to cause. Fourteen years later Allan Krause, a TB specialist at Johns Hopkins and the editor of the *American Review of Tuberculosis*, wrote of such observations: "Out of a single fact numerous writers have built up a rather stiff doctrine that avers an exceptional lack of innate resistance of primitive peoples to tuberculosis. The basic fact is the common observation that the introduction of tuberculosis among less civilized populations is followed by excessive mortality. . . . The fact is conceded; the conclusion stated is not denied; yet it is submitted that it need not follow from the premise; and it is maintained that the premise does not prove it."[38] What troubled Krause was that a theory with little evidence to support it had become so readily accepted. Yet tubercularization and virgin soil only gained in popularity—and continued to be based on supposition. George Bushnell made tubercularization central to his 1920 book, *A Study in the Epidemiology of Tuberculosis with Especial Reference to Tuberculosis of the Tropics and of the Negro Race*. The rapid spread of TB in the Dutch East Indies confirmed for one researcher that the population was virgin soil. That American Indians were either virgin soil or had not become tubercularized was dogma by the 1930s; in Australia, too, no other explanation was available for alarmingly high rates of the disease among Aborigines. Based in part on what appeared to be a spike in cases, but was likely an increase in reporting in the Belgian Congo—a common phenomenon—another writer considered it incontrovertible, in 1935, that TB was a racial malady.[39]

The appeal of such ideas proved hard to resist. Despite misgivings, and admitting that there were no comparative studies of susceptibility to TB among American blacks, whites, and Indians living in similar conditions, the Cambridge TB specialist L. Cobbett was one among many who succumbed to the seductions of virgin soil theory. It just made too much sense. "When all the circumstances are duly weighed it seems to me that, though no conclusion is possible, it is nevertheless difficult to believe that the innate susceptibility of both Indian and Negro is not far greater than that of the white races in the United States."[40] Others succumbed as well. Charles Wilcocks, before doing serious epidemiological work, considered racial susceptibility to be the "accepted view," and assumed the "natives have less power of resisting infection." By 1921 South African doctors concerned with Rand miners accepted lack of immunity as the principal cause of TB among miners. And by the end of the 1920s virgin soil and tubercularization had become part of the lingua franca. While Cummins admitted that more research was necessary, his ideas caught on and cast a shadow over all subsequent inquiries into the epidemiology of TB.[41]

But what's so striking about virgin soil and tubercularization is that they are ideas that caught on at a time when little was actually known about the epidemiology of the disease among the populations who bore the brunt of the conclusions that these ideas sought to describe. American Indians, for example, were thought by many, Cummins among them, to be a prime example of virgin soil. Yet well into the 1930s the epidemiology of TB among Indians was so poorly understood that they could hardly be used as an example of anything definite about the disease, much less as a model of a virgin soil population. How could they be when complaints in the early 1930s regarding lack of data only confirmed what had been known for decades: nationwide, no reliable statistics, if any, were kept at all for the incidence of TB, or other diseases, really, among Indians.

In the early decades of the twentieth century, research on TB among Indians was elementary at best.[42] And when combined with rampant misdiagnosis and poor record keeping, leading to both overreporting and underreporting of disease, getting a true picture of the epidemic was all but impossible. Most health inspectors, physicians, and reservation superintendents were, like Walter West at Fort Belknap, ill informed about the incidence of TB. In 1918, West reported, in the characteristically vague fashion of all reporting on TB, that "there appears to be a large amount of tuberculosis and deaths from this cause are numerous." Others, like J. R. Collard, the BIA's special physician at large, lamented in 1924 that the "massive infection of tuberculosis among infants is frequently misdiagnosed as pneumonia."[43] Reservation superintendents, too, reported that assessing the health of Indians, in any systematic way, was all but impossible. Echoing others, C. C. Hickman from Yankton noted in 1931, with obvious frustration, that it was his belief "founded upon sufficient evidence, or lack of evidence, that . . . the health situation at this jurisdiction is even more acute than is possible to realize from any data that is now available."[44] And even though the district medical officer, M. V. Ziegler, knew it was high, when he came to survey medical conditions at Yankton he could only hazard a guess as to the incidence of tuberculosis.[45] The same could be said of the Warm Springs Agency, where, according to the agency physician, no TB survey had ever been done.[46] Others, like the superintendent at Rocky Boy in Montana, found that when they began to take a look at the incidence of TB in the early 1930s the numbers were "alarming."[47]

It was not until the 1930s that large-scale surveys were conducted. Montana was typical: it was 1932 before any effort was made to understand TB among one of the West's largest Indian populations.[48] The Southwest was the same: in 1935, L. R. Jones reported that "neither the death rate nor the incidence rate of the disease are known because of the impossibility of gathering data among these people."[49] In the Canadian provinces with large Native populations, fears were rampant that TB was spreading from Indians to whites. But as the authors of the first survey of Manitoba Indians noted in 1937 regarding the actual amount of TB: "Upon this point there has been endless speculation but no statistical knowledge to temper the impression that the Indian was still overwhelmingly scourged by the disease."[50]

No systematic TB surveys had ever been conducted, yet a powerful idea about Indian racial susceptibility was firmly in place.

That virgin soil caught on when there was so little known about Indians is remarkable enough, but added to this was another dimension: the racial purity of Indians. At a time when American Indians were becoming the archetypal virgin soil population was it even possible to say who was and was not a "pure blood" Indian? The BIA had been focused on this question for decades, meticulously attempting to assess the "blood quantum" of all Indians.

Blood quantum had the paradoxical effect of both hardening and softening racial ideas. It was, certainly, a mechanism for reifying the connections between race and disease. But using it—because of inconsistent and inaccurate reporting making it so hard to quantify and thus so problematic—also undermined in the eyes of TB researchers the connections between race and the disease. Bright-line biological markers of identity based on blood were difficult to find; attributing susceptibility to TB based on something so slippery as blood quantum was impossible. Further muddying the waters, some began to conflate culture, disease, and blood into a confounding matrix.

The BIA's commitment to categorizing Indians based on degree of blood had been in full flower since the 1887 General Allotment Act and the imposition of tribal rolls on Indian communities. From the BIA using blood quantum as a way to determine who was and who was not capable of holding private property to insurance companies denying services to Indians with high degrees of Indian blood, blood quantum made its way into Indian life.[51] And consideration of its effects on susceptibility to TB was a common feature of TB talk by the turn of the twentieth century—TB was "in their blood," as one commentator noted.[52]

Interest in blood quantum took on a new dimension in the 1930s as a consequence not only of the increased surveillance of TB. It also had a political component. The interest in, at times obsession with, blood quantum came as a result of the BIA's concerns regarding support for the Indian Reorganization Act and other New Deal reforms. "Full bloods," feared as less progressive than "mixed bloods," were mired in cultural intransigence and were a barrier to political change on reservations. In terms of "progressive" values, including support for the Indian Reorganization Act, starkly drawn differences between full bloods and mixed bloods, historians have shown, were a fiction.[53] Nonetheless, as TB researchers became more and more interested in getting an accurate picture of the disease they began, at the insistence of the BIA, to track its presence among Indians based on degree of blood. Indeed, at least one researcher noted how much could be learned about "race mixture and relationship to environment and health" by studying Indians of varying degrees of blood.[54]

Many found a direct connection between the amount of Indian blood one possessed and the likelihood of having TB: full bloods had higher rates of TB; mixed bloods had lower rates. In what he claimed was the first study of its kind, H. J. Warner, who worked jointly for the BIA and the U.S. Public Health Service, set out to discover whether or not there was a link between blood quantum and TB. He found one. While he allowed for the possibility that "social and economic factors" might also be at work, his research led him to believe that the "Indian has an inherent susceptibility to tuberculosis," as evidenced by the higher rates of TB among those with more Indian blood.[55] Esmond Long declared in 1937 that a "definite correlation exists between the tuberculosis mortality and the degree of intermixture with white blood."[56] This idea became so fixed that when epidemiological research revealed that a high degree of Indian blood did not correlate with TB on the Turtle Mountain reservation in North Dakota, James Townsend, the BIA's director of health, registered surprise, as it contravened conventional wisdom.[57]

Some, like Forrest Clements, who wrote in quite blunt terms about race ("No support can be given the idea that an increased pre-disposition, or increased resistance, to tuberculosis is inherited, and the notion of innate racial susceptibility to the disease is fallacious"), began to suggest that their culture explained Indians' diseased lives. Racial difference was not embedded in the body, he argued in 1931; innate racial differences did not exist. In his view, culture explained disease. "Racial differences . . . are for the most part reflections of differences in culture, that is, differences in housing, sanitation, medical treatment and economic and social conditions."[58] When research began to call into question racial explanations, but TB nonetheless remained highest among full bloods, an explanation was necessary. Two surveys from Montana, one in 1932 and the other in 1945, are illustrative. Both rejected strict racial susceptibility to TB, but both considered blood quantum. The authors of the comprehensive 1945 study declared that "no people have a racial characteristic which makes them peculiarly susceptible to the disease because of genotypic traits. Lack of exposure of any group, regardless of race, produces an extremely high incidence of tuberculosis." Yet because they found that TB was highest among those with a greater degree of Indian blood the authors suggested that there was something in the way they lived—poor housing, bad diet, lack of hygiene—that made full bloods more susceptible to TB.[59] In short, the "culture" of full bloods predisposed them to TB.

But when blood quantum began to be factored into the quest for the cause of high rates of TB, especially when combined with the paucity of good data discussed earlier, the issue of race became truly confusing, making clear to some that it was a useless category when thinking about incidence of TB.[60] For example, Charles Walton, in a 1935 article titled "Racial Incidence of Tuberculosis in Manitoba," found that misdiagnosis and overreporting (nearly half of Indian deaths attributed to TB were reported by nonphysicians), as well as poor record keeping were responsible for a fuzzy picture of the incidence of TB in the province. But what was responsible, too, were fuzzy ideas about race. That is, in cases where Indians were not obviously "full-blooded"—how that was determined went unsaid—there was no clear definition for who was and who was not an Indian, nor was there anything resembling consistency in calling mixed-race peoples Indian over, say, German or Italian. As a result, when the Canadian government tried to assess the TB problem among Indians "nothing [was] accomplished but confusion." Walton might have possessed rather rigid ideas about race, and might have believed Indians were a separate one, but this did not lead him to suggest that Indians, as a race, were more susceptible to disease. Ironically, it was the rather rigid ideas of the time—ideas that suggested the Irish or the Scandinavians, for instance, were separate races—that made it so difficult for Walton to assess Indian racial susceptibility to disease. He could not even be sure who the Indians were![61]

Assessing blood quantum was a confusing business. Indian agents, reservation physicians, and Indians themselves used different criteria for assessing both its quantity and value.[62] Joseph Aronson, until he was hired to lead the BIA's TB control unit, had had little experience with Indians, much less with the BIA's preoccupation with blood quantum.[63] Early on in his work, wanting to be thorough in documenting all pertinent epidemiological data, he wondered how precise he should be when calculating blood quantum. Writing to the director of health, he asked: "Will you please advise me how to classify the degree of blood of those who have more than one-quarter and less than one-half and more than half and less than three-quarters. I am anxious to have the classification which I am using agree with that which is officially used by the Department." Aronson was told to calculate down to the "sixteenths when necessary to express the proper degree." But what he was not told, and remained unclear to him, was just how one went about doing that! How did one determine if an Indian possessed one-sixteenth Navajo blood or one-eighth? What was the proof, he wondered, of someone being a full blood? The answer from the BIA: there was none. Blood quantum was simply accepted as stated at the time of enrollment on tribal rolls.[64]

But for many Indians, like the Arapahos with whom Aronson was working, culture, behavior, and family ties were more accurate markers of Indianness than blood. When people from other tribes, and in some cases whites with no Indian blood at all, ended up on the Arapaho tribal rolls a set of circumstances was created in which determining blood quantum for the purposes of discerning susceptibility to TB was all but impossible.[65] In the early 1920s, reporting from the Norway House Agency on the far northern shores of Lake Winnipeg in Manitoba, the agency doctor, E. L. Stone, all but gave up on the idea of race when he noted that after two and a half centuries of contact between Indians and whites "many have as much white blood as Indian."[66] Long-term contact, if not extensive "racial mixing," also characterized the Hopi reservation in Arizona, where Senior Physician Albert M. Wigglesworth also wondered about the tenets of virgin soil theory. After quoting at length from Maurice Fishberg's discussion of virgin soil in his popular and influential textbook *Pulmonary Tuberculosis*—which followed Cummins and Bushnell— Wigglesworth wrote that "possibly, however, the Hopi have been in contact with the white man for so long that none of the above applies to them"— meaning TB among the Hopi must be explained by other means.[67]

Stone and Wigglesworth were noting what many others did and would: even if virgin soil theory were sound—neither argued for or against it— American Indians in the twentieth century were not virgin soil populations.

Yet, with great tenacity, some still held to the notion of racial susceptibility. In the small fraternity of TB researchers R. G. Ferguson was one of the most important—when it came to race and TB he was second only to Cummins in influence. And as we'll see below, his influence lingers. Ferguson conducted research for many years in Canada. He did clinical work among Indians in Saskatchewan on the Qu'Appelle reserve—what he called the Qu'Appelle Research Area—and, rare for a doctor, researched the history of TB from historic records. His research was much more thorough and involved than Cummins's ever was, and it led him to insist, well into the 1930s, that race-based *inherent susceptibility* was the primary explanation for high rates of TB among Canadian First Nations between 1882 and 1926. Ferguson wrote that "to explain these indescribably fatal epidemics of tuberculosis among primitive peoples in known environments requires the admission of increased susceptibility to the disease [among virgin soil populations]."[68] His repeated claim that lack of immunity was the principal cause of TB was an impossible one to make; by that late date neither Ferguson nor anyone else was capable of factoring out poverty or malnutrition or overcrowding and posit one single cause.

Ferguson, like Cummins, was very interested in the problem of resistance. Unlike Cummins, he compiled data on the problem from both historical and clinical sources. He and his team scoured libraries; dug into the records of the Canadian Indian Department; wrote to old settlers; and tracked the disease in real time on the Qu'Appelle Reserve in Saskatchewan. His work began in the mid-1920s and by the end of the decade he had become so well known that William Charles White—director of medical services for the U.S. Bureau of Indian Affairs—declared Ferguson's data "so carefully laid out that I am sure it offers the best opportunity in the world today for studying the epidemiology of TB in man." White hoped Ferguson's work could be the basis for similar work in the United States.[69]

But it is important that we understand Ferguson's method. And not simply to point out that Ferguson was a wrongheaded racist bent on finding what he assumed was there, for that's not who he was. I actually think he was open, as far as he could be, to reporting what he found, even if it disagreed with his assumptions. Nor am I suggesting TB was not serious among the Plains Cree people he studied; it was, and it was devastating. Yet Ferguson's data had some serious flaws. For example, to determine that the rate of TB between 1884 and 1894 was ninety-five cases per thousand people Ferguson looked at vital statistics contained in the treaty annuity books. But he does not seem concerned with their veracity. Under the kinds of field conditions in which the records were gathered, as well as the well-known problems of accurate diagnosis and lack of complete vital records on Indians, it seems likely that the figures were, at best, a reflection of the problem rather than an exact rendering of it.[70] For instance, Ferguson reports that the epidemic's worst years came between 1884 and 1900 and that mortality was highest, overwhelmingly so, in children under five. But how does he know? It's well known that small children are more susceptible than adults to all manner of pulmonary infections; TB is of course among them. But far more common—and easily mistaken for TB—was pneumonia. Could there have been a pneumonia epidemic? It's possible. Also, why did this alleged TB epidemic so affect children and not the elderly or other nontubercularized people?[71]

What's also noteworthy about his work is that Ferguson, over and over again, resisted changing his mind about susceptibility. In this he was as stubborn as Cummins. Living conditions, nutrition, and infection control—all of these had improved over the decades. Yet Ferguson remained committed to the idea that Indians were simply more biologically susceptible to the disease than whites. In the early 1930s he proposed launching a large-scale study of health and disease on the Fort Qu'Appelle reserve. Fort Qu'Appelle had been the site of his TB research, and now he wanted to take a careful look at all aspects of Indian health. His goal was noble: if he understood all aspects of the problem, he'd be better prepared to solve it. The Indians were making progress, but their inability to resist TB still did not match that of whites.[72]

Virgin soil appealed to many, but not everyone. In 1933, the well-known TB experts Wathena Myers Johnson and J. Arthur Myers synthesized what was then known about TB in the "primitive races." They digested a good deal of what had been published about TB in so-called virgin soil populations and concluded that "numerous reports of great destruction among primitive tribes and races have been made, but in most of them no present-day methods of determining facts, such as the use of the tuberculin test, X-ray films of the chest, or even postmortem examples were available." In other words, most studies did not have enough evidence to back them up. But an absence of diagnostic tools did not prevent a series of, according to Myers and Myers Johnson, "absurd" views from gaining credence. But now, they wrote, real research "has begun to revolutionize our views concerning tuberculosis." The authors hoped that finally, untested, epidemiologically unsound ideas concerning susceptibility to TB in "primitive races" could be put to rest.

Rigorous research could begin, and a true picture of the TB epidemic among "primitive peoples," including American Indians—the population Myers and Myers Johnson singled out as having been the least understood and the most burdened by fallacious theories—could at long last emerge.[73]

In addition to the outright skepticism of Allan Krause and Myers and Myers Johnson, there was a simple lack of consensus. Before survey work was done there were a variety of opinions on African and American Indian susceptibility to TB. Kenya's director of medical services, C. J. Wilson, and W. D. Inness, director of medical services for the Gold Coast, were diametrically opposed on the question. While Wilson noted the extraordinary ability of Kenyans to resist the onset of full-blown TB, Inness lamented the ease with which Africans in the Gold Coast contracted TB and died.[74] The medical secretary of the Colonial Advisory Medical and Sanitary Committee notes in 1932 that the "freedom from tuberculosis is not an expression of inherent resistance of man living under natural conditions, it is due rather to lack of opportunity of infection with the tubercle bacillus."[75] Such differences in opinion were just that—opinion, for no good data existed.

Steadfast claims regarding the veracity of virgin soil were further weakened when more systematic research commenced. Almost universally researchers proclaimed, echoing Krause and Myers and Myers Johnson, their ignorance of the epidemiology of the disease. A major shift took place. What began to emerge from these studies was a more fine-grained picture TB—of where and whom it struck and why.

2. The Fall of Race

TB was a disease that bred much speculation. But what was really known about the disease among indigenous populations and those in the developing world? As we've seen, for decades, not a lot. But by the end of the 1930s that had changed. This was the decade of surveys. In New Zealand, Canada, the United States, Tanganyika, Sudan, and Burma, among other places, a clear picture of TB began to emerge.[1]

In New Zealand, an extensive survey of the Maori population revealed the seriousness of the disease to be, much to the surprise of the investigator, "alarming"; the Maoris were worse off even than American Indians.[2] The disease was a well-known problem among American Indians—and certainly much discussed—but there had been nothing but superficial epidemiological studies before the 1930s. And virtually nothing had been done to combat TB. Most of what was known about TB among Indians was anecdotal; little was known for sure. In late 1934, long after the disease had been labeled a major killer, the director of health of the Bureau of Indian Affairs (BIA), J. G. Townsend, wrote L. R. Jones, the doctor in charge of surveying the TB problem, and charged him with devising a solution. Townsend confessed that it was "a big order." But the bureau simply had to "attack . . . a health problem that heretofore we have neglected,— that is, as far as field studies are concerned." Jones's work was critical; Townsend needed to have an accurate picture of the TB problem. He suspected lots of TB but didn't really know, and if Jones could show this to be the case, then Townsend would have an "unrefutable argument in [favor] of expanding the [tuberculosis] program."[3]

37

Jones turned up more TB infections than anyone imagined existed—and a lot had been imagined. After testing more than seven thousand Indians in the American Southwest with an average age of thirteen, Jones found that about 75 percent tested positive for TB. On the Pima reservation, Joseph Aronson found that 100 percent of the population over twenty tested positive for TB.[4] In Canada, TB was responsible for 70 percent of deaths from communicable diseases and 29 percent of all Indian deaths in Saskatchewan.[5] Likewise, research done in Tanganyika—the site of more research than anywhere else in Africa—in the early 1930s led TB specialist Charles Wilcocks to conclude, "Tuberculosis has before now played a dominating part in the destruction of Native races, and in this country, the process would seem to have begun. . . . [T]hat it will be a matter of the deepest gravity may be taken as certain."[6] The Tanganyika Medical Department's 1932 report on tuberculosis sounded a gloomy note: the disease was ravaging nonwhite populations around the world, and the "American Indians and northern Eskimos are gradually becoming exterminated, largely through its influence."[7] Taking the tropics as a whole, H. Harold Scott, of the British Colonial Medical Research Committee, could safely report that tuberculosis was on the rise—and in East Africa was becoming a "menace."[8] Despite not having reliable figures, the director of medical services in Kenya claimed by 1945 that TB had become the number one killer in the colony—of 1,884 recorded deaths, more than 28 percent were due to TB.[9]

Figures like these—figures that showed the majority of a population was infected with the tubercle bacillus (though not necessarily afflicted with active disease) and many were dying—became common. What was happening?

Before the 1950s, TB was a well-known disease in Europe and Anglo-America, but it was not, as we've learned, well understood among "native" or indigenous populations. Almost no epidemiological work had been done; drug treatment did not exist; vaccine work was only just beginning. Despite the prevalence of the virgin soil theory and the confidence with which its proponents wielded it, modest declarations of ignorance peppered just about every report on the disease. After surveying district medical officers and visiting hospitals, C. J. Wilson, the director of medical services in Kenya, wrote in 1927 that one had to "admit at the onset the most unfortunate lack of knowledge of facts . . .; the aetology of native tuberculosis offers a fine field for speculation; but, until we have much more information, it is a difficult matter for scientific discussion."[10] Ten years later things were no different: the colony's Annual Medical Report for 1937 noted that the almost fourteen hundred cases recorded that year were "no reflection of the general incidence, which it is impossible to estimate."[11] Kenya was not an outlier. The deputy director of medical services for the Gold Coast admitted in 1928 that because figures were so hard to come by, "extraordinary differences of opinion . . . are to be met with when consulting various medical officers and past reports as to the prevalence of tuberculosis amongst the general population."[12] Joseph Aronson and Esmond Long, the two well-known American TB experts responsible for the BIA's TB control work, surmised in 1939 that the rate of morbidity brought on by TB in Alaska was the highest they had ever seen, "including those of the South African natives." But Aronson and Long, like so many others, hedged when it came laying out the numbers: "Here again, however, we cannot make a flat statement in the absence of any reliable records from the primitive peoples of the rest of the world."[13]

But things were changing. While TB specialists like Aronson and Long were reluctant to make any firm claims, systematic research on TB had been on the increase since the late 1920s. The picture was by no means complete, but there were large-scale surveys in several African countries, among North American Indians, and among the Maoris in New Zealand. The era of modern TB research began in these disparate places.

The foothills of Mt. Kilimanjaro, at about forty-five hundred to six thousand feet, have been home to different peoples for centuries. The north-facing slopes are dry and inhospitable and mostly uninhabited. But the west-, south-, and east-facing slopes of the mountain see enough rain and have fertile enough soil to have sustained people for hundreds of years. They are also places where there is abundant TB—a disease first uncovered in the mid-1920s by Dr. H. N. Davies, who ran a TB clinic and dispensary in Moshi. By the late 1920s Tanganyika's director of medical services characterized it as "the tuberculous bearing belt."[14] And within the TB belt Davies made an interesting discovery: TB was not a new disease, nor was this isolated region virgin soil. Before Davies's work it was thought that tuberculosis, in East Africa, was confined mostly to towns and coastal regions. The thinking went that at those places "the native was more in touch with infection from other sources, namely immigrant tubercle carriers, and that the indigenous population was practically tuberculosis free. But here we have the Wachagga and the Wapare, at a considerable distance from the coast, isolated from any recent reservoir of infection, living in the midst of a wide infective field. It cannot hardly be questioned that a total of 894 cases discovered under difficult conditions for investigation, in less than two years, at numerous villages throughout the districts investigated, is a definite indication of a long-established nidus of infection."[15]

Thus, what Davies had discovered in Tanganyika was not a virgin soil epidemic but, rather, a well-established endemic disease. His was the first discovery of its kind in Africa and began the gradual dismantling of the idea of virgin soil. The notion of the director of medical services that a "tuberculosis bearing belt" actually lay across much of East Africa at about forty-five hundred to six thousand feet raised the possibility that TB was not a new but a very old disease. Uncovering the TB belt, and realizing that the disease did not, at least in the case of a large part of Tanganyika, follow the virgin soil model developed by Lyle Cummins, prompted Tanganyika to apply for a Colonial Development Fund Grant to explore the disease's reach across other parts of the colony.

In 1930, in preparation for surveys to be carried out in Tanganyika, Sudan, and Zanzibar, the Medical Research Council put together a "Draft Scheme for a Tuberculosis Survey in an African Native Community." Many questions needed answering: Was TB was on rise? Was it an old or a new disease in Africa? How widespread was it? Whom did it affect and why? Where did it come from, and how long had it been around? And the council wanted to answer the following question: "Is there, or not, any unusual liability to severe types of the disease amongst the natives as compared with Europeans or others? . . . If a marked liability to severe types of tuberculosis is found to exist, it will be desirable to ascertain, as far as possible, whether this is due to inborn susceptibility, want of 'acquired resistance,' defects of native hygiene, under-nourishment, overcrowding, or to a combination of several of these factors." To answer this question one could look at how long it took someone to succumb to TB after initial infection. From autopsy records one could learn what types of tuberculous lesions were present at death—were they different in Europeans and Africans? It would also be important to look for healed tuberculous lesions because their presence would indicate an ability to resist.[16] If these questions sound familiar it is because the "Draft Scheme" was, if not written by Cummins, certainly conceived with his aid and influence.[17]

The Medical Research Council proposed to answer these questions through a variety of means. To determine whether tuberculosis was a "disease of old endemicity or recent introduction" the investigators would turn to history. They would search for references to TB in the accounts of travelers, soldiers, missionaries, and others. They would also ask the "natives." Was TB new or old? Were there songs or stories or myths in which TB figured? Was it a disease recognized by their "wise men or elders," by their "'Witch Doctors' or magicians"? Tribal history would be important too: What was the history of contact with outsiders? Were the people in question nomadic or settled? What was their "spitting habit and disposal of sputa"? The investigators would need to make ethnographic inquiries designed to determine "attitudes towards contagious disease and theories as to its nature."[18] They could also answer the question of TB's endemicity by looking at its present profile. Where and whom did it strike? Was it more prevalent "amongst the natives living close to government centers, military posts, trading stations, Missions, etc." than among those in "more remote and isolated native districts"?[19] In other words, did TB affect only those in contact with civilization or everyone?

There was—and would remain in various degrees for decades to come—an interest in looking beyond biology and at history and ethnography and related matters. Doing interdisciplinary work, in other words.[20] Unlike during the eradication campaigns of the Cold War, when the control of diseases like malaria was considered by many to a purely technical problem, those working on TB in the 1930s knew that much more than science went into understanding and tackling TB.[21] With very few exceptions, TB was never considered apart from the social and environmental circumstances in which it was found. That is, almost never would one find reference to the disease simply as a germ stripped of its human context. The "Draft Scheme" was clear on this. "It is hoped that the workers charged with the duty of a tuberculosis survey amongst African natives will make full use of the opportunity afforded not only for the investigation of tuberculosis as such but also for a study of the natives themselves, their ambitions, their limitations, their customs, traditions and possibilities." This was certainly the case in Tanganyika, where Charles Wilcocks led one of the first, and most thorough, surveys. Indeed, Wilcocks wrote early on in his research that "it will be seen that purely scientific research was not the main object of the investigation."[22] To what end was all of this ethnographic information collected?

The Colonial Development Fund hoped it would be "through the sympathetic adaptation of native ideas and methods to the uses of modern hygiene, rather than by the abrupt substitution of European regulations for native customs, that success is most likely to be attained."[23]

Within a year of dissemination of the "Draft Scheme" Charles Wilcocks was in Tanganyika, John Burrows was in Sudan, and R. J. Matthews was in Zanzibar working to learn the contours of the disease. Wilcocks began right away to look into a series of questions that had been at the forefront of TB work for a generation but had not been adequately researched. Among them was, of course, looking into the question of immunity. "The theory that tuberculosis in African Natives is a more acute and fatal disease than in Europeans is of interest, and an attempt has been made to determine if this is the case in this Territory. A subsidiary question is whether or not the Natives can be regarded as virgin soil, and to what extent they have been infected with the Tubercle bacillus."[24] From his tuberculin testing and inquiries into the history of contact with a wider world Wilcocks determined, echoing Davies's previous findings, that "the figures we have found corroborate the historical probability that this territory has been in contact with Tuberculosis for many years."[25] Four years later, Wilcocks declared, after conducting 13,313 tuberculin tests, that "no part" of Tanganyika could be considered virgin soil.[26] Matthews, in his report on Zanzibar, published in 1935, also strayed from Cummins. He wrote that the "prevalent view accounts for the marked liability of primitive races to tuberculosis by the theory of disease newly introduced to non-immune stock. This may be true, but it is scarcely to be regarded as finally proved."[27]

The work of Wilcocks and Matthews and others began to chip away at the virgin soil theory. By the end of the 1930s, many members of the small fraternity of African TB specialists had dismissed virgin soil. They embraced the notion that epidemic TB was brought on by the transition to industrialization and was, essentially, what we now call a disease of poverty. Even Cummins joined the chorus, comparing Africa, in his 1937 essay "Tuberculosis and Empire," to England at the "time of the arrival of Julius Caesar on our shores"; India was where England was at the "time of the invention of 'Spinning Jenny.'" The colonial empire was undergoing a radical shift as more and more people moved to cities and more and more people were doing the hard work of bringing Africa and India into the modern world. TB thrived in these conditions—conditions in which, so Wilcocks lamented in the early 1950s, "there is little care for human dignity in the life that breeds these conditions, and become, not so much individuals as units of production."[28]

One of the most forceful proponents of this new view was South Africa's top TB expert and soon to be chief tuberculosis officer, B. A. Dormer. Despite their still being in wide circulation, by the early 1940s he considered racial explanations for the high prevalence of TB bankrupt. "It is stated in all the books that primitive races are more susceptible and less resistant to tuberculosis than the so-called civilized people. The disease tends to run a much more rapid course in primitive people, and this is ascribed to a racial susceptibility or a racial lack of resistance. We are loth to subscribe to this, as in the South African Bantu in the Native reserves, there is the problem of the high rate of infection combined with a low rate of disease in the same area to explain away. Why do not the tuberculin positive Natives in the reserves (Transkei, Natal, etc.) die of the disease?" Race, Dormer and his colleagues emphatically stated, was not a factor in one's susceptibility to TB. "We believe that if we exposed Europeans to the same degree of malnutrition and sustained physical effort as Natives at a time when they were highly allergic, they would succumb to the identical type of disease."[29] This kind of thinking began to seep into other parts of Africa as well. Arthur Williams, who would soon go on to spearhead the first antibiotic trials in Africa, relied on the work of Wilcocks and Dormer to "effectively dispose of the 'virgin soil' theory, as an explanation of the ravages of tuberculosis in African communities," in a report he submitted to the director of medical services in Uganda at the end of 1945.[30]

By then a similar view prevailed in United States. James Townsend, director of health at the BIA, made a similar point when wondering about discussion of race in a recent paper comparing TB in various races. Rather than simply comparing races, "would not comparisons between races be of more value if we could in some way compare races at the same economic levels?"[31] In 1936, when Aronson began his work leading the BIA's TB control unit— work that would last nearly twenty years and eventually make him one of the world's leading experts on the BCG vaccination—he found the racial susceptibility argument compelling. It was not until he had begun what he called the "trailblazing project" of TB surveying and vaccination that he even *began* "to question the validity of the claim that the Indian is peculiarly susceptible [to TB]."[32] Four years later, after surveying thousands of Indians on four reservations and in southeastern Alaska, he and his colleagues concluded that social and economic conditions, or what they called "bionomic" factors, were responsible for the high incidence of TB. "The establishment of slum areas in rural districts, rather than . . . a peculiar racial susceptibility to the disease," they wrote, was responsible for rates of infection.[33]

Opinion was thus beginning to shift. But Cummins would not let it go. Two years after Dormer and his colleagues began the South African assault on virgin soil theory Cummins responded by flipping Dormer's conclusions. He claimed that black South Africans were, as Dormer noted, "highly allergic" to TB not because, as Dormer argued, the conditions in which they lived rendered them highly allergic but because they were biologically susceptible. Cummins simply refused to believe—I can, after a point, see no other explanation—that South African TB and European TB were the same disease and that there might be factors more powerful than biology at work.[34] Cummins's view also prevailed in other quarters in South Africa, such as the mining industry. Well into the 1940s, Frank Retief, the chief medical officer for the Witwatersrand Native Labour Association—the body responsible for recruiting mining labor across southern Africa and beyond—claimed that "in the native there is a comparative inability to develop acquired immunity, which in the European so markedly alters the course of the disease." The "low racial immunity" of natives led to an altogether more serious form of the disease in native miners than it did in Europeans generally. Like Cummins, Retief—who, it must be said, acknowledged that poverty, overcrowding, and malnutrition also contributed to TB's success—believed there was something inherent in the biology of those he called "tropical natives" that made them different.[35]

And so, of course, race did not disappear. For Cummins, and others (such as Lucien Hoebeke in his work on the Belgian Congo), race transcended all. Virgin soil had outlived its usefulness, to be sure; such populations no longer existed. Yet race remained, and Cummins was unable to look at other factors, such as overcrowding and malnutrition, as paramount; no matter how he calculated it, his common denominator was race. The notion put forward by Dormer and others that environmental conditions were more responsible than race called into question the essence of Cummins's beliefs. When, in 1935, he introduced the special issue of the British journal *Tubercle* devoted to the three Colonial Development Fund studies from Wilcocks in

Tanganyika, Burrows in Sudan, and Matthews in Zanzibar, Cummins allowed that Africans were capable of resisting the disease. "Under the familiar conditions of home life, the African native, so child-like in respect to mentality and outlook, appears to receive tuberculous infection like a child: developing a 'natural' type of disease in which the larval lesions, caseous and non-fibrotic, are well tolerated, provided no adventitious factor of aggravation becomes operative." But when risk factors, such as hard labor and "the excesses and self-indulgence to which these child-like, pleasure-loving beings almost always give rein when opportunity offers," were factored in, Africans developed active disease. In terms of their ability to resist active TB Cummins likened adult Africans to European children—both were equally unable to fend off active disease if the conditions were right. But Africans were different still. "For, behind the child type of tuberculosis seen in Africans, lies a real inborn lack of power to develop the resistance to tuberculous lesions commonly observed in Europeans." For Cummins, the balance of evidence "points to a biological dissimilarity in the average response to tuberculosis infection as between the black and the white races." Lucien Hoebeke, too, thought there was something essential in Africans predisposing them to TB that went beyond virgin soil. That is, virgin soil could be plowed over; race formed the bedrock. And something had to explain what Hoebeke considered a rising tide of TB. One of the essential differences that he considered was black skin. The sun's purifying ultraviolet rays could not penetrate it, thus denying blacks one of the benefits of white skin.[36]

Yet more evidence—scientific evidence—kept appearing that made Cummins's claims look less and less likely. Myers and Myers Johnson noted in their 1933 review of TB research among children and "primitive races"— the review that found so much research wanting—that many conclusions had been reached without the benefit of modern tools like x-rays. But by the early 1930s that was changing. Of special interest was research on healed lesions—research possible only with the widespread availability of x-rays.[37] And what this research revealed was fascinating. As early as the late 1920s, R. G. Ferguson was looking into the question of the relationship between healed lesions and resistance. And, as we've seen, while he did not shake off completely his belief in racial susceptibility—he wrote in 1929 that innate lack of resistance "appears to outshadow any effect of predisposing factors, such as food, housing, and sanitation, in survival and recession of the epidemic"[38]—he did, because the evidence was undeniable, come to believe that Indians were able to resist tuberculosis. X-ray evidence of healed lesions proved it. For Ferguson TB among Indians fell into two different types: acute and quickly fatal and found among those individuals not yet tubercularized; and chronic TB characterized by a quiescent infection in resistant individuals who appear to be able to resist TB much like the "older races."[39] Ferguson's work both buttressed and battered the notion of racial susceptibility. On the one hand, his research showed that North American Indians could resist TB; some individuals became infected but never progressed to active disease. On the other hand, high rates of active TB among Indians as compared to whites convinced Ferguson that there was a difference in the ability of the two *groups* to resist TB. The latter finding was, in the end, speculation, while the former—proving Indians could resist the active disease— was rock solid. And contrary to Cummins.

Ferguson was not alone. By the end of the decade Wilcocks was the leading expert on TB in Africa. It had been a productive time. Not only did he come to the conclusion that virgin soil could not be applied to Tanganyika, he also, more or less simultaneously with, but independent from, a number of studies on American Indians, made the more important claim, possible as a result of extensive x-raying, that Africans could resist TB as "efficiently" as Europeans. Having found "undoubted evidence of chronicity and protective reaction" in early work in Tanganyika, Wilcocks had suspected this was true since his work in the late 1920s and early 30s.[40] In fact, speculation that Africans could resist TB as well as anyone had been circulating in Africa for decades. In Kenya, several medical authorities claimed to have found both high incidences of infection but very little disease and many examples of Kenyans who had become sick and recovered. As early as 1910, when answering a general inquiry regarding the presence of TB among the Kikuyu in central Kenya, John Arthur, the doctor at the Church of Scotland Mission in Kenya, wrote that "it seems to me that there is existing in the Kikuyu people to-day an immunity to this disease and also that the germ itself is not so virulent as one would find it at home." The deputy director of medical services, in 1928, also claimed that Kenyans had unique powers of resistance.[41]

And when evidence of resistance was finally supported with clinical evidence at the end of the 1930s Wilcocks concluded that whites and blacks could, under the same conditions, resist TB equally. This was, as he put it, not only of "theoretical interest." It was a major claim with significant real-world value. If true it would contradict, and provide a useful counter-point to, an increasingly popular application of Cummins's ideas about acquired immunity and tubercularization that suggested that Africans, rather than benefit from control measures, would have to wait for evolution to render them resistant. As Wilcocks noted, his finding would give "ground for the hope that adequate treatment can be made effective, and that the alteration in the conditions of life and education, which is the subject of all public health work, can help to control tuberculosis."[42]

Others agreed. American Indians, according to those who had abandoned racial reasoning, could not be helped to overcome TB if it was assumed they were racially susceptible. H. F. Schrader, a doctor among the Blackfeet in northern Montana, had little patience with such explanations. "The idea has developed that [susceptibility] is a scientific characteristic of the Indian and very seldom do we hear that the Indian exposed to Tuberculosis under ideal conditions for acquiring and spreading [the disease] may have something to do with it." On the Blackfeet reservation, a place where the high incidence of TB in 1935 was "like a knockout blow on the chin," Schrader considered explanations that blamed high rates of TB on Indian bodies to be a barrier to treatment and prevention. Because Indians were exposed to TB under conditions most favorable to its spread, he concluded, the "notion that the Indian per se is unusually apt to acquire the disease should be discarded."[43] In a similar vein, Louis Dublin, a well-known statistician and frequent adviser to the BIA, wrote: "It seems to me very poor grace, in the light of these obvious facts, to pull in by the legs abstruse and unproved assumptions about the unfavorable genetic constitution of . . . Indians to explain away the bad health conditions that persist among them."[44] Alaska's territorial epidemiologist, J. A. Carswell, lamented the lack of reliable data on Indians and disease—too many laypeople misdiagnosing the cause of death, for example, skewed statistics—and its effect on treatment and prevention. To Carswell the preponderance of the evidence argued in favor of a very high rate of tuberculosis among the Alaska Native population. But race was not the reason. "Excessive and continuous infections with the human tubercle bacilli and undermined resistance" combined to ensure that tuberculosis ravaged Alaska Native people. Carswell did not suggest that Indians were unable to resist tuberculosis. He argued that Indians in fact had the same capacity to resist TB as anyone else, but that their ability to do so was diminished by malnutrition, overwork, and crowded living conditions.[45]

In Manitoba, one doctor reported in 1936 that "we have been accustomed to think of the Indian's lack of resistance to tuberculosis as entirely racial." But ideas were changing. Now, it had become clear, "there is no doubt that a great part of the Indian's low resistance to tuberculosis is due to his abject poverty. Like most other social problems this one is less medical than economic and educational."[46]

The claim made by these doctors, all of whom had considerable experience in TB-ravaged communities, that poverty was at the root of TB was almost the exact converse of claims made in South Africa by Cummins and the Chamber of Mines Tuberculosis Research Committee. In a country where evolutionary ideas regarding native peoples were especially well developed, the logic of tubercularization—that immunity to TB was a natural process unable to be speeded up unnaturally—was easy to apply. The Tuberculosis Research Committee downplayed the possible efficacy of control efforts, believing, under the direct influence of Cummins, who served as the committee's adviser and consultant, that tubercularization must run its course. Evolution could not be speeded up. In a climate where people were so prone to believing in race-based theories of disease causation, B. A. Dormer, South Africa's chief TB officer, recalled in 1956 that Cummins "sold" his notion of racial susceptibility to the Tuberculosis Research Committee.[47]

Charles Wilcocks claimed that *right now* Africans were capable of resisting TB; Cummins argued that this would not happen for generations. Until Wilcocks's work in Tanganyika and the several simultaneous studies of American Indian reservations, most believed that "primitive" peoples were not only highly susceptible to TB but also likely to die soon after they caught it. At the end of the 1920s, one TB authority in the Gold Coast wrote that all cases of TB he had seen "proved rapidly and invariably fatal."[48] But Wilcocks and the American Indian researchers found substantial evidence of healed lesions—strong evidence of an ability to fend off death from TB—that made clear this was not true. On the File Hills reserve Ferguson found in 1934 that a substantial number of children had evidence of previous tuberculosis, now healed, "indicating a pulmonary reaction approaching that of immunized individuals."[49] James Townsend, the director of health at the BIA, wrote in 1941: "It is our belief that the Indian race, as a race, is no more susceptible to tuberculosis than the white race. In other words, given the same low economic level malnutrition, in some instances, and poor housing, the tuberculosis morbidity rate among whites would more closely approximate that of the Indian. In the thousands of X-rays that have been taken throughout Indian county, it has been found that the pulmonary pathology in the Indian's chest is practically identical with that of the white tuberculosis subject. This picture shows a tendency to heal."[50]

Finding healed lesions, as well as evidence of chronic TB, signaled that "primitive" peoples were not doomed to die. This was a monumental shift in thinking. The revolution in ideas led Esmond Long to write in 1941 that although the "current conception until recently has been that Indians were unusually susceptible to tuberculosis" he could now cite a number of studies that refuted such claims.[51] And by the late 1940s TB researchers in the United States had reached an alternative consensus based on surveying and vaccination that involved tens of thousands of Indians—by the end of the 1940s, for example, more than twenty-eight thousand x-rays had been analyzed; seventeen thousand five hundred children were vaccinated in the spring of 1949 alone.[52] The epidemiological research carried out in the 1930s and 40s led Arthur Myers and Virginia Dustin—Myers was one of the giants of TB research at mid-century—to conclude in 1947 that "tuberculosis is simply a contagious disease. Wherever it is permitted to exist, it spreads to all races of people. Ideal conditions for its spread have obtained among the so-called 'primitive' human races. This fact has been largely ignored while tuberculosis workers have ascribed the disease to such poorly understood factors as low resistance, high susceptibility and lack of immunity."[53]

Though few would say so as boldly as he, Dormer declared in 1958 that the environment caused TB. At the British National Association for the Prevention of Tuberculosis conference that year he stated, "At some point or other in the battle of life one must 'nail one's colours to the mast' and I will do this here and now when I speak my conviction that if any nation with limited resources at its disposal, be they financial or human, were to put its money into good food for every citizen, proper housing for every citizen, clean safe water for all, proper disposal of sewage and waste for the whole community—it could safely ignore the ever increasing demand for the provision of expensive hospitals, clinics, physicians, chemicals, antibiotics and vaccines in the campaign against tuberculosis."[54]

And yet. While Myers and Dustin and the accumulated research of people like Wilcocks, Aronson, and Dormer made it clear to many that malnutrition and living conditions, for instance, were at the root of the TB problem among "primitive" people, the salience of race would not disappear. Late in his life Wilcocks reflected on this in his unpublished memoir. He wrote: "We (including myself), had the feeling of superiority to all coloured races, part-ly because we confused technology with intelligence. . . . We did not govern by fear, but by the thoroughly British sense of effortless superiority, innate in our race and largely due to our upbringing. We should know better now."[55] By the early 1960s, when Wilcocks wrote his memoir, most did know better. It did not get in the way of research or planning; no one used race to stymie work on TB control. Pondering the point had largely disappeared. Race, however, did occasionally creep in at the margins.

There were prominent voices, particularly in African TB control, who still considered race, if not critical, at least noteworthy. W. S. Haynes was one. He conducted the first survey of TB in Kenya in the late 1940s, opened and then ran the Port Reitz Chest Hospital in Mombasa, and was generally considered the doyen of Kenya TB specialists until the late 1950s. And while there's no evidence that race compromised his commitment to TB control—and committed he was—Haynes remained firm in his belief in racially spe-cific susceptibility to tuberculosis. For example, in 1959, when trying to figure out why Kenyans from Nyanza had less TB than Kikuyus from the Central Province, he could only offer a racial explanation. Because the "Nyanza tribes" were more isolated, he knew that their exposure history could not explain their relative immunity to TB and thus there must another explanation. But this was neither surprising nor a novel explanation; to the contrary: it was well known that some races simply had greater "natural im-munity." As Haynes noted, "It seems there really is a greater degree of natu-ral resistance to TB amongst them [Nyanza tribes] than amongst the purely Bantu. As in the UK, the English and Scottish have higher immunity than the Welsh or Irish."[56]

Nobel laureate F. M. Burnet, one of the century's most prominent bi-ologists/geneticists, was a firm believer in the genetic basis for differences in susceptibility to TB. In his formulation race came first, then genetics. That is, when writing about TB Burnet took the category of race as his starting point; race was fixed until certain conditions changed the genetics of a given race. For example, the "Red Indians" and the "Negroes of Mauritius" had once been hypersensitive to TB, but in a few generations that sensitivity gave way to resistance. Burnet's explanation was that "it is reasonable to believe that in a race free for many centuries from tuberculosis, genetic combinations associated with very low resistance to tuberculosis may appear and be transmitted widely. When tuberculosis is encountered and the conditions are apt for its free dissemination, bearers of such genetic combinations are selectively eliminated and there is a premium for survival of other combinations making for resistance."[57] Others, like F. Marian Macken, who surveyed Aboriginal TB in Australia in the 1950s, considered that "mixing of race by the addition of more resistant white blood is a good thing."[58]

Into the 1950s some TB workers used race as a way to explain the differing rates of TB in seemingly similarly situated populations. For example, J. C. Buchanan of the Medical Research Council, wondered why Indians and Fijians, two different races in his view, both living in Fiji, had differing rates of TB. Allowing that differences in lifestyle might account for the differences in TB rates—Fijians were afflicted more frequently—Buchanan noted that it *seemed* to him that the higher incidence of TB in Fijians was explained by Indians' "hereditary immunity." For some a racial explanation just made too much sense.[59]

But claiming that racial susceptibility explained higher rates of TB was just cover for not doing anything about TB, argued J. Tenret, the medical director for what was then called Ruanda-Urundi. Racial susceptibility had no basis in the truth, he claimed; the rapid progress of tuberculosis in Africa was best explained by malnutrition and poor hygiene.[60] This was of course Dormer's position. Others in Africa agreed. In the late 1950s, a former colonial medical officer in Nyasaland, A. C. Bruce Singleton, wrote a review of TB control measures in Africa and noted that in the past the "racial aspects" of the disease may have been overstated. Myers's work led him to see that TB in Africans and whites was really the same disease.[61] By the early 1950s ideas about American Indians, race, and health had been so shaken that two TB and public health experts declared that the entire category "Indian" had become so mired in confusion—in part as a result of the ever-shifting, inconsistent, and inaccurate, blood quantum reporting—that "for public health purposes and methods as well as in comparable disciplines . . . it has little value."[62] As those involved in American Indian health were beginning to realize, some in the global community too were discovering that worldwide there was no connection between race and TB. In 1955, Johannes Holm, the director of the World Health Organization's TB control efforts, declared that the disease was explained by conditions of poverty.[63]

The change in thinking regarding race and TB did not arise in a vacuum. To the contrary, beginning in the 1930s ideas about race more generally began to change significantly; immutable racial characteristics, many began to think, did not exist. At mid-century, Alfred Kroeber, the Berkeley anthropologist, wrote that the greatest achievement of the previous fifty years of cultural anthropology had been the profession's abandonment of race as a way to explain behavior; TB researchers were doing the same as a way of explaining disease. The 1950 UNESCO statement on race was the culmination of a half century of thinking on the subject. Culture—something that was in flux—came to replace race—something that was fixed.[64] At the time, TB workers and anthropologists rarely, if ever, had much to say to each other. But they were reaching similar conclusions: race was becoming a dull explanatory tool.

By the 1950s it was still possible to find, here and there, TB workers clinging to a supposed connection between race and TB. But mostly the connection had been severed.

Yet even now, in the second decade of the twenty-first century, race has still not disappeared. It turns out that the ideas developed in previous decades concerning virgin soil and racial susceptibility to TB have remarkable tenacity. In the past, the connection between American Indians, race, and TB had great explanatory power. To many it was self-evident that high rates of the disease must be caused by Indians' unique susceptibility or lack of immunity. Making that connection is still common. David S. Jones has shown how ideas concerning Indians as virgin soil—a term made famous among historians by Alfred Crosby in 1976—have been accepted uncritically by historians unable or unwilling to challenge medical research. It has become common practice, Jones argued, for historians to accept claims of "no immunity" without interrogating the meaning of the term or trying to understand the multitude of causes that make populations susceptible to infectious disease.[65] The easy acceptance of virgin soil theory with regard to TB is troubling because virtually none of the peoples affected by the disease could be classified as constituting virgin soil. By the end of the nineteenth century and the beginning of the twentieth, when TB first became epidemic, almost all North American Indians had had significant contact with the outside world. They were no longer living in circumstances that resembled precontact life—both prerequisites for virgin soil.[66]

There was not necessarily anything natural about their acquiring TB.

Virgin soil theory is not a thing of the past, nor is the search for racial susceptibility to TB over. A recent spate of research, some made possible with advances in genetics, makes it clear that the connections between race, TB, and virgin soil is still of interest. And what's troubling about some of this research, among other things, is the easy acceptance of outdated, historical ideas concerning Indians, and others, as virgin soil for TB. That is, outdated, overturned ideas are relied on in current research as evidence for the validity of virgin soil theory. To take one example, Ferguson's work on Canadian First Nations' experience with TB ca. 1880–1930 is routinely cited as proof that North American Indians were virgin soil for TB. But, as discussed above, the population Ferguson studied was not "virgin" at all.[67] Contemporary TB researchers make no attempt to take into account the context in which Ferguson's research was carried out—the ever-increasing marginality and ill health of Indians—nor do they question his methodology. One group of researchers considered Ferguson's study of virgin soil to be the one that "best characterized" racial susceptibility to TB among, according to the authors, "North American Indians"—a category entirely too large to have much meaning.[68] Another TB expert considered Ferguson's work to be the instance in which racial susceptibility to TB was "most strikingly observed." Indeed, he surmised that when the epidemic subsided and the death rate slowed down, this must have been because only those naturally selected for resistance to TB were left alive.[69] Still another recent paper has argued that Indian virgin soil TB epidemics—which, again, did not begin until the late nineteenth century—slowed down only "upon the elimination of susceptible individuals and survival of random resistant mutants." This paper's conclusions concerning Indians were also based on Ferguson's work—and based on that work the paper claimed that by the end of the nineteenth century the TB rate for American Indians generally was nine thousand per one hundred thousand. This is a misleading claim; TB never came close to reaching such proportions among most Indians. TB affected different tribes differently at different times. And, even more important, Ferguson *himself* never made this claim; he argued that on the Qu'Appelle Reserve in Saskatchewan the TB epidemic *peaked*, during an epidemic, at this number in 1900 and then steadily fell.[70]

Modern medical research into the genetics of TB immunity—and disease more generally—is concerned with ethnic/racial susceptibility just as

TB workers were in the early decades of the twentieth century. In light of recent discoveries in genetics, researchers have reopened debates (if they were in fact ever closed) concerning the connections between race and susceptibility to disease and demonstrate a continued interest in categorizing people by race—indeed, within the discipline of epidemiology race-based research increased in the 1990s.[71] Contemporary biomedical discourse surrounding race and disease continues to try to connect the two, echoing the earlier discourse on TB and Indians and perpetuating the naturalization of disease in various populations.[72] And while there may indeed be a genetic explanation for TB—some recent research suggests this is a possibility—the ethnicity of the populations affected varies so greatly—Han Chinese, Taiwanese aboriginals, Koreans, West Africans, Canadian First Nations, and possibly others—and the social history of mixing among the populations is simply not considered by most biomedical researchers that the groups' ethnic (or racial) makeup might be of little value.[73]

One particularly striking example of biomedical research not accounting for context comes from a 2010 paper. When reviewing the state of the field on susceptibility to TB, the authors made the following claim: "The idea that a genetic influence is present in susceptibility or resistance to tuberculosis has long been established and differences in susceptibility to tuberculosis in diverse populations were recognized even 100 years ago."[74] This is, to a historian, a problematic statement. While I do not expect that microbiologists will do historical research when writing about the genetics of disease, I do think it's entirely reasonable to expect a scientist not to commit elementary flaws in historical methodology *when employing history as evidence and pedigree*. In this instance, the authors consider that the age of the claim is what makes it valid. But they of course do not consider that ideas about race might have changed over the course of a century, nor do they interrogate the veracity of the original claim. From where did this conclusion come? A study from 1998 that validates its claim by citing work from the 1960s that cited Ferguson. What Ferguson showed was that a lot of Indians had TB; he made a claim about *those Indians at that time*; others observed differing rates of TB among different "races"; and in 2010 a group of geneticists can use this material as evidence for a claim about susceptibility to TB.

Of course, without taking into consideration the context in which massive numbers of American Indians acquired TB, contemporary researchers are making spurious claims. Imagine the following claim, stripped of all context, that might be made one hundred years from now: in the 1990s and 2010s rates of TB soared among South Africans; this shows that South Africans are uniquely susceptible to TB. This is a ridiculous claim, of course. But it's little different from contemporary geneticists, or whoever, making similar claims about American Indians in the past. This is not to say that there's no place for genetics in explaining susceptibility to TB. Indeed, recent work in the genetics of TB in Canadian French and Native populations argues that the bacillus spread, at very low levels, from French Canadian fur traders to Native communities from the early eighteenth to the middle of the nineteenth century. As time went on the bacteria percolated below the surface until environmental and social conditions caused it to boil over into active disease on an epidemic scale in the late nineteenth century—much like what has happened, as we will see later, with the reactivation of TB in HIV-positive people. The argument, in short, is that the epidemic Ferguson identified occurred not in a virgin population but in one already infected.[75]

Further complicating matters is the frequent conflation of race with ancestry: race (or ethnicity) becomes a simplification of and stand-in for the complexities of an individual's ancestry.[76] The genetic component of the search for TB's mysterious hold on some populations and not others might be buried deeper than current ethnic or racial identities are capable of revealing. Other work, based on geography and not at all on race or ethnicity, shows that there may be a connection between susceptibility to TB and helminthic infection.[77]

Continued research on both genetics and environment might advance the long struggle to combat TB effectively. It might not. Whatever the outcome of that work, the notion that American Indians' previously high rates of infection are proof of the existence of a genetically predisposed race, and the use of that idea as a historical pedigree for contemporary research showing a connection between race or ethnicity and TB, ought now to be discarded—as it was decades ago.

Despite all that was written about tuberculosis in the decades before World War II very little was actually done to combat the disease in the developing world. In part, this was because there was not much that could be done: there were no drugs to cure the disease, and a reliable vaccine was elusive. While most began to see the disease as a problem of poverty, they knew too that curing the world of its economic ills was not going to happen anytime soon.

Before World War II the major breakthrough was not biomedical. It was a change of outlook. Widely accepted, but not well studied, ideas about race and susceptibility dominated, and then they did not.

One consequence of this change in outlook was a major push to try finally to do something about TB among American Indians. Both a vigorous control program and a large trial of the BCG vaccine, the work among American Indians was a major break with the past and the beginning of a global move to tackle tuberculosis.

PART TWO

Control, 1935–1975

3. The Challenge of TB

Little that happened in the developing world in the decades before World War II could have led one to predict that in the early 1950s the recently formed World Health Organization (WHO) would make TB the target of what it called the "largest mass action the world has ever known against one single disease."[1] Or that by 1960 the WHO's Expert Committee on Tuberculosis would claim, because of progress being made in the fight against malaria, that "tuberculosis is generally conceded to be the most important specific communicable disease in the world as a whole, and its control should receive priority and emphasis both by the WHO and by governments."[2]

This new era—an era marked both by extraordinary energy, commitment, hubris, and discovery as well as by disappointment, frustration, humility, and resignation—started in American Indian country when, in the half decade before the United States entered the war, the Bureau of Indian Affairs began the first large controlled trial of the BCG vaccine. Publication of the results of that work coincided with the founding of the WHO and the push toward global development and the improvement of the world's health. After the war things moved fast. The year that the WHO targeted TB the director of the Eastern Mediterranean Office of UNICEF marveled at the "rapidity of postwar developments." Things were moving at such a pace, in fact, that he worried that "organizational success has been so great that it has been difficult for the progress in knowledge and technique to keep pace with this development."[3]

Take a look at Kenya. In the 1930s little was known about TB there; by the early 1950s the colony's director of medical services declared that "tuberculosis is now and is likely to remain the most difficult communicable disease for which to evolve a policy of prevention and treatment on anything like a comprehensive scale." He considered it "perhaps the most intractable public health problem in the country." According the East Africa High Commission, TB was "rapidly increasing" in all of East Africa. Paul Hutton and his colleagues at Makere University in Kampala, Uganda, warned that TB might become the "most important of the infectious diseases."[4] In 1950, when the East African Bureau of Research in Medicine and Hygiene, under the auspices of the East Africa High Commission, released a study that determined TB was on the rise in the region, the U.S. State Department thought that the disease presented a "sufficiently formidable problem to cause considerable anxiety."[5] TB could not be ignored.

And then, within a few more years, Kenya was the site of some of the most pathbreaking international research in TB—research designed to answer critical questions. Were Africans susceptible to the newly discovered TB antibiotics? Would the BCG vaccine work in "primitive" populations? Would anti-TB antibiotic drugs work in African conditions? Could cheap, but effective, drugs be developed and deployed in East Africa?[6] The answer to all of these questions was yes. In a very short time Kenya went from being a place where TB was little known to being the home to a wide-ranging and sophisticated international research agenda—research that would forever change how TB is treated. And, in an even shorter period of time, Kenya went from this vaunted position to being saddled with a serious drug-resistant-TB problem, a burgeoning, virtually impossible to control TB epidemic that would eventually become intimately entwined with a new, even deadlier disease: HIV/AIDS.

Mass TB control was rolled out very quickly into a world where knowledge of TB was hard to come by. With a few exceptions, little was known about TB in most of the developing world. In 1951, Hugh Stott, TB expert and a longtime resident of colonial East Africa, wrote the TB section of the East Africa High Commission's East African Medical Survey. Few had been more involved than Stott over the years in the control of TB in the region. Yet despite his expertise he found himself admitting that "little is really known about tuberculosis in the African and it is only comparatively recently that any determined attempts have been made to investigate the question on a scientific basis."[7]

TB control on such a scale was so new, so novel, that the WHO and UNICEF dreamed up the imaginary country of "Hypothesia" and designed mock plans for a mass campaign in this nonexistent South Asian land.[8] In 1953, the doctor who carried out the WHO's first African TB survey wondered in amazement at "how much the Organization and the world in general would profit scientifically and practically from such work in the 'terra incognita' of Africa."[9] The WHO leadership took note: campaigns against Africa's "traditional" diseases like yaws and malaria were, because of postwar economic development, beginning to "meet with success." Tuberculosis, on the other hand, was getting worse because of industrialization and the rapid change from rural to urban life. Yet so little was known about TB in rural areas that opinion ranged: some observers considered it "Killer No. 1" while others claimed "it is of little importance."[10]

Thus, the WHO and UNICEF launched what was to become the largest medical intervention in world history—the mass BCG vaccination campaign—and the Medical Research Council and the WHO set to work on pioneering antibiotic research in "Hypothesia" and "terra incognita." As we will see in Kenya, the health system was weak; shoring it up to manage the burdens of TB control was never done. Pushing quickly into places not ready to embrace and take full advantage of medical technology, however, was not limited to TB control, nor has this approach gone away. It's been a feature of malaria control efforts for generations: from the WHO's malaria eradication program, launched in the 1950s and dead by the late 1960s, to the more recent Roll Back Malaria campaign, programs to control the disease have been foisted upon places unable, because of weak health systems, to implement them properly.[11]

Still, in the 1950s and 60s especially, there was will and there was money and there was growing expertise mixed with hope and hubris on the part of planners. And so began the most productive period in the history of TB control known to the world before or since. The push to control TB that began in Indian country in the mid-1930s was a turning point in the history of medicine rarely seen. A disease that had seemed unstoppable was now, in the minds of many, finally up against two formidable foes: the BCG vaccine and antibiotics. In developing countries, however, resources were limited; so too was local expertise. For these reasons, among others, the WHO saw fit to devise, as early as 1953, "simplified, inexpensive, cruder techniques, equipment and institutions for tuberculosis control which will be more suitable for the actual conditions encountered." While realizing that "such methods will be less 'sensitive' than those used elsewhere, they will be realistic and thus far more effective. For they will be within the economic and technical possibilities of these countries and can be extended for large-scale, country-wide mass tuberculosis control work."[12] Thus, from the beginning reality tempered ambition. The search for the most "suitable" methods could mean many things.

American Indian reservations, India, and East Africa were of particular interest. Nowhere was TB taken more seriously, and nowhere were more resources directed at the disease, than in these three places. The Bureau of Indian Affairs in the United States began a TB control program and a large-scale BCG trial among the country's most TB-addled population. The Kenyan and Indian governments, UNICEF, the WHO, the British Medical Research Council (MRC), and to a lesser extent the International Union Against Tuberculosis (IUATLD) attacked TB in Kenya and India as in no other place. Experimentation, innovation, failure, enthusiasm, inertia, hubris, and humility—all of these things characterized their work. The American Indian BCG trial alerted the world to the possibilities of controlling TB in developing countries. The projects in Kenya and India pioneered many of the modern treatment techniques, such as mass vaccination, domiciliary care, and antibiotic treatment. Once interest was piqued the pace of research moved at such a rapid clip that only two years after Richard Neubauer declared Africa terra incognita, the secretary of health for Kenya noted that the "eyes of many of the underdeveloped countries of the world are on Kenya waiting for a constructive lead in tackling this tragic human problem."[13] Research on the efficacy of antibiotics in East Africa had become so routine by 1957 that one doctor involved in setting up early antibiotic trials confidently claimed that "the machinery is so well oiled in East Africa that we do not envisage any additional difficulties in getting the trial to run smoothly."[14] India, a country that before independence in 1947 was doing next to nothing about the disease, became, less than a decade later, home to the world's largest mass vaccine campaign—tens of millions of Indian children submitted their arm to the needle—as well as the site of pathbreaking research in domiciliary care. Kenya and India, and American Indian reservations before them, became living laboratories for testing TB control methods.

All of this work was designed to be exported. The American Indian BCG trial—for a time the largest and most influential trial—was not simply for domestic consumption: the world was watching. The chemotherapy research in Kenya, which resulted in shorter antibiotic treatment and cheaper drugs, was from the beginning seen as an export product. And the mass vaccination campaign in India was explicitly designed as a test case. The work among American Indians and in Kenya and India made clear that TB control was possible in the developing world. TB workers did not think of these places as simple stand-ins for other developing countries; their particular problems were considered at most stages of the research. But they were all considered proving grounds for novel TB treatments. The methodology developed in each place, it was hoped, could be applied elsewhere. Speaking of one trial planned for East Africa in 1956 a principal investigator at the MRC hoped that the "findings will be of considerable importance not only to the treatment of tuberculosis in East Africa, but also for undeveloped territories throughout the world."[15] Several years earlier, when writing about the BCG vaccine demonstration project in India, Johannes Holm, the director of the International Tuberculosis Campaign, wrote: "India is in a key position as regards BCG vaccination in the Far East. If a mass campaign could be successfully carried out there, neighboring lands would realize that campaigns were possible in their countries too. On the other hand, if a mass campaign failed in India, it would be most unlikely that other countries in that part of the world would embark on mass campaigns for many years to come."[16] In the mid-1960s, when planning future research projects, Wallace Fox of the MRC argued that by carrying out research in both places TB workers would be able to test what worked in the one place in the other.[17]

TB workers in both India and East Africa were keenly aware of what the others were doing—at times, they were even the same people: beginning in the late 1950s Indian TB experts, for example, spent months in Nairobi working with Kenyan TB experts. Kenya was the epicenter of TB research in Africa. For a time the WHO considered it to be the ideal place to train all of the WHO's fellows in TB work from South America, Africa, and the Mediterranean.[18] In 1964, Indian researchers in New Delhi published results of a new drug combination directly inspired by work done with similar drugs in East Africa.[19] Questions asked in one place were being asked in the other. But the answers could vary; finding a one-size-fits-all TB treatment regimen was never the goal. Thus, when the WHO and the MRC demonstrated, in 1959 in Madras, that domiciliary care could be as effective as hospital care, this did not mean that these findings would, or even could, be replicated elsewhere, much less in the general population outside trial conditions.

And TB workers at the time, like William Stott, the Kenya-based coordinator of the MRC trials, knew this. He wrote in 1959 that "it is certain that the methods used will have to vary from population to population."[20] Alternative methods had already been considered, for instance, in British Somaliland. In a place with a highly mobile, really nomadic, population domiciliary care was something of an oxymoron. Thus, UNICEF attempted to build what it called "TB hostels." These were temporary structures designed to accommodate Somalis' seasonal movements: "they substitute for the home, responding more to social than medical needs."[21] Several years later researchers in both India and Kenya found that thiacetazone worked well in Madras and East Africa but not as well in Bombay and West Africa. Thus the MRC embarked on a trial in East and West Africa, India, Pakistan, and China to determine just which populations responded to this drug and why.[22] There was, of course, a desire to be develop some sort of universal norms of treatment, treatment that could be applied broadly—why do otherwise? But TB workers were not trying, because they knew it was impossible, to flatten the world into an undifferentiated mass.[23]

The American Indian BCG trial that began in the late 1930s signaled the beginning of an extraordinary time in TB control. When the Second World War ended and the American Indian BCG results were published in 1946, three decades of pathbreaking work on TB control commenced. The BCG vaccine made its way around the world and into hundreds of millions of bodies; antibiotics cured TB. But it was a bipolar time, full of both lofty highs and deep, deep lows. For this reason, TB workers in India, Kenya, and elsewhere were never so naive as to be lulled into thinking they were creating, much less inhabiting, what has been called a "techno-utopia."[24] In public forums there were some, like the president of the East African Public Health Association, who cheered the victory over TB long before the game was over.[25] But in private—in correspondence, memos, meeting minutes, quarterly reports, and publications in specialist journals—most TB workers were worried. For despite the breakthroughs, despite the urgency most felt regarding TB, research was carried out in a "hand-to-mouth existence." Guaranteed funding did not exist, and by 1963 the MRC lamented that it was "clear that the research being carried out in East Africa is barely viable on the present basis."[26] Research sponsored by the WHO was in trouble too: donor nations, by the early 1960s, were already growing weary of spending more money on TB research and were beginning to place restrictions on their do-nations.[27] Halfdan Mahler, chief of the TB section at WHO, worried that should research in the developing countries be curtailed a tremendous amount of research potential would be lost.[28] The WHO and the MRC had moved into Kenya with high hopes and, for a time, a commensurate level of commitment. The projects were cause for celebration too. In 1963, the WHO and the BBC teamed up for a radio documentary called the "Right to Health" to commemorate the fifteenth anniversary of the U.N.'s Universal Declaration of Human Rights. TB control efforts in Kenya were show-cased.[29] But the commitment to TB work withered under financial pressures, institutional rivalries, and different visions of what TB control should be. By the late 1960s, Dr. Brandon Lush of the MRC found TB research to be in "near chaos"; the WHO especially had "too many cooks" in Kenya.[30]

Yet very little of this—the worry, the paltry funding, the specter of drug resistance—seeped into the history of TB, much less colored the opti-mism and hubris of some at the time. In public pronouncements and in the mainstream press, in the 1950s and 1960s especially, there was a buzz in the air about disease eradication and wonder drugs, beginning perhaps with Selman Waksman winning the Nobel Prize in 1952 for his work discovering streptomycin, an antibiotic that could cure TB.[31] And there was tremendous excitement over TB's new miracle worker, isoniazid, in the early 1950s; cov-erage of its Lazarus-like effect on tuberculosis patients was featured in pub-lications like the *New York Times* and *Time*. Was it now time to cheer the death of TB? After all, a cure had been found.[32] Isoniazid was not alone. Other drugs would be discovered too: over the course of about twenty years, from streptomycin in 1944 to rifampicin in 1963, with PAS, pyrazinamide, cycloserine, and ethambutol coming in between, this was the golden age of TB drugs. It was the climate in which infectious disease specialist T. Aidan Cockburn claimed in *Science* in 1961 that "we can look forward with confi-dence to a considerable degree of freedom from infectious diseases at a time not too distant in the future."[33] He went on to write a book about it: *The Evolution and Eradication of Infectious Diseases*. William Stewart, the sur-geon general of the United States, is even said to have claimed in the late 1960s that "it is time to close the book on infectious diseases, and declare the war on pestilence won."[34] Many in malaria control shared these views and were dedicated to technological fixes, inflexible in their approach, and unin-terested in local social and ecological circumstances.[35] Some believed medical technology would foment the leap from primitive society to modern civilization. Purposeful programs led by outsiders to fundamentally change the way people interacted with medicine were not uncommon. As Walsh McDermott, a prominent TB and international health expert, noted in the first International Lectureship given at the National Institutes of Health in 1963, biomedical research and interventions were crucial to what he called "planned modernization."[36] For McDermott, and others, "purposeful modernization," was "the major social movement of our times."[37] At the end of the decade McDermott had concluded that the technology available to control TB was so effective that this "is one of the few instance to date in which a major disease can be decisively altered *without* having to await improvement in the social infrastructure."[38]

Biomedicine was at the heart of the movement: formerly sick people made well could then become productive citizens. They would learn the benefits of modern, preventive, miracle medicine. And along the way, for example, they might resist communism and embrace democracy. In a 1954 memo entitled "Health Programs as a Factor in Accomplishing United States Objectives in Asia," Henry Van Zile Hyde, chief of the U.S. Public Health Service's Division of International Health, argued that the "mass diseases sapping the productive energies of the Asian population yield readily and rapidly to modern techniques. At the same time, programs aimed at the control of disease provide an almost unique vehicle for wide diffusion of the concepts and social technology of democracy."[39] Health was, of course, tied to economic development, too; until diseases like TB and malaria were controlled, the reasoning went, workers would remain unproductive and markets would lie untapped.

Alongside schemes to use medicine to modernize countries or to promote democracy was the push for disease eradication. While the push for eradication of TB was never adopted as policy, as it was for malaria and smallpox, some thought that the technology available to control TB, especially after it was decided that the BCG vaccine was efficacious and antibiotics were discovered, could actually eradicate the disease. In 1962, Fred Soper—famous for his efforts to eradicate malaria—declared that TB could be wiped off the face of the earth. When people finally accepted that TB "was no longer a social and economic but rather a public health and medical administrative problem," Soper wrote, it could be done away with.[40] Others, like Carroll Palmer of the U.S. Public Health Service and chief of the

WHO's TB Research Centre, and James Perkins, president of the National Tuberculosis Association, were not as convinced as Soper regarding the social and economic aspects of TB. But they, too, talked about eradication. Perkins challenged the WHO at an international symposium on TB to take on the task of tackling TB, just as it was doing with malaria.[41]

It's clear that some in the world of TB control were fixated on technology, dazzled by its promise, and hopeful that it would take care of tuberculosis. And it's true that after World War II narrow, biomedical approaches to disease control became dominant.[42] This is certainly, as we will see, what some were convinced was happening in India: techno-fixes were being offered instead of significant structural change. This constellation of ideas concerning medical modernization was part of the intellectual universe in which TB control was designed.[43]

But neither the mass BCG vaccination campaign nor, even less so, antibiotic treatment attempted, as some would argue for modernization more generally, to harness the power of the state and the power of technology to forcibly reorient traditional societies into modern ones.[44] BCG and antibiotics were not aimed at restructuring traditional into modern life. They both, to be sure, infiltrated daily life as a conduit for modernity. They both worked, though not necessarily purposefully or consciously, to reorient peoples' relationship to medicine. Yet, although BCG and antibiotics entered the bodies of hundreds of millions of people in the developing world, these two interventions don't fit into the conceptual framework that scholars have built up around modernization and development. Neither involved any large-scale social, economic, or environmental engineering schemes. In fact, home-based TB care worked best when daily life was interrupted as little as possible and people were allowed to simply carry on. Indeed, they are in some respects the opposite of modernization schemes, as they involved not even the attempt at large-scale social or economic engineering. Doctors, rather than patients, had to change their behavior. Soper—one of the principal architects of the postwar malaria eradication scheme—had no doppelgänger in TB control. His remarks regarding eradication, alongside those of Carroll Palmer—who was normally so sober—and James Perkins were not at all representative of the vast majority of those involved in TB work.

On the ground and in the field, and even, at times, at higher levels of planning, rather than be dazzled by the promise of new drugs and seduced into thinking medicine would make "primitive" people "modern," or that the technology of TB control would tackle poverty, many TB workers were, at best, cautiously optimistic—and more often they appeared, in the face of drug resistance, escalating rates of TB, and costs, to be frustrated with the lost promise of medical technology. In 1957, when addressing a joint meeting of the British and Scottish Tuberculosis Associations, Johannes Holm, the director of the WHO's TB office, warned those in the world of TB control that, even with antibiotics, there was still a long way to go: not enough was known about the drugs, and few TB workers had much experience with them. The WHO, he said, "is not so optimistic . . . [as] to believe that the availability of these drugs means that the problem of tuberculosis is almost solved."[45] The following year, P. D'Arcy Hart, in charge of TB research at the British Medical Research Council, reviewed the state of his art. Impressive gains had been made; antibiotics were becoming better understood. This was all to the good, as Hart recognized that TB "is paramount as an epidemiological problem in the underdeveloped countries of Asia, Africa, and South America." It is, in fact, "the principal infectious disease." But there was no bluster; there were no predictions of eradication. Rather, Hart admitted gravely that "inroads on its prevalence have hardly begun."[46]

A year later, once the MRC's East African work was well under way, little had changed: Hart imagined research in East Africa continuing indefinitely—there was, after all, no adequate mass treatment of TB, and "pretreatment isoniazid resistance continues to increase yearly as a baffling problem."[47] The European director of UNICEF declared, in 1962, that establishing "adequate tuberculosis control programs in these developing countries is no more than a dream, since even the most rudimentary organization for public health protection is lacking, and that tuberculosis control in these countries can only be considered within the framework of more broadly based and strengthened public health services."[48] And in Kenya, where Africa's most robust TB control program was running at full steam, Kent Pierce, director of TB programs, mournfully reported in 1961, that after five years of hard work, "it cannot be claimed with any degree of confidence that the problem shows signs of diminishing."[49]

If one were looking for a much more realistic and well-thought-out prognosis in the annals of eradication literature one could do no better than Georges Canetti's. In 1962, Canetti, a prominent French TB researcher at the Pasteur Institute in Paris, published a landmark article outlining the hurdles that needed to be jumped over before anything approaching eradication could be achieved. Eradication, according to Canetti, meant "literally the total suppression of the disease." While this was a noble goal—who would not want to achieve it?—Canetti was no Fred Soper. "Eradication," Canetti cautioned in the very first few sentences, "cannot be discussed as a realistic possibility, that is to say as an objective that can be achieved in the relatively near future, except in certain rare countries in which the reduction of endemic tuberculosis is very advanced and the anti-tuberculosis organization particularly effective." Which was to say: nowhere in the developing world. Malnourishment and what Canetti called "super infections" with TB and other diseases made eradication a distant possibility. So, too, did the problem of resistance, warfare, and migration. Canetti knew that if eradication is truly a goal, to achieve it "there is one absolute priority: the perfecting of chemotherapeutic methods adapted to conditions of 'developing' countries."[50] This, as we will see, was the priority of the MRC and the WHO in East Africa and India. But they never spoke of eradication, nor did most others. Canetti might have used the word eradication but the conclusions he reached certainly don't help flesh out the caricature of the era.

Hope and despair characterize the era. Hope fueled by the technology available, and despair brought on by the difficulties of getting that technology to work in the real world. It's on American Indian reservations, in India, and in Kenya where both promise and failure are most vividly on display. But hope is not the same thing as hubris, and despair is not the same thing as resignation. Having hope did not mean doctors thumped their chests as they chased TB back into the ground; and despair did not mean they gave up, resigning themselves to defeat. Most in the world of TB control were well aware of the formidable challenges they faced. They did not think infectious diseases were becoming a thing of the past; they were not under the sway of technology.[51] The Fred Sopers, the MacFarlane Burnets, and the T. Aidan Cockburns of the world of disease control might have crowed about ridding the world of infectious disease, confident in their claims that the scourge of contagion was becoming a thing of the past. But spend some time with Wallace Fox or Pierce Kent, the director of TB services in Kenya. They would have found Soper's or Cockburn's optimism misguided, even naive.

The chapters that follow are detailed examinations of the challenges of controlling tuberculosis that look at the American Indian BCG trial; the spread of the vaccine around the globe; and the considerable challenge of making antibiotics work in the real world. They tell a story that will reorient historical thinking on the history of tuberculosis. There were breakthroughs, to be sure. Antibiotics worked. The BCG vaccine showed promise. And there was commitment from the Bureau of Indian Affairs, the WHO, the British Medical Research Council, UNICEF, the Kenyan government, and others. Yet BCG was found wanting; antibiotics proved hard to control; and institutional commitments waned. Paradoxically, the period of greatest scientific progress and most robust institutional engagement in the fight against TB was also the time when the disease became more and more difficult to control.

4. Preventing TB
American Indians and the BCG Vaccine

As the notion that American Indians were uniquely susceptible to TB began to fade, as people like Joseph Aronson began to see that the disease wreaked such havoc not for racial but for economic reasons, TB control among American Indians was revolutionized. It happened in a very short time. During what's come to be called the Indian New Deal—a period from 1933 to the Second World War when almost all aspects of Indian affairs were turned upside down—tuberculosis control efforts in Indian country were completely overhauled. For the first time TB was taken seriously. During the tenure of Commissioner of Indian Affairs John Collier, keeping Indians healthy became a priority. It's hard to overstate the importance of the almost overnight change in outlook regarding Indian affairs. For those in TB work, like L. R. Jones, the first "special physician" in charge of TB at the Bureau of Indian Affairs (BIA), it was about time. From where Jones stood, "tuberculosis is still the greatest of evils [with] which we will have to contend." He went on to cite alarming figures—prevalence among Indians in the early 1930s was fifteen and twenty times that among the white population in Montana, for instance—to convince anyone who "entertain[s] the slightest doubt that this disease is still the greatest reaper among the Indian population." Convincing people of this, Jones worried, would not be easy. His first task, then, was to make certain that Indian Service employees became "tuberculosis minded." (That they were not already is symbolic of the state of affairs.) Jones aimed to focus on children, for they could be saved; it was too late for the present generation.[1]

But before anything could be done, something more needed to be known about TB. As we've seen, not knowing much about the disease did not stop ideas about Indians and race and TB from hardening into dogma despite little data. But a control program would fail utterly if such a situation were allowed to continue. Some knew this. In 1928, the Institute for Government Research (now the Brookings Institution) released *The Problem of Indian Administration* (commonly referred to as the Meriam Report, after its principal author). The Meriam Report considered the paucity of data on Indian health to be one of the BIA's most significant failures, going so far as to say that it was "absolutely impossible to effectively plan or direct a constructive health program" without adequate data.[2] Those in the field came to the same conclusion: in 1931 the reservation physician at Yakima complained that the lack of data on TB resulted in poor, infrequent, and inconsistent treatment; disease surveys, of which there had been none, would change that.[3] As late as 1947, two TB experts correctly claimed that the "unfortunate fact is that until recently little was done to detect tuberculosis among Indians before they were desperately ill and when treatment is of little help among the people of any race."[4] It took decades for those interested in TB among Indians to realize, as a team of specialists noted in 1942, that "in order to combat a problem through a program of control, the extent of that problem must first be known." Simply knowing about the incidence of TB, they argued, has "been of tremendous value in awakening interest and stimulating a desire for treatment."[5] As Bertram Kraus quite sensibly suggested in his 1954 survey of Arizona Indian health, not knowing the incidence of disease kept it from being treated. He considered the primary reason that the Indian death rate from preventable diseases like TB was so high was because they "remain undetected and untreated for a much longer period of time in Indians than in Whites."[6] "Undetected and untreated" disease remains one of the central challenges of TB control in the twenty-first century.

Not only was little known about the disease, little was done about it. The two were of course directly related. The BIA had little control over the epidemic for myriad material reasons—little funding, too few reservation doctors, not enough hospital beds, and extreme poverty on Indian reservations. Before the 1930s, there were, here and there, successful efforts to combat the disease. At Pine Ridge James Walker reduced TB between 1896 and 1903 via education, case finding, and working closely with medicine men. His success was short lived.[7] Indian agents, reservation doctors, and bureaucrats in Washington tried to improve sanitation and to segregate tuberculous Indians in sanatoriums and hospitals. These were mostly half measures. There were never enough beds for sick Indians: by 1914 the Phoenix East Farm Sanatorium—the largest TB hospital run by the BIA—could only accommodate one hundred tuberculous patients; by the mid-1920s it was chronically underfunded and overcrowded.[8] The Meriam Report made clear that not only was TB the number one Indian health problem, almost nothing was being to combat the disease. The report, too, documented extreme, nationwide Indian poverty. Malnutrition was rampant in children, but Indian schools spent only about eleven cents per student per day on food—the report advocated an immediate, emergency appropriation of one million dollars for food. The report largely blamed the BIA's land allotment policy for creating such conditions. Thus BIA policies were both creating the conditions for the rise of TB and doing virtually nothing effective to combat it.[9]

By the end of the 1920s, the treatment and prevention of TB had come only a short distance from the "neglectful murder" described by J. M. Woodburn in 1889; in fact, according to Fred Ford, director of health at the BIA, in 1950 the prevalence of disease in general was as great then as it was at the turn of the century.[10] J. C. Hancock, who worked among the San Carlos Apaches, was quite blunt about the consequences, writing in 1933: "It seems that, in time, tuberculosis may exterminate the tribe."[11]

When the BIA embarked on a multipronged strategy to control the TB epidemic—a series of TB surveys conducted all across Indian country, an ambitious program of vaccination, and the deployment of public health nurses—it signaled the beginnings of the first concerted effort to understand the disease among Indians and stem the tide of TB.[12] Intervention was sorely needed. In 1936, on the eve of the BIA's ambitious plan to combat TB, Elinor Gregg, in charge of the BIA's public health nursing program, summed up what many doctors, nurses, and others in the field felt. "Nothing has given me more genuine distress than our utter lack of adequate care and control of tuberculosis in the Indian Service."[13] In 1935, Esmond Long and Joseph Aronson, both of the Phipps Institute in Philadelphia and both TB experts, determined that the time had come to do something. Working under the auspices of John Collier's "Indian New Deal," Long and Aronson determined that the "high mortality and morbidity from tuberculosis among the various Indian tribes in the United States makes it highly desirable that a program dealing with the epidemiology, prevention, and control of tuberculosis be instituted among these people."[14] Looking closely at families with multiple tuberculous members, identifying "spreaders," honing in on the source of the disease—all these were innovative practices when it came to Indians and TB.[15] So too were technologies of surveillance and detection like spot maps and increased use of x-rays on the Navajo reservation, as well as a standard test for TB. It was a difficult task: to locate cases on the Navajo reservation, for example, from December 1937 to July 1938 nurses and doctors made more than nine hundred home visits and traveled more than seventeen thousand miles.[16] And while no method of surveillance was as invasive and distasteful to modern readers as Long's suggestion that Navajos who had been tested for TB be tattooed, all of these changes in the management and control of TB were a radical departure from past practice.[17]

Writing to Aronson, James Townsend declared that "you and I and all of us are engaged in one of the most important studies in the control of tuberculosis that has ever been conducted in this country and you know full well is being watched with considerable interest."[18] The TB program among American Indians was the only serious control effort among Native people anywhere in the world. While Charles Wilcocks might have been able to get a handle on the TB problem in Tanganyika, almost nothing was achieved in terms of control. The BIA's control program was far ahead of any other—both by virtue of being the only one and by virtue of actually being well run and well funded.

It was the BCG vaccination that was the most novel intervention.

Bacillus Calmette-Guérin—named for the two French biologists who developed it in 1908—is a live, attenuated vaccine. More people have received the BCG vaccine than any other. Since it first began to be used in France in the 1920s an estimated 4.5 billion people have received it. Millions still receive it today. It's the only TB vaccine. No other viable vaccine has ever emerged. Go almost anywhere in the world outside the United States—where it was only used on a limited basis, as most public health specialists considered TB rates to be low enough not to warrant its use or doubted its efficacy—and you'll find people with the telltale scar. The geographical reach of the vaccine is impressive; no corner of the populated world has been spared. The mass vaccination with BCG is, without doubt, the most far-reaching and longest-lasting prophylactic medical campaign in world history.[19]

Doubt and hope have been features of the vaccine's history since the beginning—doubt about its efficacy and hope that those doubts were wrong.

Reflecting on fifty years of BCG's use and thinking hard about why trials had produced such wildly varying results (ranging from zero to 80 percent efficacy), British TB expert Ian Sutherland wrote in 1971 that if "artistry is needed to estimate the benefits of BCG, clairvoyance is required beyond that point."[20] Controversy has dogged the vaccine since the beginning. In 1930, less than a decade after it was first used, a contaminated strain of the vaccine killed seventy-six infants, out of a total two hundred and fifty vaccinated, in Lübeck, Germany. For many years, the tragedy cast a dark shadow over BCG; the memory of it was invoked anytime one needed reminding that BCG was less than perfect.[21] So deep is its impact—or so often repeated a story—that still today, close to a century afterward and long since the vaccine has been deemed safe, the WHO must explain away the anomaly of the Lübeck tragedy, and only the Lübeck tragedy, when discussing BCG on its website devoted to TB vaccines.[22] Ever present though the specter of Lübeck was, what fueled a perpetually smoldering, sometimes raging, debate was and would remain the controversies over whether or not BCG even worked, and not its safety. Already in 1933, a review of its use in Western Europe claimed that few subjects had had as much written about them as BCG—including "regrettable sheets of invective."[23] Fifty years later, after failing to show any protective value in the largest controlled trial to date, another researcher characterized much of the debate over the vaccine as "acrimonious."[24]

And why wouldn't there be controversy: the vaccine's value has been tested and tested, yet results range from zero to 80 percent efficacy—of course there was vigorous debate over such wildly divergent results. Unleashing such a vaccine into the world, on a scale that almost defies de-scription, was a guarantee of controversy.[25] But people wanted it to work. Broadly speaking, two camps emerged: the skeptical and the faithful. There were some who ardently believed that BCG was useless and who never let go of that belief. There were, too, those who were convinced, with just as firm-ly held convictions, that the vaccine had value. Sometimes views overlapped. But when it came to actually using BCG, testing its efficacy, and so forth, zealotry was not generally a feature of the landscape. A skeptic could doubt the vaccine's efficacy but still be willing to try it; and like most thoughtful people of any faith, those who believed in BCG at times questioned their commitment. Faith was shaken. Thus, while there were, to be sure, invective and acrimony and heated debate, there was also oscillation. In a world where TB was killing millions every year and there was no way to stop it medically, if the possibility existed that a cheap vaccine could reduce the world's burden of TB, why not try it?

The story of BCG is emblematic of much in the history of TB control. There's the search for an affordable solution to a massive, seemingly intractable, problem. There's both the hubris and the uncertainty of science and the difficulty of translating trial results to the real world. There's the innovation and the inertia in which a period of great activity is followed by one of stasis and inflexibility. There's hope followed by despair. And in the end there's still a tremendous amount of TB.

Desperation brought BCG to Indian country. Doctors had no effective treatment, too few hospital beds, and lots of tuberculosis. BCG might work. And some doctors, not knowing what else to do and appalled at the high rates of TB on their reservations, began to clamor for it. For Charles Nagel, the reservation doctor at Fort Belknap, TB care had "become an obsession," and he was keen to try BCG on newborns. His obsession got the attention of M. C. Guthrie, then director of health for the BIA. Guthrie, appalled by the "terrible scourge" of TB but intrigued by the "investigational possibilities," wrote to the director of the National Tuberculosis Association to inquire about BCG.[26] Once the BIA's interest was piqued, the pace of momentum picked up quickly. The new director of health, James Townsend, made BCG his mission. Within a year, the BIA went from simply tossing the idea around to figuring out how to carry out a trial in Indian country. The excitement was palpable. L. R. Jones, a TB specialist working for the BIA in the Southwest, wrote in 1935, "It is my feeling that we should congratulate ourselves and commend the Office [of Indian Affairs] for furnishing us this opportunity to take part in one of the greatest movements in Public Health and Preventive Medicine that has ever been attempted."[27] Jones hoped that if they could devise a proper experiment BCG might become the "deciding factor in our control program."[28] But he also knew that BCG had its problems. When he surveyed the Southwest he revealed that 75 percent of Indians reacted positively to tuberculin—that is, three-quarters of the population were already infected. To be effective, Jones made clear, the BCG program had to be directed toward children.[29] Despite its uselessness among the huge portion of the population *already infected*, R. H. Heterick, the district medical officer in the Southwest, was anxious to get the BCG program up and running: considering how "comparatively little we are achieving at present" it was a plan, it was action, it might help future generations.[30] Jones agreed: BCG will not help those suffering from TB now, but it "will no doubt prove its worth in the future." He felt compelled to caution, though, that "if anyone is hoping that visible benefits will be reaped on a large scale in the near future they should be disillusioned."[31]

The desperation borne out of the depths of TB's seeming intractability; the hope and optimism that BCG just might work; and the fact that there was just nothing else out there—all of these would come to characterize the use of the vaccine for decades to come.

Much had to be worked out. Concerns over the safety of the BCG vaccine, the ethics of running an experimental trial on Indians (whether couched and carried out in humanitarian terms or not), logistical difficulties, and political problems—all of these had to be considered in getting the program off the ground.[32] In the beginning, some were so nervous about BCG's unsafe reputation that its use was to remain a secret.[33] Consent, too, was initially something Esmond Long wanted to dispense with. Under normal circumstances consent would be sought, but Long claimed that "our clients would not understand our explanations and it would only arouse their suspicions."[34] Indians were not the only suspicious ones. Oliver La Farge, the Pulitzer Prize–winning author of the novel *Laughing Boy: A Navajo Love Story* and director of the American Indian Defense Association, was outraged over the possibility of what he worried, with good reason, would be a ham-fisted experiment run by the BIA. Though La Farge knew a study of BCG might provide good data on its efficacy, he still worried. First, he did not think the BIA was capable of running a proper trial or that Indians were proper subjects. "The Indians, an underprivileged people, complicated by malnutrition, abysmal sanitary conditions, having a staggering death rate, are absolutely *not* proper subjects for experimentation of this type," La Farge fumed.[35] Fueling his concern was the fresh memory of a failed trachoma control experiment run on the Navajo reservation in the 1920s. As a result of that botched campaign, many Navajos who had undergone a novel trachoma treatment left the hospital worse off than when they arrived. For this reason Matthew Sniffen of the Indian Rights Association declared that "the Indians should not be used for experimental purposes."[36]

While Sniffen's and La Farge's concerns were quickly allayed by assurances that BCG was safe, the BIA still proceeded with caution, as this was all so new, and, frankly, so experimental that nervousness and secrecy in addition to excitement and hope prevailed.[37] At a meeting regarding BCG on the Navajo reservation concerns were raised over the source of the vaccine—and the Lübeck tragedy was mentioned. As a result of fears over BCG, at the beginning of the program only a few knew exactly what was going on; the BIA followed a policy of official secrecy, not even telling all reservation doctors what they were planning.[38] Esmond Long knew that the history of the vaccine demanded it: while BCG showed promise, it had not been thoroughly vetted for efficacy, and, despite it having been used on millions of children, concerns over safety were still quite high.[39]

The first step was choosing the appropriate reservations and populations. Joseph Aronson spent a month, in the fall of 1935, traveling the West looking for the right site.[40] Some, like the Pueblos of New Mexico, were considered and quickly dismissed. James Townsend thought there were too many other projects under way among the Pueblos and decided "not to burden the Pueblos with the B.C.G work at this time." Other locations, most notably the Navajo reservation, were carefully considered and then abandoned. The Navajo reservation proved too much of a challenge—it was too big, the population too spread out and too mobile, and the leadership too angry with John Collier over his disastrous sheep-reduction program. Carrying out a controlled experiment there would be all but impossible.[41] The reservations chosen, then, were picked as much for their high incidences of TB as they were for their qualities as ideal laboratories.

And this was important: because the vaccination and epidemiology program was an experiment to be carried out in the hopes of finally showing whether or not BCG was a viable vaccine, conditions had to be ideal. When the BIA settled on the Pima and Wind River reservations in, respectively, Arizona and Wyoming, eventually expanding to Turtle Mountain in North Dakota, to Pine Ridge in South Dakota, and to southeast Alaska, they did so because these places appeared to provide stable, relatively sedentary populations who had good relationships with medical personnel and who could remain under surveillance for a number of years. They were also settled more densely than other places and had a medical infrastructure staffed by doctors and nurses eager to participate in the program. Tribal councils bought in, too. There was also the comparative angle to consider: with a study spread far and wide, and showcasing a variety of housing, dietary, and environmental conditions, researchers hoped to show that BCG could work anywhere.

Finally, each of these places also had very high rates of TB. All of these qualities were essential, thought Director of Health Townsend, as well as Aronson and Long, if they were going to be able to test the efficacy of BCG and begin to understand the epidemiology of TB.[42]

Controlling TB was of course a central concern. But just as important were the research aspects of the program; this was, after, all a trial. Because no controlled trial had ever been done—attempts to do so in Europe had been unsuccessful—the work was especially important.[43] And American Indians, to some, were perfect subjects. One early supporter of the BCG work, the director of the Minnesota State Sanatorium, wrote that "the Indian, without his knowledge or consent, offers us a human experiment in immunology which we can ill afford to ignore. The material is conveniently located, they are or should easily be made available for record and study, and the results applied to regulative measures for control."[44] Right from the start, Esmond Long, in particular, recognized that running a well-controlled trial was essential if the BIA's efforts were to have any impact on the international community of TB researchers—a community that was relatively small and well aware of the BIA's pioneering trial.[45] The BIA considered the research program launched in 1935 that revealed TB as it was rather than as it was imagined so important that in the face of wartime budget cuts in 1943, Townsend recommended that research continue unabated, and with full funding, for another ten years. If the program were curtailed the loss of knowledge would be insurmountable.[46] Others were indeed watching. Less than a year into the program, Kendall Emerson, the director of the National Tuberculosis Association, hoped the BIA could double the number of research subjects "because of the worldwide interest" in the question of BCG's efficacy.[47] The work in Indian country became so well known that observers from outside the United States came to visit. Dr. Ali Shah, a TB expert from India visiting the United States on a fellowship from the Rockefeller Foundation, spent time in the spring of 1939 with Aronson in Arizona.[48] Nearly four years after the program began, the Pasteur Institute in Paris invited Aronson to present his work before the French Academy of Medicine.[49] Just after the war, on the cusp of the newly formed WHO's adoption of BCG for a mass vaccination campaign, Johannes Holm, soon to be the director of the International Tuberculosis Campaign, toured Indian country to learn about Aronson's work.[50] A year later, in 1947, Long finally got his chance, at the Tuberculosis in the Commonwealth conference in London, to tell the world about Aronson's success with BCG.[51] The world was indeed watching.

Commissioner of Indian Affairs John Collier, and others, initially considered Aronson's plans overambitious and ill considered. Aronson's conviction that he could carry out case finding, vaccination, and follow-up work with existing personnel, Collier thought, was misguided. Initially, Collier and Townsend were so uninterested in doing more than testing the efficacy of BCG that without the intervention of Long on his behalf Aronson might never have been able to carry out basic epidemiological research—research he and Long thought critical to understanding the disease and the long-term effects of BCG.[52] By many accounts Aronson was tough to work with: he was demanding and impatient. He found the bureaucracy at the BIA absolutely maddening. As Long said, "He has a lot of faults, but when all is said and done, he has made a mark which won't be lightly erased. He is something new out here, and it is my humble but earnest belief that he will leave a lasting impression. He has a lot of steam, some of it working against him, but it will be worth our while to keep our hands on him and he won't blow up."[53]

Once the work got under way in early 1936 Aronson and his staff moved fast. By the spring of 1938 they had their test population: 1,559 children had been vaccinated (with thirteen different lots of BCG), and 1,460 had been designated as controls.[54] Then, they waited. There was at one time talk of expanding the sample size to forestall criticism over what could be perceived as a small study population. Moving into the southern United States to study the Cherokee in North Carolina and the Choctaw in Mississippi, heading toward the Mexican border to include the Papago or to the Hopi mesas—these were all considered. But staffing, money, and the difficulties of finding a pliable population—it was difficult enough keeping tabs on three thousand children scattered across four reservations and southeastern Alaska, and it would get worse as time went on, they got older, and people migrated for work and war—all combined to ensure that the five locations settled on early in the planning remained the extent of the study area.[55] Even so, this was the largest controlled study the world had yet seen.

But it was not perfect. Three years into the trial, once the intake had been done, at the yearly meeting held in Washington, D.C., Miriam Brailey of Johns Hopkins leveled some criticisms against the BIA's work. Fair and well reasoned, Brailey's critique is important not just for what it said about the BCG work at the time. It's important for two other reasons as well. First, it might help in understanding the results of the Aronson trial—results not published until 1946. And second, Brailey's concerns are some of the first signs of a strain of skepticism regarding BCG that would never be eradicated. Brailey made several points: the study population was too small (this would be echoed by other researchers commenting on other trials in the years to come); she did not think TB was as prevalent among American Indians as most others did; and, finally, all-cause mortality, as well as mortality from TB, was very low among the study population and thus gauging the efficacy of BCG as measured by its effect on mortality, which is what Aronson was doing, would be difficult.[56] Aronson and Townsend listened patiently and did their best to assure Brailey that her concerns, while they raised good questions, did not trouble them. The study was well designed; the study population was well chosen. They carried on.

Fast-forward to 1946. Aronson's results have been published: BCG worked. Aronson found a "marked protection against the development of tuberculosis" in the vaccinated group.[57] But what of Brailey's concerns? Aronson offered a reply of sorts in 1948 when he published a comprehensive overview of the BCG program that included, among other things, some noteworthy numbers. Aronson's figures for all-cause mortality and deaths from TB tell an interesting story—but not the story Aronson wanted to tell, and it's one that makes it hard to be certain of the protective effects of BCG. For example, in 1935 on the Wind River reservation the death rate from TB was 657 per one hundred thousand; all-cause mortality was 2,375 per one hundred thousand. The total population was 1,979. Ten years later the population had increased to 2,376—not a huge gain—but the TB death rate fell to 246 and the all-cause mortality to 1,851. While the TB death rate was still high in 1945 it was much lower than it had been, and the population had increased. There certainly were bumps along the way, but generally speaking the year the BCG program began marked the beginning of a steady, and quite remarkable, decrease in the annual TB death rate. This decrease cannot be attributed to BCG alone because of course it included those already infected and toward whom BCG was not directed.[58] Aronson knew this and was not claiming otherwise.

If tuberculosis was steadily declining among American Indians, was it declining naturally?[59] Aronson anticipated this question. He knew the TB rate was falling and had been "for many years." The point I made above—

that by looking at mortality figures one could clearly see that BCG could not account for the rapid and dramatic decline of TB—is not the point at all, according to Aronson. He wrote that "an evaluation of the effectiveness of BCG cannot be made by comparing current mortality and morbidity rates from tuberculosis with former rates." If one were to do that the point I made would be easy to make. Aronson argued that his study was valid because the controls and the vaccinated in his population were so similar that comparisons should be made between them and not between the current population's and past population's historical epidemiology.[60] Considering the similarities between the controls and the vaccinated and the fact that there were fifty-three TB deaths among the controls and only six among the vaccinated, Aronson regarded BCG a success. That is, even in a climate of generally reduced TB mortality the risk of infection and death was greater among those unprotected by the BCG vaccine.

But in places where TB rates were falling Aronson's findings were not definitive. Aronson knew this. To really understand the protective effective of BCG in such a population one would need to know not only the number of new cases of TB but also the number of new *infections*. That is, if most TB is coming from people already infected then all that's been shown is that they've developed TB disease; it says nothing about new infections. And *new* infections were what BCG was designed to prevent. The six cases of TB among the BCG group and the fifty-three among the controls were new cases;[61] neither group had been infected before the trial. In 1940 Aronson reported that the annual average rate of infection for the five thousand American Indians he had tuberculin tested was 8.9 percent. Of note, too, was that in most places—Alaska was the exception—there were no cases of latent TB in anyone under fifteen.[62] In 1955, after retesting the same populations, Aronson documented a sharp decline in TB in school-age children. But Aronson, cautious and realizing that the decline in TB was very likely caused by many things, wrote that the "data presented in this study do not provide direct evidence that BCG vaccination was a contributing factor in reducing tuberculous infection."[63]

What we don't know much about from Aronson's work is the social and economic profile of the vaccinated and the controls. When he divided the groups in the late 1930s he made an effort to ensure that all were "of the same age and sex, living in the same area and under precisely the same conditions."[64] In the intervening decades, as he conducted his follow-up studies, we don't learn whether social circumstances changed or not among the two groups. Were those in both groups who died of TB at special risk of infection? Did they live with infected relatives or attend a boarding school where students had active TB? Aronson was acutely aware of the effect social and economic conditions had on one's risk of TB. Indeed, when doing the follow-up work in 1955 he admitted that time did not permit the kind of fine-grained work needed to tease out the effects (or not) of social conditions.[65] To assess the efficacy of BCG in the context of low rates of infection it would be helpful to know a bit more about those who did get TB. For example, were those who became infected living in households where an older family member had active TB? In a 1945 survey of TB among Indians in Montana, two BIA researchers found that the highest number of TB deaths was among infants and children under five. Why? Because they lived in homes where the risk of infection was high.[66]

When reflecting on two decades of BCG work among American Indians, Aronson went a step further, if not into the camp of skeptics then certainly out of the church of true believers. While remaining committed to the efficacy of BCG under the tightly controlled conditions of his trial, he also recognized that sharply declining rates of infection made it very difficult to assess the efficacy of any prophylactic measure—it was simply too tough to sort out cause from correlation.[67]

Considering all this, would Aronson's work be replicable under different conditions? Assuming for the moment that BCG did work on Indian reservations and in native villages of southeast Alaska (an assumption not completely warranted), were the conditions in these places similar enough to conditions elsewhere that it was reasonable to expect that such results could be repeated? The 80 percent efficacy rate Aronson achieved became something to strive for, repeatedly cited as proof of the possibilities of BCG. Yet even he knew it was no magic bullet. "Under no condition," he wrote, "should BCG vaccination be regarded as a substitute for approved prophylactic measures used in control of tuberculosis"—by which he meant better sanitation, better living conditions, and more to eat.[68]

Aronson's concerns notwithstanding, the pioneering work he and his colleagues did in Indian county blazed a path for the vaccine. BCG's value soared, and hope rose along with it. And over the next decade BCG would spread across the planet to become the most widely used vaccine in history.

5. BCG Goes Global

The American Indian trials were an important stop on BCG's global migration. Since Joseph Aronson's study was the vaccine's largest controlled trial, Aronson knew his results were being keenly awaited in the United States and abroad.[1] The 80 percent efficacy rate that he claimed to have achieved would have a life of its own, trotted out anytime one needed to garner support for the vaccine. The number became a symbol of what was possible with BCG. One need only watch for that number, as it appears again and again almost anytime BCG is being contemplated, to gauge the impact of Aronson's findings. The figure of 80 percent became a shorthand for the Aronson trial; a shorthand for hope.

The success of Aronson's trial buoyed BCG's prospects.[2] In East Africa, for example, Aronson and Palmer's paper piqued interest in BCG. Hugh Stott and Charles Wilcocks—by then two of the most prominent British TB workers, with considerable experience in the region—came around to the possibilities of BCG upon reading the results coming out of North America. According to Stott, there was now good evidence finally available that BCG was effective in "primitive" populations.[3] Others in Africa also knew about the American Indian trial and were encouraged by its results. When considering a TB program for Uganda, the author of a countrywide survey found Aronson's trial results very promising. What's more, he saw "some similarity with the tubercle bacillus of these Indians and the Africans of Uganda."[4] Dr. Frank Retief, chief medical officer of the Witwatersrand Native Labour Association—charged with attending to the health of workers in South Africa's mining industry—attended a session on

BCG at a TB conference in Durban, in 1952, where he was encouraged by Johannes Holm and Carroll Palmer's discussion of Aronson's pioneering work.[5]

At the most basic level what was so important about the North American Indian trials was, simply, that they had been done at all, because until then nearly nothing had been done to test BCG's efficacy, especially where the disease was highly prevalent.[6] By the late 1940s France, Spain, Eastern Europe, and Russia had adopted BCG to various degrees. It was in the Scandinavian countries that the vaccine was most widely and enthusiastically used.[7] Other countries, too, had been deploying BCG for decades. Japan, Jamaica, China, Peru, Vietnam—all had been vaccinating with BCG, to varying degrees, since the 1930s. But no one really knew if it worked.[8]

In Africa, too, BCG was in use, but what good it was doing was unknown. While Peter Allan in South Africa and Charles Wilcocks in Tanganyika had considered running BCG trials in the 1920s and 30s, before World War II only the French, and in the Congo the Belgians, were using it on the continent.[9] But none of this work was helpful in determining the vaccine's efficacy; BCG was used indiscriminately rather than in a controlled fashion. When considering the mass application of BCG in British East Africa in the early 1950s Wilcocks did not place much stock in the French experience with the vaccine, writing that "the recording of results is so incomplete that little reliance can be placed on the work. In general, the French have adopted the attitude that the value of BCG has been proved, and that all that remains is to apply it to their colonial people. In this they may be right, but for the British colonies a more critical and experimental approach would be preferable."[10]

The French use of BCG was part of their somewhat haphazard, unfocused approach to TB. Richard Neubauer, in his 1953 WHO survey of TB in Africa, learned from officers of the Colonial Medical Service and from Pasteur Institute doctors that "no reliable data about the tuberculosis problem in this part of the world are really known and no reliable statistics exist," because "no proper antituberculosis service exists in either West or Equatorial Africa." Neubauer knew that the French had taken an interest in TB long before other colonial powers had. But he also knew, after meeting with Pastorians in places such as Dakar, that apart from some sporadic testing and a mobile x-ray unit in places such as Niger, "little has been done so far in the way of a systematic attempt at tuberculosis control. There is practically no antituberculosis service, nor any antituberculosis institution in any of the territories" of French Africa.[11] In Algeria a more robust TB service existed, and a large-scale BCG trial had been under way there since 1935—the results of which were unpromising and not known until 1960, long after BCG had made its way around the world.[12] But south of the Sahara TB control was either nonexistent or sporadic or, as in South Africa, directed at high-risk groups like miners.

The American Indian trials were thus a breakthrough. Not only did they provide evidence that BCG worked. They also primed people like Holm, Wilcocks, and Stott—prominent people involved in the burgeoning international push to control TB—to roll out BCG on a massive scale.

Research showing that BCG might work was crucial. Of critical importance, too, in BCG's migration around the globe was the International Tuberculosis Campaign (ITC). Called by the *New York Times* in 1948 "the greatest medical crusade in modern history," the ITC was an unprecedented attack on TB. With the "tentative conclusion" that it "can reduce new cases of tuberculosis by about 80 percent," BCG was foremost in its arsenal. Focused initially on war-ravaged Europe, the ITC was jointly run by the WHO, UNICEF, and several Scandinavian relief agencies. It would eventually expand its operations to India, North Africa, parts of the Middle East, and Latin America. The campaign vaccinated seventeen million children. TB needed to be attacked on a global scale, as the ITC put it, because the disease is "a true internationalist; so must be the means to combat it."[13] The ITC was the precursor to, and to a great extent the model for, the WHO's mass vaccination campaign.[14] Holm ran both. In 1951, when the ITC shut down, the WHO and UNICEF took over mass vaccination.

By the time the ITC closed its doors there was no place on the planet where BCG was not in use. It was remarkably universal. But what's especially remarkable is that it traveled the globe at all. For it did so freighted by considerable doubt that it would work. But for a long time uncertainty was no match for the faith in its possibilities and the hope that something had finally been found to stem the tide of TB. BCG became unstoppable. As early as 1947 G. S. Wilson of the British Medical Research Council wrote that "vaccination with B.C.G. is now so universally applauded that any attempt to question its value is regarded almost as heresy."[15] Why? Because so many believed that *something* had to be done, there was nothing else out there, and there was no harm in trying. This rationale had prevailed since the 1930s and would for decades. G. Gregory Kayne, a British TB authority, wrote in a 1936 review of the vaccine's use across Western Europe that "where the tuberculosis mortality is high, the economic conditions poor, and dispensaries and sanatoria inadequate (as in Spain, for instance), BCG clearly appears to offer a simple method of prevention *faute de mieux*."[16]

Considering the severity of the TB problem in much of the world, the possibility of an effective vaccine was a powerful force. It's hard to imagine a different path: of course the believers won. To the believers the skeptical offered nothing but doubt, and doubt was not going to slow the spread of TB. Outside the United States—where skepticism and doubt and concerns about BCG's efficacy, combined with what appeared to be the naturally falling rate of TB, meant its use was limited to high-risk groups like American Indians—the skeptics did not do much more than point out problems.[17] Other than in India in the 1950s, as we will see, BCG encountered very little opposition. Those who voiced doubt with anything resembling vehemence were considered naysayers and cranks determined to undermine a promising and heroic international effort to rid the world of a dread disease. How could the faithful not win?

What's more, in the twenty years or so after World War II the two organizations most invested in global health—UNICEF and the WHO—pushed BCG. There was really no competition. At least in public, UNICEF and the WHO more or less unequivocally, and largely uncritically, supported BCG—no one could have stopped them even if they had wanted to. Poor countries were desperate. As Niels Brimnes has shown, momentum turned into inertia, and in the 1950s and 60s, especially, BCG spread across the planet even though there was no clear idea whether or not it worked. Studies suggesting it did not work were tossed off as methodologically unsound—indeed, any evidence with the least bit of ambiguity was seen as reason to push on, not to slow down.[18] BCG had become, within less than a decade of its mass rollout, almost impervious to criticism. For a time, and to a point, that faith was admirable. BCG was, at a minimum, safe. No one would be harmed. Taking swift action with the tools available against a global killer was bold. It was also, especially compared to the dithering in the decades to come, unique. Virtually every other intervention in TB control would be studied to death. BCG, on the other hand, was found to be safe, and in some circumstances—enough, it turned out—to be effective, and so why not release it into the world. At some point, however, that hope blinded people to the realities of BCG.

In 1950, as those running the ITC debated who would assume responsibility for mass vaccination work—the WHO or UNICEF or the two together or anyone at all—and whether or not the campaign would extend to the developing world, Brendan Frasier, UNICEF's man in Copenhagen, wrote a confidential memo to Maurice Pate, the executive director. Frasier exemplifies the hope and faith people put in BCG. He knew well the controversies over BCG; he knew UNICEF would face considerable skepticism about the value of mass campaign with a vaccine that still posed many questions. But for Frasier the simple fact that BCG was in use was enough. "If WHO had not approved BCG as it has done, if medical opinion did not overwhelmingly endorse it as it does, and if assisted countries did not share in campaign costs so strongly as they do, one might question the value of BCG. But UNICEF has not doubted its merits, and it has to my knowledge no reason newly acquired to drop it now." Admitting that it might take some time to learn whether or not BCG will have done any good, Frasier nonetheless declared that "if there were any fundamental doubt of its efficacy, this issue—rather than who shall handle the work and how—would be foremost." That the question of efficacy wasn't at the fore was enough for Frasier. While they hoped, but could not yet promise, that BCG was 80 percent effective—that magic number from the American Indian trial—"such evidence as has been forthcoming is giving medical authorities in many countries the confidence underlying their attention to mass campaigns."[19]

Frasier was of course not alone. In the tight-knit, small world of international TB control he was joined by other people with power. Holm was on board. So too was Carroll Palmer, one of the giants of the TB world. Palmer had cowritten with Aronson the paper on the American Indian trial, and now, charged with compiling and analyzing BCG's effects around the world, he ran the WHO's Tuberculosis Research Office in Copenhagen. Palmer was not a true believer, not by any means, but nor was he an outright skeptic. His view, for now, was that although BCG's long-term epidemiological effects were still unknown this should not stop its use. With that in mind, in early 1952, while preparing a statement on BCG for U.S. Congressional hearings on UNICEF funding, Palmer wrote to Pate, "There is still a good deal of skepticism about BCG. Perhaps it is even increasing, especially since there are no striking indications that tuberculosis has been dramatically influenced in the countries where large mass campaigns have been done." It was of course too early to expect results, but Palmer knew people were impatient. He took comfort in being able to say to the skeptics, "'We never thought it [BCG] was any final solution—but it was the best we had, it was all that could be done for TB, where something had to be done.'" The doubts over BCG were getting a lot of attention now that UNICEF and the WHO had launched the mass campaign and were getting ready to head into the developing world. But Palmer was prepared. "There is great strength, I believe, if we together meet the storm now brewing about BCG with equanimity and a quiet firm confidence that while BCG may not have been all that we hoped, we are trying energetically to make it all that it can be."[20] Palmer did not of course believe in the power of BCG on blind faith; he knew its promise was as yet unfulfilled and did not know if it ever would be. But, like others, he knew nothing else existed.

That nothing else was out there motivated Hugh Stott in Kenya as well. In 1950 Stott, one of the few actively pursuing TB in Kenya, reflected on the possibilities of a BCG trial and vaccination scheme. Deeply frustrated over the claims and counterclaims regarding BCG's efficacy, he argued that the constant battles over the vaccine ensured it would not be used where it was most needed. Despite the fact that "no absolute statistical proof is available to prove the efficacy of B.C.G.," he still wondered: "Is it not essential to investigate any method which has the remotest possibility of lowering morbidity and mortality from tuberculosis to any extent?, and which, if proven to be effective, can be put into operation relatively quickly."[21]

When the WHO took over the BCG program in 1952 from the ITC, it was willing to roll it out based not on certainty—because it could not—but largely on the promise BCG held. Early that year the WHO's director, Brock Chisholm, mulled over the unknowns. He knew that there was considerable variability in the vaccine, depending on where it was produced; its potency, dosage, and protective value had not been "accurately determined"; there were significant differences in its behavior based on geography; and with more production facilities coming on line "existing problems will become even more complex." In other words, "the vaccine in its present form by no means fulfills the requirements of an ideal prophylactic and must be improved and perfected."[22] Considering all this was important—Chisholm and the WHO, for instance, recommended that unapproved BCG production facilities be discouraged—but not nearly enough to slow down the mass campaign. Caution was called for, to be sure. But this cup was half full, not half empty.

Faith mattered most in the field. Running a pilot program in India in 1953, Halfdan Mahler, thick in the mire of day-to-day operations—dealing with broken-down vehicles, exhausted staff, poor roads, uncertain supply chains—admitted that it would likely never be known exactly what role BCG would play in reducing TB in India. But to make the program work, to inspire workers and the public, people had to *believe* it worked.[23]

Palmer and Mahler, Stott and Chisholm—they were not naive optimists, convinced that BCG worked because no one had proven it hadn't. They were down-to-earth realists deeply committed to easing the world's TB burden. To do that they knew some amount of faith was involved in getting BCG out into the world. Palmer needed to convince Congress that investing in UNICEF and its BCG program was not a waste of money—we must try, he knew. And Mahler, hard at work in the field and faced with all manner of problems that kept morale low, had to believe in BCG, and so did his staff. Otherwise, why bother? Stott looked at the amount of TB in Kenya, and, like doctors on American Indian reservations before him, was desperate for *something*. Chisholm ran a global organization—one of the first of its kind—an organization that needed to take action, to prove its value, and launch the war on TB. They, and many others, were all willing to take a chance on BCG. Faith in its promise sustained them.

That faith would be severely tested in India.

6. Questioning BCG
Mass Resistance in India

India, where TB was rampant, was of particular interest to those launching the global assault on tuberculosis.[1] Shortly after independence, in November 1948, it became the first developing country to enter into an agreement with the International Tuberculosis Campaign. For three years the ITC ran a BCG demonstration project in India. In 1951, just as the BCG campaign was set to expand across the country, and the ITC's work was drawing to a close, Johannes Holm, director of the ITC, wrote: "India is in a key position as regards BCG vaccination in the Far East. If a mass campaign could be successfully carried out there, neighboring lands would realize that campaigns were possible in their countries too. On the other hand, if a mass campaign failed in India, it would be most unlikely that other countries in that part of the world would embark on mass campaigns for many years to come."[2] India was a proving ground, a test case.

The presence of lingering fears about the vaccine's safety, doubts about its efficacy, and uncertainty that a mass vaccination strategy was right for India plagued the program from the beginning. The very public battle over BCG in some quarters of India—one cannot use this story as a stand-in for the entire subcontinent—brought to life the divisions between the skeptics and the faithful. The doubts and fears expressed in India—some well considered and others ill conceived—were manifested in a robust Indian response to the campaign. And while opposition elsewhere to the mass campaign was not unknown—there was resistance in Iraq, Vietnam, and Mexico—the

anti-BCG movement in India became more significant than any other opposition. It lasted longer and reduced the number of vaccinations significantly.[3]
To try to derail the mass campaign, the protest's protagonists focused on
BCG's unknowns. To do so, the leaders of the resistance steeped themselves
in Western biomedicine, routinely citing the medical community's doubts
about BCG's efficacy. They were angry and frustrated—angry that India
was being used as a living laboratory and frustrated that, rather than focus on
the conditions that gave rise to TB, Indians were being offered a cheap and
unproven vaccine. Uncertainty surrounding the vaccine, as we have seen, did
not generally lead to using it less. Uncertainty in the face of desperation in
fact led in the opposite direction: the widespread rollout of BCG around the
world. But in India uncertainty provoked vigorous opposition. Those in the
developed world consistently thought: BCG is safe, and since we have nothing else, why not try it. India—and of course everywhere else BCG
traveled—was on the receiving end of that uncertainty.

The anti-BCG forces that emerged in India were neither the first nor
the last eruption of antivaccination sentiment in the country; India appears
to have been rarely willing to simply accept vaccination. In fact, so cowed by
antivaccination sentiment were colonial medical officials that fear of potentially violent resistance to cholera vaccination in the 1930s—when the British
and the Congress Party were in deep disagreement over the party's civil dis-
obedience campaign—forced the British to abandon plans for compulsory
cholera vaccination.[4] There was frequent resistance to smallpox vaccination
that was mostly local and episodic.[5] In postcolonial India compulsory smallpox vaccination sparked off local and spontaneous, rather than national or
regional and well-planned, resistance linked to larger political debates, particularly in the 1970s. Cholera vaccine trials from the 1970s to the 1990s as
well as vitamin A supplements also sparked periods of fierce opposition—
opposition that mimicked the opposition to BCG, challenging the science
and protesting that cheap fixes were no substitute for structural change.[6]

Good timing brought about a major change in India's tuberculosis control
strategy in the late 1940s: political independence and new possibilities for assistance in international health put India on the path to a major assault on the
disease. During the first half of the twentieth century, Indian and British
public health authorities gradually identified tuberculosis as a major health
concern. By the middle of the century there were an estimated 2.5 million

active cases of tuberculosis and half a million deaths annually.[7] Before 1947, tuberculosis control was based on educating the public in hygiene and treatment through dispensaries, while the number of tuberculosis sanatoriums was vastly insufficient.[8] In the late 1940s, when the BCG vaccine appeared, the Indian government found it appealing: it was cheap and seemingly effective. In a May 1948 press note announcing the ITC's mass campaign, the government explained that such a scheme "will be a cheap and effective method of reducing the incidence of tuberculosis which is assuming epidemic proportions at the present moment in the country."[9]

With the emergence of organizations designed to promote international health, BCG had now become a realistic option. With support from the WHO the government of India established a BCG laboratory at the King Institute in Guindy just outside Madras. It began producing vaccine in August 1948. The first BCG vaccinations in India followed in Madanapalle, a rural location a few hundred miles from Madras.[10] And in November, India became the first non-European country to enter into an agreement with the ITC. The agreement marked the beginning of a two-and-half-year-long, countrywide demonstration campaign. Controversy quickly followed.

The BCG campaign was set to begin in Madras in early 1949. Resistance immediately appeared. A. V. Raman, a former sanitary engineer, began to publish editorial after critical editorial in his monthly publication *People's Health*. And over the next two years, the ITC's international staff and the authorities in Madras faced crippling counterpropaganda from Raman and his supporters.[11]

Raman was already a vocal critic of the government. In the November 1948 issue of *People's Health*, before ITC personnel had even set foot in India and possibly before the agreement between ITC and the government of India had been officially signed, Raman attacked the Union government's general health policy.[12] He accused the government of favoring "technical" solutions, arguing that the government ought to give priority to sanitary reforms: clean drinking water, proper housing, and sewage. Among the vilified "technical" solutions was BCG: "Much is talked about BCG vaccine and its effect. Some months back, a foreign expert contacted us to do some publicity in favour of BCG vaccination. We had a straight talk with the expert. We put it to him plainly[:] 'Of what earthly use is BCG in the present living condition of the Indian masses; every moment of their lives, they take a dose of infection; they continue to take in heroic doses of it day in and day out.' The expert confessed 'unless the living conditions are improved, BCG cannot be expected to yield the desired results.' The Minister of Health can just as well pass a resolution that every home should be a BCG factory and every hospital a tuberculosis hospital."[13] To Raman, BCG vaccination was nothing but a cheap and inferior pseudo-solution, or, as he phrased it: "If in this way we devise what are triumphantly devised to be short cuts through which to eradicate diseases, we would be deluding ourselves and deluding the public. Cheap things are not always good or safe. Cheap things are mostly nasty."[14]

The formal inauguration of ITC's campaign in Madras was planned for February 15, 1949. But as the date drew near news of Raman's opposition to BCG vaccination began to appear in Indian newspapers.[15] On February 4 Raman addressed a scientific society in Madras, where he targeted BCG and invoked the uncertainties surrounding the vaccine, declaring "'I strongly protest in the name of India . . . against our boys and girls being made a sort of cannon-fodder and treated like guinea-pigs for the sake of experimentation.'"[16] By referring to articles critical of BCG from scientific journals in Britain and the United States, Raman adroitly exploited the existing disagreements over the vaccine's safety and efficacy—a tactic particularly well deployed in a lengthy piece published on the eve of the rollout in the important regional newspaper the *Hindu*. Finally, he doubted the good results with BCG in the Scandinavian countries.[17] Raman ended his article by quoting the Swedish professor Arvid Wallgren—a renowned tuberculosis specialist and a member of the Coordinating Committee of ITC—to the effect that Sweden would not do trials with BCG because it would be too risky to leave any children as an unvaccinated control group. Instead, such tests had to be undertaken in areas " 'where BCG vaccination was not prevalent and looked on with suspicion.' "[18] While Wallgren's statement supported Sweden's strong belief in BCG, Raman misrepresented him. He linked Wallgren's comments about a Scandinavian trial to the fact that BCG trials had been conducted on American Indians in the United States and concluded that Indian children were intended to be guinea pigs for a dubious vaccine: "The research workers in BCG had conducted experiments on guinea-pigs, calves and on American Indians. What the research workers are now after is to get a wider field for conducting their experiments! . . . I am driven by the irresistible conclusion that the authorities are exposing the people of this country to be utilised by research workers for their benefit. Guinea-pig experiment is no good; man is necessary."[19]

With its allusions to ill-conceived foreign schemes, Raman's rhetoric was compelling in a country that had recently won independence. P. V. Benjamin, tuberculosis adviser to the Union government, had to urge people to treat the foreign experts with more dignity. They were—as he put it—"on a mission of mercy."[20]

People's Health continued its campaign against BCG by bringing to its readers the latest information on BCG—made possible by fast transmission of medical information to southern India.[21] Especially important was research conducted by the internationally known American tuberculosis expert Carroll Palmer. Especially valuable ammunition in the fight against BCG was Palmer's admission that "strict scientific proof of the effectiveness of BCG vaccination in the control of human tuberculosis is not available." To this Raman readily added that Palmer's "opinion cannot be brushed aside as 'uninformed criticism' nor [can] the expert advisers of the Ministries of Health, Provincial and Central, continue to assert that BCG vaccination has transcended the stages of experimentation."[22] The uncertainties surrounding BCG among medical scientists allowed Raman to assert that BCG was still in the experimental stage. By deploying expert opinion to support his claim, Raman hoped to convince his readers that the vaccine should not be introduced in India except for limited and controlled experiments.

Raman used his extensive references to the scientific literature to position himself as a believer in Western scientific medicine. As early as 1946, Raman considered ill advised the demands from various quarters of the nationalist movement that India design its future health system according to indigenous traditions like ayurveda. Raman critiqued modern medicine, yet he warned against "rushing to the other extreme." He advised: "A great deal of spectacular progress is being achieved by modern systems of research today, which we can ill afford to ignore. The path of wisdom would therefore lie in our keeping in step with the latest developments of modern thought without necessarily fouling our own nest."[23] Raman also wrote approvingly about streptomycin, the newly discovered anti-TB drug.[24] Clearly, he could not simply be dismissed as an irrational critic of Western medicine.

Raman's anti-BCG campaign overshadowed the program's formal inauguration. Instead of celebrating the beginning of a new era in tuberculosis control, the speeches and addresses from the Indian medical authorities became defenses of the campaign.[25] Staunchly supporting the scientific merits of BCG, the speakers nonetheless admitted that BCG had to be part of a broader effort. Thus P. V. Benjamin agreed that better housing and general sanitation would be the ideal way to tackle tuberculosis in India, but he also argued that "as our resources are limited, it will take many years before we could carry all these out. It is because of the consciousness of our limitations that we are advocating the BCG vaccination."[26]

While Raman's critique took both Indian and Scandinavian TB workers by surprise, his position was based on well-known arguments in the public debate over health in late colonial India. In his rejection of BCG, Raman took inspiration from the Bhore Committee and Gandhi: "In view of the above considerations, we wish to make our position beyond doubt. We would give the first and foremost priority to the improvement of the nutritional and environmental conditions. The Bhore Committee has said so. Long before the Bhore Committee, Mahatmaji has said so. The fact, however, is that there is hardly a single Health Minister in any Province today, who is troubled by the disparity between official policies and Mahatmaji's teachings."[27]

The Bhore Committee, established in 1943 under the chairmanship of Sir Joseph Bhore, made recommendations for the postwar development of the health system in India. Having consulted with some of the world's most renowned advocates of social medicine, the committee's report was deeply influenced by this doctrine.[28] Adopting a broad, inclusive definition of health as "that positive state of well-being in which mind and body are able to function to their fullest capacity," the committee considered environmental hygiene essential: "Without these our towns and villages will continue to be factories of disease, which will help to maintain undiminished demands on the curative side of the medical services."[29] But the committee knew resources were limited. In the communiqué that led to its establishment the committee had been advised to plan boldly, not extravagantly, and in its recommendations the committee noted that financial limitations could not be overcome immediately.[30] The disagreement between Raman and Benjamin in February 1949 echoed the predicament of the Bhore Committee: Raman desired ambitious long-term environmental and social engineering schemes; Benjamin recognized the immediate, short-term economic realities.

The committee eschewed technological fixes. It warned that the "new health order" could not be achieved through "a bottle of medicine or a surgical operation" and declared: "There is no magical wand to wave these changes into being overnight."[31] Although BCG was a well-known prophylactic at the time, the report took no notice of it, focusing instead on isolation and treatment of TB patients. Financial constraints meant that priority went to the development of an organized domiciliary TB service, supplemented by clinics and hospitals.[32]

Raman and the Bhore Committee not only agreed on how to tackle tuberculosis. They also shared views on the role of the state. The committee unambiguously endorsed the "idea that the State should assume full responsibility for all measures curative and preventive, which are necessary for safeguarding the health of the nation."[33] Raman agreed. Writing about the futility of seeking parental consent before vaccination, he declared: "It should not be forgotten that the State is the parent of the country, parens patriae, and that it is bound to accept full responsibility in the matter without shifting it on to uninformed and ignorant parents of our college boys and girls."[34] Thus Raman reminded his audience of the expectation, prevalent in the years immediately before independence, that India would develop a "welfare" state that intervened in its citizens' lives in a much more ambitious way than with an injection of a questionable vaccine.[35]

Raman also looked to Gandhi. Gandhi was positioned in direct opposition to the current health regime, a regime personified by the adamantly pro-BCG Union Health Minister Rajkumari Amrit Kaur. Raman's November 1949 *People's Health* editorial referred to Gandhi's famous remark about Western medicine as "the essence of black magic" and then challenged the minister: "Come, come Rajkumari don't these words form themselves again on your memory, well? India was made the scene of a mass vaccination campaign, almost immediately after his death." According to Raman, Gandhi had realized "that diseases can be eradicated by improving the living conditions of man, not by injecting products of western vivisection."[36]

The figure of Gandhi was an enormously powerful rhetorical reference. However, neither man was simply opposed to Western medicine.[37] While Gandhi often criticized it as inadequate and immoral, he was also eager to position himself as a believer in science, if this was understood as the method of scientific inquiry. In 1921, after having reiterated his statement about Western medicine as black magic, Gandhi wrote: "Having said this much I would like to pay tribute to the spirit of research that fires the modern scientist. My quarrel is not against that spirit. My complaint is against the direction that this spirit has taken."[38] Gandhi did not entirely reject Western medicine; he identified specific practices that he found particularly objectionable.

Chief among these were vaccination, a "savage custom" and a "sacrilege," "tantamount to partaking of beef."[39]

Gandhi endorsed certain elements of Western medicine, such as sanitation, which he repeatedly described as a science.[40] On one occasion in 1929 Gandhi positioned vaccination and sanitation in direct opposition to each other. Arguing that he rejected vaccination on religious grounds, he admonished: "But those who do not get themselves vaccinated ought to know and follow the rules of sanitation."[41] It was precisely this opposition that Raman latched onto—though without its religious associations—when he emphasized that India needed sanitary measures and not vaccination schemes.

When Raman invoked the Bhore Committee he gave his support to the doctrine of social medicine and hoped for a powerful and interventionist state; he used Gandhi to bolster his claim that vaccination was a particularly problematic medical technology. Combining these two well-established positions allowed Raman to offer a forceful argument against vaccination and in favor of sanitation as the TB control strategy for India.

While Raman and others continued to argue against BCG in *People's Health* up to 1951, it was in the spring of 1949 that the opposition was most energetic and visible. The Scandinavian experts in ITC noticed the opposition against BCG in Madras. From New Delhi Svend K. Svendsen, ITC's chief medical officer in India, reported that the anti-BCG campaign had begun unexpectedly and that Raman had managed "to fill most of India's newspapers with counter propaganda, particularly in Madras and Bombay." And while Svendsen remained hopeful about the success of the campaign, he cautioned that "we must not, however, expect that BCG in the near future will run triumphantly through the Indian masses. It will take a lot of hard work."[42] In other locations the campaign seemingly went on without facing extensive opposition; the problems in Madras did not prompt any soul-searching within ITC. Neither was Rajkumari Amrit Kaur shaken. In April she delivered a speech in which she unconditionally supported BCG and assured the public of the benevolent intentions of the Western countries.[43]

But Raman's protests caused the Madras government to postpone mass vaccination. Following the controversy in February 1949, politicians' and bureaucrats' early enthusiasm for BCG waned. In June 1949 the provincial government informed the Union government that, considering the significance of the opposition, it preferred to train only one team instead of three as originally planned. When opposition died out more teams could be trained.[44] In autumn 1949, when Benjamin wrote to the minister for public health in the Madras government, Dr. T. S. S. Rajan, and asked whether the province was interested in participating in the next phase of the BCG program, the provincial government opted out of the Union government's plans to intensify BCG vaccination.[45] For Madras, this phase would mean training another ten vaccination teams. This proposal did not, Rajan informed the authorities in New Delhi, have the support of the Madras government.[46] The internal memorandum behind Rajan's rejection of the plan (written by an "additional secretary" in the Public Health Department) directly referenced the opposition radiating from the pages of *People's Health:* "It will be seen that, progressively, B.C.G. vaccination is being sought to be made a common garden affair like vaccination against small-pox, and as though the efficacy of B.C.G. vaccination and freedom of danger therefrom are established facts! Actually, an anti B.C.G. campaign is raging throughout the world and in Madras; in the last month's issue of 'People's Health,' the arguments against B.C.G. have been clearly marshalled in an article."[47]

With Madras turning its back on BCG, and Raman's resistance at its height, the campaign was in trouble. At the same time, because of logistical difficulties and ambition outweighing commitment to the campaign, the WHO's Indian representative characterized the campaign as a "flop" and the results so far "extremely disappointing."[48]

In early 1950 another attempt was made to convince Madras that it should join the intensified vaccination campaign; the regional director of ITC wrote specifically to offer assistance to the Madras authorities. The provincial government remained adamant and declined the appeal. Explaining that "the time is not yet ripe for any mass B.C.G. Vaccination before public apprehensions have been allayed," it also promised that "additional provision for more teams will be made if it [is] found that the results have been satisfactory and the considerable public opposition obtaining in this state has been overcome."[49]

The campaign in the south was a mess, and the ITC was moving on. Nonetheless, when vaccinations were to be carried out across the entire country the momentum gained by the ITC appeared unstoppable. Indeed, in the general "Draft Plan of Operation" for the years 1952 and 1953, the Union government thus declared that it had decided to carry out an extensive campaign of BCG vaccination of the total population of children and young adults.[50] The new international health regime and the government of India put an unprecedented amount of resources into assuring its success. But it all threatened to come apart once again as the WHO and UNICEF launched an even bigger campaign.[51]

For a time, opposition seemed only a minor concern. To be sure, here and there it was a nuisance; in a few places it was serious. But even so, well into the WHO's mass campaign, in the spring of 1955, Halfdan Mahler, the WHO's senior officer—who would go on to both lead the WHO's TB office and become the WHO's most powerful director-general—wrote a lengthy report on the ups and downs of the program. Toward the end of his report, after noting various successes and quite a number of setbacks—the indifference of doctors (as he noted: "BCG is a word by which medical directors threaten unruly doctors in the departments"), the lack of interest in public health demonstrated by certain sectors of the government—Mahler declared that "no really dangerous country-wide opposition has ever appeared so far towards the BCG vaccination. The press, radio, cinemas and the campaign's own publicity units have all contributed in consolidating BCG's popularity."[52] Mahler noted that many people were suspicions of outsiders, especially regarding the unprecedented nature of such a public health campaign. Nor was he oblivious to protest. A year earlier, in April 1954, he had reported "rather serious anti-propaganda . . . in several of the big states." Protests ranged from the use of the popular slogan that referred to BCG as "Birth Control Government-guarantee" to "dramatic features" in the vernacular press in Orissa that harked back to the Lübeck disaster and cited the major European scientists opposed to BCG. One of the Danish nurses, Inger Mundt-Petersen, reported people fleeing from vaccinators in Orissa, claiming BCG meant "Birth Control Germ." Further, there was such serious resistance in Madhya Bharat, combined with "incapable personnel" and too little money, that Mahler considered the program there a failure.[53]

Considering the suspicions, Mahler knew that winning over villagers and city dwellers, by educating them about the harmlessness of BCG and the dangers of TB, was critical to the campaign's success. Relating the story of the conversion of one village in Madhya Pradesh from hostility to openness by replacing scolds and threats with smiles and jokes, Mahler noted that the "BCG team had learned an embarrassing but fruitful lesson—To tell everybody once more that this is the biggest show on earth."[54] Indeed, he believed from the beginning that the BCG campaign was creating a new public health consciousness among rural and urban Indians as well as doctors.[55]

The pockets of resistance to the campaign did not dampen enthusiasm, nor did they foment worry about its ultimate success. Opposition appeared to be isolated—even the fatal resistance in Madhya Bharat did not spread. Perhaps most encouraging was that all seemed well in Madras, where the mass campaign got off to a good start. Raman's voice had been silenced: likely due to financial constraints and lack of energy, he stopped publishing *People's Health* in 1951.[56] Dr. Sangham Lal, director of medical services for Madras state, and previously a staunch opponent of the mass campaign, had been converted to the cause. He officially launched the program.[57] Indeed, when the WHO/UNICEF mass campaign began in Coimbatore, in November 1954, Mahler thought it a smashing success: "This explosive inauguration of the campaign caught the anti-propagandists asleep on their previous laurels; and some last minute efforts by them had no effect whatsoever." By then, January 1955, Mahler had good reason to be optimistic: "30 million people [had been] tuberculosis indoctrinated through the campaign's health education units."[58] There were challenges, but he considered one of them well on the way toward being met: people were coming around to the value of BCG. He was pleased that people with little or no experience with vaccination—the smallpox campaign was still nascent; most large scale public health interventions were responses to crises not sustained efforts—were responding favorably to what then was the largest vaccine effort in world history.[59]

But then, seemingly out of nowhere, things took a turn, and the campaign was under severe threat. In August, the *Indian Express* reported that, according to the Madras minister of health, the BCG teams were creating "mass hysteria" wherever they went.[60] A month later, the *New York Times* reported that the program in South India was in jeopardy.[61] A mass resistance movement had erupted. By September, UNICEF's field agent wrote that "the effect of the anti-propaganda is not to be underestimated, and it will influence the test-totals of the Indian BCG-Campaign."[62]

Radiating outward from the epicenter of resistance in Madras, across many parts of India the number of tuberculin tests plummeted from highs above 90 percent to in some cases zero.[63] One doctor reported from Uttar Pradesh, in the far north, that the resistance in Madras had "created a panic in the minds of the general public." Tensions were so high that he warned "there will be a public beating on the arrival of the [BCG] party."[64] In Andhra Pradesh UNICEF's BCG field nurse wrote that while the mass campaign had been lax in getting educational materials into the hands of local people the opposition had been active—and successful. Anti-BCG pamphlets were in every house in Chittoor.[65]

Across the Bay of Bengal, in Rangoon, Burma, the Reddy Young Men's Association requested copies of the movement's Bible, "BCG Vaccination: Why I Oppose It."[66] In Chittoor, Andhra state, the field nurse reported that about half the parents of school-aged children requested that they be exempted from vaccination—the other half were outraged that their children were vaccinated without parental consent.[67] Still farther north, in Punjab, one man termed the BCG doctors' LMS (Licentiate in Medicine and Surgery) degrees "License for Murder and Slaughter."[68] And, finally, the resistance in Madras fanned the flames of the antivaccination movement in England, where M. Beddow-Bayly, one of the movement's stalwarts and already on record as being against BCG, took great pleasure in seeing massive resistance to BCG.[69]

The man most responsible for this resistance was Chakravarti Rajagopalachari—the first governor-general of India, chief minister of the Madras government from 1952 to 1954, one of the founders of modern India, and the man whom Gandhi called the "keeper of my conscience."[70] Popularly known as Rajaji, he was an old friend of Raman's; they frequently socialized, spending most evenings together during this period.[71] Sympathetic to Raman's anti-BCG sentiments, Rajaji warned the Indian health minister in 1952 that the "the atmosphere is not favourable for plunging into a mass campaign"; in fact, the campaign against BCG should be taken seriously, he intoned, when devising vaccination policies. While chief minister of Madras, he kept his thoughts on BCG private.[72] But by mid-1955, he was becoming an outsider. He had been forced to resign his post as head of the Madras government. He began to develop more and more antistatist views, which led him to disagree more and more with the policies and practices of the Union government in New Delhi—policies he perceived to be bolstering central state power.[73] His protest against BCG was in part a protest against the modern Indian state. And for that he picked the perfect target—a more powerful symbol of Prime Minister Jawaharlal Nehru's modernist pretensions would have been hard to find. Mass BCG vaccination was a scheme largely devised by outsiders in league with the central government that would require Indians to submit to a medical practice many found objectionable.

Rajaji successfully tapped into a popular and deep-seated vein of suspicion, resentment, and nationalism that had been brewing since Raman's earlier protests. Like Raman before him, Rajaji and his supporters opposed BCG for many reasons. They were angry over what appeared to be experimentation on children; they had lingering worries over BCG's safety and questioned its efficacy. Profound doubt that a single technological solution would solve India's entrenched TB problem also stoked the protest. Distrust and disdain of expert outsiders made many suspicious of the campaign. An allegiance to ayurvedic over allopathic medicine characterized some of the opposition. Rajaji embodied this spirit. As one of his many correspondents put it, "The sage of the East ... refuses to bow to the West and the Westernized."[74]

But the anti-BCG forces did not possess a facile anti-Western medicine stance. The opposition's characterization by one WHO doctor, P. Mohamed Ali, as "medical Rip Van Winkles" was not apt.[75] In fact, Rajaji and his supporters readily deployed the opinions of British and American TB specialists—especially when they meshed with their own views. The people with whom Rajaji corresponded, and Rajaji himself, were anything but medical Rip Van Winkles when it came to BCG. They had a firm grasp of the global literature on the vaccine. They knew well the controversies surrounding it. When the *British Medical Journal* published its skeptical assessment of BCG in April 1955 those opposed to the vaccine in India seized on it. Two months after its publication N. K. Iyengar, a woman from Calcutta, published a letter to the editor in the *Statesman* citing the *BMJ* article as support for the anti-BCG movement.[76] Rajaji and his supporters did not object to Western medicine; they cleverly used it against the mass campaign by showing the uncertainty of BCG. Iyengar, and others, used the doubts raised by the *BMJ* to express her worry over the "serious danger" India would face if "blind adoption" of BCG proceeded and Rajaji's warnings went unheeded; if "advanced countries," she wondered, were hesitant about BCG, why should India accept it?[77]

Rajaji and his supporters opposed what they perceived to be a scheme hatched by foreign experts and an increasingly powerful strong central government bent on imposing its will on Indian bodies. A member of the Bahawalpur State Relief Committee in New Delhi wrote Rajaji in September and characterized the medical profession in India as being trapped in "mental slavery" to the West; the government was "fast becoming a terror creating machinery."[78] A correspondent from Madras, who freely quoted from some of the giants of Western medicine, made his outrage clear when he wrote, referring to the indiscriminate use of BCG, that the campaign had gone too far—"the Britishers would never have done it even in Kenya."[79] When one man learned that Rajaji favored a legislative solution to the introduction of BCG into India, he wrote of his vehement opposition: if the legislature gets involved then mandatory vaccination is all but assured—"no amount of public protest will be heeded."[80] Frustrated that their concerns were, according to one correspondent, "set aside as the blabberings of an ignoramus," Rajaji's supporters worked hard not to appear as simply reactionaries or antimodern cranks.[81] They did so by supporting their views with citations to the literature on BCG. The protests against BCG became a contest over who could better marshal scientific authority—Rajaji and his supporters or the government of India and those in the WHO and UNICEF.

But Rajaji's faith in Western medical science also had limits. While chief minister of Madras, Rajaji first voiced his uneasiness with BCG to the Union health minister, Rajkumari Amit Kaur. Despite assurances to the contrary—in the spring of 1952, he wrote: "I am a believer in modern medicine and scientific methods and particularly the great results derived from Pasteur's discoveries"—Rajaji was deeply troubled by BCG.[82] But Kaur was disheartened by what she perceived to be Rajaji's irrational opposition to the vaccine, especially given her conviction that science supported BCG. Of course, she wrote, improving living conditions, isolating carriers, and providing adequate treatment were essential to combating TB. But in 1952 India was unable to implement adequate TB control measures. A vaccine was the best hope. The rest of the world had accepted BCG; she wondered why Rajaji had not. She wished he would change his mind, for Madras was missing what the rest of India was benefiting from. "I can only hope," she wrote to Rajaji, "that the example of the rest of India will in due course make the people of Madras demand vaccination."[83] She could certainly hope.

When Rajaji began to challenge BCG in public, he continued to claim that his criticism was thoroughly scientific; he expressed no doubt about technological solutions in general. Indeed, he advocated the use of antibiotic "wonder drugs"—drugs that at the time were much more experimental than BCG.

Referring to promising results with isoniazid in actually curing the disease, he could not understand why the use of antibiotics was so limited, while vaccinations continued on a mass scale.[84] At one meeting, according to the *Hindu*, Rajaji not only "narrated the vast progress that had been made in the science of tuberculosis treatment," he went to great lengths to assure the audience that he was not blindingly opposed to vaccination—indeed, he declared himself a firm believer in smallpox vaccination. He just wanted a vaccine that worked.[85] He quoted Francis Bacon, whom he saw as a key figure in the development that had led to the "remarkable success of modern science," and declared that his opposition was not "emotional" but based on "what might be called scientific reasons."[86] He labeled BCG "quackery." In a key passage from *B.C.G.: Why I Oppose It*—his widely distributed, much admired, and much reviled pamphlet—he forcefully laid out his position, claiming that proper science was on his side: "I am not against modern 'western' therapy or modern science. B.C.G. has nothing to do with modern western medicine. . . . [M]y conclusions are not based merely on my a priori fears and doubts, but on the definite pronouncements of most eminent and illustrious medical men of the civilized world. The Indian medical men that have been recruited by the Health Ministry to conduct and speak for this campaign, the biggest among them, are not as eminent as any of the medical men, on the basis of whose observations and opinions, I have come to the conclusion that this mass campaign of inoculation with live tubercle bacilli is wrong and must be given up."[87] Rajaji demonstrated his knowledge of Western medicine by peppering his pamphlet with a liberal dose of quotes from renowned international medical journals.

Rajaji's attack on BCG demanded a response from the campaign's supporters. And in a volley of editorials and articles published primarily in the widely circulated *Hindu* newspaper, a very public debate ensued. First coming to the aid of P. V. Benjamin in defending the scientific basis of BCG was Dr. K. S. Ranganathan, director of the national BCG laboratory in Guindy just outside Madras and a supporter of the BCG campaign from the beginning.[88] In the middle of June 1955 Ranganathan called the opposition "a relic of the past" and (erroneously) claimed that the efficacy of BCG was established through proof "that was irrefutable and statistically sound."[89] In early July, J. Frimodt-Moller, the respected superintendent of the Aryogavaram Sanatorium, described BCG as "one of the latest gifts of medical science to mankind for effective protection against the disease."[90] Three weeks later, however, Frimodt-Moller again addressed the issue—but more cautiously. While convinced that BCG was harmless, he admitted that it would take some time before the efficacy of BCG could be established.[91] Rajaji immediately seized on Frimodt-Moller's equivocation. He quoted him to suggest that "the BCG campaign in India was really an experimentation on an unjustifiably large scale rather than a prophylactic measure of proved value."[92] Frimodt-Moller, now forced to publicly clarify his position, published a statement in the *Hindu* on August 3. While admitting that it would take time to produce sufficient data to determine the degree of immunity conferred by BCG, he asserted, like all the faithful, "This need not hold us back from applying B.C.G. as a general measure in this country. We have sufficient evidence from experiments in animals as well as from observations in human beings to know that B.C.G. affords considerable immunity."[93]

Rajaji's pamphlet was so successful at galvanizing opinion against BCG—it circulated all over India, and people in Burma, England, Canada, and likely elsewhere, read it—and so adroit at using Western medical research to buttress the case against the vaccine that the government was compelled to respond in kind. *The Truth about B.C.G.: Why Government Have Launched a Mass Campaign*, published by the Madras government in mid-August, specifically took issue with Rajaji's misuse of the evidence and experts. Rajaji's claim that he based his opposition "on the definite pronouncements of most eminent and illustrious medical men of the civilized world" galled the campaign's supporters.[94] The government's pamphlet highlighted this sentence to show that the eminent medical men, such as Frimodt-Moller, referred to by Rajaji actually supported BCG.[95] "Whoever may be the 'most eminent and illustrious medical men of the civilised world' who endorse the views of Rajaji," the pamphlet trumpeted, "Dr. Frimodt-Moller is not one of them."[96]

Rajaji's arsenal, like Raman's before him, included Carroll Palmer. At a meeting in October 1955 Rajaji praised Palmer as the " 'Shri Krishna' of the 'BCG Gita.' " Rajaji claimed Palmer opposed BCG.[97] But the *Truth about B.C.G.*, as well as Palmer himself, countered this claim.[98] Throughout his pamphlet, and in his correspondence, Rajaji turned doubts about the efficacy of BCG into hard-held opinions regarding its worthlessness. And in this regard, he willfully distorted Palmer's work. Palmer rebutted, writing that to summarize his work as anti-BCG "is obviously to distort and misquote my views."[99] Rajaji readily invoked the experts of modern medical science: when he agreed with them, they were reliable; when he did not, he was dismissive. For Rajaji, and Raman before him, to say nothing of those in support of BCG like P. V. Benjamin, it was a question not of believing in expert knowledge or not but of which experts to believe in.

While Rajaji relied on Western medicine to criticize the mass campaign, he did not have an especially well-developed position on Indian versus Western medicine. His followers did. Some who supported Rajaji did so because they considered the mass campaign, and the Indian government's support of it, a reproach to ayurvedic medicine. From the earliest days of the mass campaign ayurvedic and naturopathic practitioners and supporters spoke out against BCG—the Delhi Naturopathic Association, for example, wrote a resolution condemning BCG.[100] Many of ayurveda's supporters did not simply reject Western medicine as much as want ayurvedic medicine to be taken seriously.[101] There were those like A. B. Parisad, president of the Institute of Ayurvedic Studies and Research in Calcutta, who thought it acceptable to incorporate the best of Western medicine into ayurveda. What concerned him was that the "central and provincial governments are after integration and seduced by strange voices from abroad."[102] The government's commitment to ayurvedic medicine was thin, some complained; Union Health Minister Kaur was accused of discounting Indian in favor of Western medicine.[103]

Some things were more alarming still. Further angering Rajaji and his supporters was their perception that the campaign was a vast experiment on children. BCG was directed at the young, and as one correspondent put it, some considered Rajaji to be "the saviour of our helpless children." Rajaji told Kaur that the BCG campaign was "bacteriological warfare against children."[104] His pamphlet and his public pronouncements against the campaign provoked such concern that A. B. Shetty, the minister of health for Madras, decried the climate of fear created by Rajaji.[105] While by the 1950s doubts about BCG's safety had largely disappeared, they proved easy to stir up—which Rajai did by filling his pamphlet with parents' and local health officials' tales of BCG-induced health problems. Rajaji used these letters to his advantage in ways that did not precisely square with the facts.

Except in two cases, Rajaji included the letters in *B.G.C.: Why I Oppose It* before he or anyone else verified their accounts. Stories about children going blind or being stricken with TB after vaccination were offered as a powerful injunction against BCG. But their inclusion also warranted investigations into their veracity. Of the fifteen letters Rajaji quoted, two were accompanied by follow-up materials—materials that made clear that the blame placed on BCG was anything but well placed. Why Rajaji included the medical reports contradicting the parents' claims is unknown. They weakened Rajaji's position and force one to wonder about the veracity of the other thirteen cases. And in fact there are four more cases of alleged BCG-induced illness in Rajaji's papers absent from the pamphlet. All four were investigated at Rajaji's urging; all four were found to be unrelated to BCG—one child, in fact, had never been vaccinated! Just as with the scientific materials, Rajaji used some of his evidence from parents selectively. He quoted at length from a letter written to him by a man in New Delhi whose son had what appeared to be an adverse reaction to BCG. The man was angry over the supposed ill effects of BCG, yet in his original letter he supported the goals of the BCG program. After describing his family's experience he wrote, "I may add here also that I have no reason whatsoever to doubt the intentions or the bonafides of the Government. The interest of the public at large is always supreme in the eyes of the Government and it is for this reason only that a large sum is being spent over the scheme in quite good faith."[106] This was explicitly edited out of Rajaji's pamphlet.[107] What Rajaji did so successfully was to tap into a general uneasiness about vaccines and outsiders with needles and create a link in the minds of the public between sick children and BCG. He did this through his pamphlet, and, in at least one case, by urging a child's father to contact all the major Indian newspapers—something the father did before his son's poor health was found to be unrelated to BCG.[108]

While the veracity of some of the stories is suspect, Rajaji included them in his pamphlet to highlight what was at the root of the entire protest: as far as Rajaji and his supporters were concerned India was not a laboratory for testing an unproven, potentially unsafe, vaccine. The possibility that the campaign—novel, untested, invasive, of outside origin—might be harming children was especially alarming. And because the WHO did consider India a lab of sorts Rajaji was not unwarranted in writing: "I cannot resist the feeling that the mass campaign in India is a vast empirical experiment in the supposed interest of scientific progress and that Indian children are being offered for experimentation on the same plan as was put in operation among the people in war ravaged areas and [referring to the American Indian trials] uncivilized dependent communities."[109] That the WHO explicitly used India as a test case for the mass rollout of BCG deeply offended Rajaji and his followers.

What's more, Rajaji and others were dismayed that the WHO appeared to be focused on a technological fix for what was so obviously a problem of poverty. This strain of criticism emerged out of the perception on the part of Rajaji and his supporters—strongly echoing Raman's earlier critique—that the WHO considered BCG to be a panacea. Rajaji was concerned that BCG would be presented as a cure-all and that efforts to improve Indian lives would take a backseat to experimental measures like BCG. It was along these lines that many wrote to Rajaji. S. R. Srinivasa Raghavan was emblematic: "It is high time that our 'Experts' felt more humble about themselves. . . . [O]ur essential disease as a society in this world is poverty and not the multifarious ailments that result from poverty. I hope you will understand me when I say that there is no point in compelling man to live in slums and unhealthy quarters with no wherewithal to buy his needs, making him contract all the diseases in the medical dictionary and suddenly discover that a mass B.C.G. campaign is manna for him."[110]

BCG was certainly not a solution for the conditions that gave rise to TB. No one claimed it was. But in a country where raising living standards was a long-term prospect and not a possibility in the short run, not at least trying to tackle TB with BCG would, according Rajkumari Amrit Kaur, to "be guilty of criminal negligence."[111]

7. Faith, Failure, and the BCG Vaccine

India in the 1950s offers a powerful, dramatic example of resistance to BCG vaccination. Scholars love acts of resistance. But mass resistance to the mass vaccination campaign was rare.[1] And so this moment in BCG's history demands our attention for other reasons. It is important because of its place in time and the richness of its documentation. It entailed both the first WHO/UNICEF-led large-scale vaccination campaign in the developing world and the first well-documented response to that campaign. It's a response that foreshadowed critiques of vertically oriented medical interventions focused on a single disease rather than on the conditions giving rise to disease more generally. It's an early example of the outcry over experimenting with drugs in the developing world that would escalate in the decades to come. It's also important because it's not out of place. When viewed in light of the doubts surrounding BCG, the criticisms leveled at the program have a familiar feel. Rajaji, especially, took seriously the doubts about the vaccine then in circulation and used them to call into question the wisdom of the entire program. While many questioned the value of BCG in medical journals and memos, and many more would in the decades to come, Raman and Rajaji attempted to turn those doubts into action and actually stop BCG. No one else even tried. The power of the then newly emerging global health superstructure made up of bodies like the WHO and UNICEF and willing national governments—governments generally ill prepared to take care of their own unhealthy populations—was greater than the power of the critique.[2] Seen in this way, Raman's and Rajaji's suspicions should not be surprising. That a novel, invasive, painful, time-consuming procedure, with a considerable shadow of doubt cast across it, provoked skepticism on the part of thoughtful, well-informed Indians seems almost predictable. Rajaji, to be sure, was not at all times careful in his critiques—on occasion he misconstrued expert opinion and misrepresented the experiences of several children—yet he also leveled a set of critiques at BCG that were in step with the decades-old skepticism surrounding the vaccine. When viewed in light of the concerns over BCG's efficacy, Rajaji's and Raman's protests seem sensible. Imagine today what the reaction would be were the WHO to launch a similar campaign—a campaign that had at its center an unproven vaccine—in the developing world. It's hard to imagine because it simply would not happen.

The decade of resistance to the BCG vaccine in India is an important moment in the history of Western medicine's migration around the globe. Raman, Rajaji, and their followers made clear that there would not be passive acceptance of the interventions of the new international organizations. Just as important, the resistance also demonstrated the power of these new organizations: their interventions certainly met with resistance, and that resistance highlighted the need to take into account local circumstances if programs were to be successful. But resistance did not stop the mass BCG campaign. Raman only managed to slow down the introduction of BCG in South India. Rajaji's effect on the mass campaign is hard to assess, but if the number of tuberculin tests and vaccinations are any indication of the campaign's progress then the balance of the evidence suggests that the impact of Rajaji's protest was over within six to nine months. In September 1955 the mass campaign appeared to be in jeopardy; by late October 1955, Dr. P. Mohamed Ali of UNICEF reported that "the active opposition is fast dying down" in Madras, and toward the end of the year Ali described the situation in Madras as being in a slow recovery.[3] Of course, there might have been intangible effects—perhaps Rajaji's opposition soured many on mass public health campaigns. WHO doctors in other countries were certainly worried that a poorly run campaign could, as one doctor in Ethiopia put it, cause "aversion to the State and the action of the great international organizations."[4]

The protest movement in India was unique but not singular. Small pockets of resistance emerged in Iran, Mexico, and Vietnam. During the early years of the U.S. Public Health Service's BCG trial in Puerto Rico, in the early 1950s, thirty thousand children refused to participate for "political" reasons.[5] Pockets of resistance emerged, too, in Lesotho in the late 1960s.[6] And BCG met not just with popular resistance. In Ethiopia the WHO shut the program down in 1956 because of perceived high costs and the "growing inpopularity [*sic*] of BCG in certain technical quarters." As the UNICEF representative in Addis Ababa put it, "The Ethiopian BCG campaign was, thus, brought to peace under the slogan: 'Good as long as it lasted but far too expensive.'"[7] Yet the march of BCG across the developing world could not be stopped. That the anti-BCG campaign in India made no impact on the steady forward march of the vaccine demonstrates the power of the hope and faith placed in the BCG vaccine; India would continue to use BCG for decades and become the site of the largest controlled trial of the vaccine ever done. Never had the world seen medical intervention on this scale, nor had there been nongovernmental organizations like the WHO and UNICEF that were truly global in scope.

In the years after the short-lived protest in India the mass BCG campaign continued. Doubts, however, would continue in tandem with the campaign—and these critiques and cautions against unbridled enthusiasm did not just come from outsiders peering in from the fringe of the TB world. To the contrary. In 1962, Wallace Fox—who was by then one of world's most prominent TB researchers—wrote: "It is an alarming thought that over 130,000,000 BCG vaccinations have been performed by the WHO/UNICEF BCG vaccination programme in developing countries (following 350,000,000 tuberculin tests in the campaign) and yet there is no satisfactory evidence that any appreciable measure of prevention has been afforded by this enormous programme."[8] Two years later, Halfdan Mahler, director of the WHO's TB program, admitted that there was no proof of the effectiveness of BCG in the tropics.[9] Further still, the WHO itself reported that

> BCG-vaccination is, according to a small number of properly controlled trials, *highly efficient under the particular circumstances of these trials;* but almost nothing has been done to investigate the general validity of this finding, either under varying epidemiological conditions or for the widely varying modes of application of the vaccine. To the extent that BCG vaccination really prevents 80 per cent. or more of tuberculosis among vaccinated persons, it would seem to be

of as much potential importance in tuberculosis control as all other control measures taken together (case-finding, treatment, isolation); and, of course, it is very much cheaper. But BCG is used today on a wide scale also under circumstances where indirect evidence would seem to raise some doubt concerning the degree of its usefulness.[10]

BCG vaccination, nonetheless, did not lose its appeal in India or elsewhere.[11] Vaccination was still, even in the era of antibiotics—and especially in the era of drug resistance—a critical resource. In 1961 UNICEF's medical director for the Eastern Mediterranean noted that in places like Pakistan, for example, BCG vaccination was of even greater importance in the face of growing drug resistance. The value of BCG "has been overshadowed by the spectacular gains obtained from tuberculosis chemotherapy, but the mounting number of reports from all parts of the world on rapidly increasing primary microbial resistance to drugs is reverting the attention of worried public health workers to the importance of BCG vaccination."[12] At a WHO-sponsored seminar on TB held in Nairobi in 1960, the delegates all agreed that there was nothing other than BCG out there, and nothing cheaper. For this reason alone how could they not use it? Despite still not knowing if it was efficacious the WHO recommended BCG's continued and expanded use across Africa.[13] By the mid-1960s, Kenya's official policy on BCG was that "this preventive procedure is the most important tool in controlling tuberculosis in Kenya." The 80 percent efficacy rate found in Joseph Aronson's trial among American Indians had by then become a magic, almost fetishized, number. And because of the high rate of new infections in children, the WHO and the Kenyan government reasoned that "vaccination must have priority over all other control procedures."[14] By the end of 1965, one million Kenyan children had been BCG vaccinated.[15]

Since its first foray into the developing world—in India, beginning in the late 1940s—the WHO had been using this same, altogether reasonable, rationale: in the absence of an alternative and in a country with lots of TB and very little money, and now growing drug resistance, BCG was a bargain and should be tried.[16] Local doctors echoed this point. Reporting on TB in rural India in 1959 Dr. P. Mohamed Ali, in a memo that he implored his correspondents to keep confidential, pushed for even greater BCG coverage, as it was the only viable preventative.[17] Georges Canetti, another TB luminary—and the brother of Nobel laureate in literature Elias Canetti—thought that advocating against the use of BCG in the developing world, simply because it had not been found unequivocally efficacious, was unconscionable and inexcusable. He knew that conditions were different in the developing world and that the best results for BCG had been achieved in the developed world, but no matter.

> It is highly probable that, on the whole, the reduction in tuberculosis morbidity produced by vaccination may be less in the conditions of "developing" countries than in those of "developed" countries, due to the unfavourable influence of under-nourishment, of repeated tuberculous superinfections, of associated diseases, etc. We are still very badly informed about the possible incidence of these factors. However, it is obvious that the *certain* data which we possess, by controlled studies, on the reality of protection in a "developed" country, outweighs the *ignorance* of the extent of protection in a "developing" country. This is a matter of common sense. . . . For all these reasons, BCG vaccination must be continued and even increased in "developing" countries. No programme in an anti-tuberculosis campaign has the right to neglect it, and every care must be taken to render it technically more perfect.[18]

Canetti's rationale was simple: first, we know more about BCG than not; and second, even though conditions in the developing world are quite different from those found in the developed world, this is no excuse to not use BCG. Reasonable and rational as this sounds, it's still based on hope and faith.

Of course, what the faithful hoped for was the prevention, maybe even the eradication, of a deadly disease. This would have been a triumph unparalleled in human history. Hope and faith can be powerful motivators. And up to a point, there *was* no harm in trying. With no medical alternatives for the prevention of TB in sight—chemoprophylaxis, we will see later, had been written off—trying BCG made sense. But where should the line have been drawn? That is, at what point should those advocating for the continued use of the vaccine have realized that a new strategy was necessary?

As we've seen, at the end of the 1950s, when looking back on twenty years of BCG research, Joseph Aronson pointed out that BCG's effect was all but impossible to discern in areas where the infection rate was in steep decline. Others voiced the same concerns. As Carroll Palmer and colleagues made clear in 1958 when analyzing two much larger trials in Alabama and Georgia and in Puerto Rico, the vast majority of cases of TB in these places arose in reactors to tuberculin. In other words, it was people not included in the trial, rather than participants, who acquired the most TB; it was people *already* infected with the bacilli who went on to develop active disease.[19] Regarding reactors, Palmer came to an important realization—a realization that would help to understand the low success rate with BCG in the years to come: "A more credible interpretation [of the seeming rise in cases] is that the incidence of disease among reactors has always been substantial and that it only seemed low and of little consequence in situations in which a large number of cases were arising as a result of new infections."[20] But in the places Palmer was looking at, the opposite was now the case: low rates of new infections. Contrast this with Kenya in 1964: there 80 percent of cases were new infections, not the reactivation of disease in those already infected. This is an entirely different problem.[21] Palmer's point was that in places where infection rates were low BCG might have no value, especially if most new cases were coming from those already infected.[22] Further, testing BCG's efficacy in areas of low infection would not necessarily tell you much about how it would or would not work in areas of high infection. Aronson's study was well set up and rigorously run, but its conclusions might not be applicable to places where BCG was most needed—those places where infection rates were high. Palmer preferred a cautious approach to BCG—an approach not uncommon in the United States.

Then came the news from Britain: a ten-year follow-up to a trial of fifty thousand schoolchildren had found that BCG had a significant protective effect. While the results were sound and the trial was well run, the same question needed to be asked of this trial as of Aronson's: were the results replicable, especially in areas where rates of infection were high—much higher than in Britain.[23]

Just as the impact of the British trial began to settle in—news that seemed unequivocally good—more bad news for BCG emerged. Carroll Palmer and George Comstock reported in 1966 on their fourteen-year follow-up to their Georgia trial. They concluded after nearly a decade and a half of observation that "the evidence indicates that the protection afforded by BCG in this population was less than modest, relatively short-lived, and least effective among the segments of the population that needed it most."[24] The news from Puerto Rico was no better. When reflecting on the poor results of the Puerto Rican trial, in 1974, Comstock acidly commented that a "major lesson of the past 20 years—that the effectiveness of BCG vaccination in various circumstances can range from 80 per cent down to 0 per cent—seems to have gone unheeded by most of the world's tuberculosis workers. Time and time again one hears that the BCG can give 80 per cent protection, with the implicit assumption that any strain used in any situation will live up to this expectation." But as had been well known since the late 1950s, there were many, many strains of BCG, all different from one another.[25] Comstock did not mince words when offering his final assessment of BCG: "Because BCG vaccination is the major method of tuberculosis control in all but a few of the highly developed nations, it is particularly tragic that the use of scarce resources to administer BCG must still be based on blind faith."[26]

Comstock's certainty notwithstanding, one still must wonder why Palmer and Comstock's results differed so much from those in Britain. In short, no one knows exactly. Palmer argued that something called nonspecific mycobacterial infection—more prevalent in warm climates—compromised BCG. P. D'Arcy Hart—the doyen of the British TB world—thought, as did others, that the potency of the vaccines differed. Both Palmer and Hart allowed that neither explanation could account entirely for the dramatic difference in the respective trials. There was, all admitted, an element of mystery.[27]

To solve the mystery, to—one hoped—answer once and for all whether or not BCG worked, in 1968 the WHO and the Indian Council of Medical Research embarked on a massive trial in South India. The trial—one of the largest ever conducted on any drug—ran for eleven years. It covered a population of three hundred and sixty thousand just outside Madras. Low-grade tuberculin sensitivity, due to nonspecific mycobacterial infection, was common. Would BCG work in such a context? The answer, which came in 1979, was unequivocally no. BCG had no protective effect. The medical world was stunned; some gloated, while others went into defensive mode. The results were scrutinized, second guessed, and judged to be sound. BCG did not work.

Yet, as Niels Brimnes has clearly shown, not even after BCG had failed on such a scale did it lose favor. Shortly after the results came in, the WHO convened a study group to explore what had happened. When the members of the group released their findings in 1980 they admitted that the "lack of protection from BCG in the study population was a complete surprise and has so far defied explanation."[28] But the Indian results, the experts said, might not apply elsewhere—conditions in India might be different enough from, say, Kenya, that BCG's lack of efficacy in one place might not be indicative of its potential for failure or success in another. Later that year the group met in Geneva to issue its policy recommendations. By now in this story the recommendations should not come as a surprise: considering that some places are low on resources and BCG might be the only thing available, there's no harm in using it. The results from the Indian trial had, it seems, no impact on BCG's continued use. What to make of the trial? Brimnes puts it well: "What appears striking here is how the universality of the BCG trials suddenly disappeared. Since the 1950s WHO and UNICEF had vaccinated millions with BCG, because it apparently worked in Europe. Now, however, the disturbing results from the Chingleput study were explained—if not entirely dismissed—simply as local."[29] Some even theorized that there was a South Indian variant of *Mycobacterium tuberculosis* not susceptible to BCG.[30] This is entirely possible, but if it's possible that there are strains so different that they don't respond to the BCG given, and if there are so many different strains of BCG, how would it ever be possible to land on the correct combination?

Over the years it became clear that BCG's problems were myriad, but at each step enough people thought they were surmountable. Light was shown to have a detrimental effect on the vaccine; different strains from different labs acted differently; nonspecific mycobacterial infection was thought to compromise BCG's efficacy; vaccination rates in some places were low and the cost was high—all of these, not to mention the failure of the South Indian trial, were reasons, if not to abandon BCG, to seriously question its continued use. At each step of the way, however, a combination of faith and futility won—the faith that the problems could be solved, and the futility that stemmed from knowing that in many places there simply was nothing else to use.

Debating BCG's efficacy continued.[31] But after the failure of the Indian trial, even though the vaccine was still in use, much of the momentum from the old days was gone. BCG was no longer the center of attention but, rather, occupied an uncomfortable position in the world of TB control. For by the mid-1990s the WHO recognized BCG's virtual uselessness in preventing primary infection and infectious pulmonary disease, while at the same time it recommended the vaccine's continued use in high-prevalence areas.[32] It became, and remains, a major component of the WHO's "Expanded Programme on Immunization" because it helps to prevent severe, but relatively uncommon, forms of the disease in children.[33]

Despite a recent review's suggestion that BCG seems to have had some protective effect against pulmonary TB when administered early in life and before exposure to either *Mycobacterium tuberculosis* or environmental mycobacteria (more abundant the closer you get to the equator), the vaccine has nonetheless done little or nothing to reduce the world's burden of pulmonary TB—by far the most common and infectious form of the disease.[34]

Did the persistent faith in BCG limit the development of viable alternatives? Of course, this is a difficult question to answer. But it's a possibility: for as long as BCG was in use, and the faithful prevailed, nothing else emerged. And, at least according to George Comstock, time and money were being wasted doling out an ineffective vaccine. There were no trials of other vaccines; there was no robust (or even lackluster) research. British TB expert Paul Fine's sharp-tongued comment from the late 1980s sums things up: "It seems as though the global BCG campaigns were more successful in eradicating tuberculosis research than in eradicating tuberculosis."[35]

The story of BCG is a chapter in the failure of TB control. Like all historical verdicts, this is a retrospective judgment. The promise of BCG buoyed a decades-long heyday of hope and experimentation and seemingly boundless energy. Failure, not to say doubt, was far from most people's minds. There were skeptics and believers, and the faithful won. Once BCG was deemed safe there was little reason not to at least try it. What's clear from our vantage point, however, is that the doubts expressed about the vaccine added up to what should have been a death sentence for BCG. However, BCG spread across the planet at a time when the regulation of such things was much less robust than it is today: during the mass campaign, for example, a country simply signed an agreement with UNICEF, and BCG was on its way. The logistics of getting BCG to where it needed to go were daunting, to be sure, but deciding to do so was pretty painless. And thus BCG traveled the globe.

No successful TB vaccine has ever been found. And because BCG does not work, no other preventive agent has been given to so many people with so little effect. It's possible that the BCG vaccine is the world's largest failed medical intervention.

8. Curing TB
Antibiotics, Drug Resistance, and Compliance in Kenya

To re-create the excitement and anxiety produced by the discovery of antibiotics for TB is all but impossible. But try to imagine it. You're a doctor in Kenya in, say, 1945. You've got a patient with active TB; she's just come in that day, having suffered at home until faced with the fact that she had no other choice: she had to visit the clinic. She has a hacking cough. During her first night in the clinic sweat pours off of her emaciated body. The sheets are drenched. Blood is splattered on her pillow. Her chest x-ray shows a lung being eaten alive by TB. You can maybe give her some cod liver oil. You can make her feel better. But she's more or less reached the point where your clinic has become a hospice. In Kenya at the mid-century mark this was the state of the art. As the director of medical services told his staff: "Until a specific bacteriocidal agent, which is both inexpensive and easily administered, is added to our armamentarium, some progress, and even arrest of the disease, may be achieved by ensuring proper rest and appropriate diet."[1]

Now you're a doctor just nine years later, in 1954. Same patient; same symptoms. But you've got antibiotics; you can save her life. Your patient will get a course in the clinic and then go home. In time, she'll be fine.

This scenario, crudely rendered though it is, reflects the rapid change brought on by the introduction of antibiotics. Their discovery was a medical breakthrough of the sort rarely, if ever, seen: for centuries, there had been no cure for TB. And then there was. Doctors like Arthur Williams, who would go on to become a pioneer in the treatment of TB in East Africa, wrote in frustration in 1945 that "no very encouraging reports have appeared on the synthetic preparations . . . so far tried out." If and when chemotherapy for TB became a reality it would "revolutionise not only the treatment of the disease but the whole social and public health problem of tuberculosis."[2] With the discovery of effective antibiotics, the revolution that Williams imagined came to pass less than a decade later.

But, as we will see in this chapter and the next, it was a revolution the promises of which went unfulfilled. Excitement over the new drugs quickly turned to worry. And the hard labor of making them work in the real world began.

Making sense of what happened in Kenya has meant sifting through a lot of paper. It was clear Kenya was crucial to the story of global TB control. Kenya, after all, was the site of the some of the most important TB research ever undertaken—before or since. Both the British Medical Research Council and the WHO launched long-running research projects in Kenya—the MRC began working in Kenya in the mid-1950s and ramped its work up considerably in the late 1950s when it began a series of pathbreaking clinical trials. The WHO came to Kenya in 1958 when the WHO, UNICEF, and the Kenyan government jointly founded and funded the Nairobi Chemotherapy Research Centre. They surveyed the country and eventually set up a mass vaccine campaign, too. For nearly two decades Kenya was the scene of an intense effort to understand and control TB. The postwar impulse to develop—that impulse that spawned the creation of the WHO, for example—was keenly felt in British colonies like Kenya. The close to two decades between the end of the war and Kenyan independence also saw the British ramp up development activities, increase scientific research, and push into rural Kenyan lives in unprecedented ways—so pervasive was the colonial state in postwar development schemes that some have called this "the second colonial occupation."[3] At the same time, urban migration to Nairobi—observers at the time and since have commented on the swelling of the city's population—continued to exacerbate the problem of TB. Inadequate housing, not enough work, and a flaccid public health sector all but ensured that the city would be an incubator for disease.[4] After independence, Jomo Kenyatta's government made access to health care, especially in rural areas, the focus of robust efforts. While these efforts were not as successful as was hoped for, it was still the case that from independence through the 1970s life expectancy rose, access to care increased, and infant mortality dropped.[5] More Kenyans became doctors; the "Africanization" of medicine was an important postindependence goal. In terms of medicine, in many respects the colonial and postcolonial states mirrored one another: both consolidated medicine into a central state apparatus that was a symbol of their power and of their weakness.[6]

It was clear: if I was going to write a book about TB control in the twentieth century I needed to consider Kenya. But what was the story? Several dozen important research papers came out of Kenya between the mid-1950s and mid-1970s. I pored over them; at times I felt overwhelmed at their technical detail; I did not really know what to make of them. What was there for a historian?

I headed to the archives in England, Kenya, and Geneva. I collected lots and lots of material. As I sifted through my stacks, reading and rereading the documents, I kept being confronted by a mass of technical detail on things like dosage regimes and budget discussions and so forth. I despaired of ever being able to transcend the details of medical research. But at some point I came across two documents that piqued my interest. Written nearly a decade apart—the first in 1952 and the second in 1961—both concerned drug-resistant TB. Though drug-resistant TB, especially multidrug-resistant TB (MDR-TB), is now such a focus in the world of TB control, I had not considered it to have been an issue so long ago. But it was, and it seemed to be serious. In the first document, a rural doctor, fearing the development of resistance, refused to use isoniazid, a new antibiotic then just on the market and hailed by many as a wonder drug; in the second, only nine years later, Kenya's director of TB services warned the government that drug-resistant TB might now be out of control. How could it be that in such a short time Kenya went from having no antibiotics at all to facing a serious drug-resistant TB problem?

From reading about drug-resistant TB in places like Russia, Peru, and South Africa, to name only a few, in the late twentieth and early twenty-first centuries I knew it was now a serious problem. Antibiotics that promise to cure TB, when used improperly, can make the problem they were designed to solve actually much worse. Had that happened in Kenya more than half a century ago? How could that be when Kenya was under the constant scrutiny of the MRC and the WHO? I decided to find out. I had my story.

It's a convoluted story. Many moving parts are at work here. There's a welter of details, but there are also significant gaps in the record. It's a story filled with unfamiliar-sounding drug names like isoniazid and thiosemicarbazone, pyrazinamide and ethambutol. There are concepts such as primary and secondary drug resistance that will be new to many readers. Shifts in policy and medical practice occur regularly and often without explanation; there's inconsistency and contradiction. Why people with TB might or might not take or be able to take their drugs, as a historical matter, will also likely be a surprise to some, yet understanding it is critical. It's an important story. As I noted in the Introduction, the *Bulletin of the World Health Organization* not long ago published an article claiming that the emergence of extensively drug-resistant TB (XDR-TB) "is evidence of a new form of regression: we have taken the curable and made it nearly uncurable."[7] The origins of how that happened are to be found in the 1950s and 1960s and into the 1970s when TB workers first sounded the alarm about drug-resistant TB and its potential to career out of control. Drug-resistant TB is not a new problem; its seriousness and causes were identified decades ago. In that regard, XDR-TB is not a new form of regression; considering the story that follows, it's an almost predictable outcome.

That this story takes place in late colonial and early postcolonial Kenya is also noteworthy—though it is not as important as one might think. Just as I was startled at finding drug-resistant TB so pervasive I was also surprised by the absence of commentary regarding the fall of the empire—the empire that employed just about all the doctors and others I talk about in the following pages. But it's clear that medical research carried on apace, barely registering what was obviously a colossal change in other aspects of Kenyan life—from the lifting of race-based employment restrictions to of course having Kenyans running the government. Such a volatile time in Kenyan history, I had assumed, would have generated at a minimum an observation or two. Indeed, some of what follows, for instance, takes place during what's known as the Mau-Mau uprising—an event that has generated a robust historiography and is well known as a critical time in the late colonial history of the British Empire. It's a time when the empire was clearly on its last legs, resorting to brutal violence in the face of challenges to its power.[8] But not only does little of what follows seem to have been affected by late colonial power struggles; almost no one talked about them. As we will see, some thought that the Mau-Mau uprising exacerbated TB, as access to care and drugs was restricted during the so-called Emergency; and afterward, when travel restrictions were lifted, patients became hard to keep track of. But, even though much of the TB research took place just north of Nairobi, in the Kikuyu homeland of Kiambu—an important site of the Mau-Mau uprising—anticolonial sentiment seems to have been a small star in the constellation of social concerns doctors looked at regarding drug-resistant TB. Likewise, independence came and went, and TB work carried on.

Of course, as a historian my job is to ferret out connections, to expose the connective tissue of events that might otherwise seem unrelated. And so surely, my historical instincts told me, British doctors working in Kenya at the end of empire would have been fretting about the colonial enterprise, its collapse, and the subsequent dire consequences for their TB work. I assumed I would find keen observers like Pierce Kent—the director of TB services in Kenya; an energetic letter and memo writer; and a frequent worrier over such governmental matters as budgets and so forth—at least wondering what the fall of the empire and the emergence of newly independent Kenya might mean for British-sponsored TB research. Back in London, certainly, those running the research would have wondered the same. But none of this is so. Why?

One possible answer is that the doctors and medical bureaucrats featured in this story carried out their work, like other researchers in the colonies, not concerned with the broader issues of late colonial politics. In an era when the Colonial Office, with a substantial boost in funds courtesy of the Colonial Development and Welfare Act of 1940, deployed a new cadre of elite researchers across the empire, especially in Africa, those working on TB were freed from worrying about anything but TB. Indeed, it was the wish of the MRC that it retain exclusive control over all aspects of medical research in the colonies and that medical researchers operate with substantial autonomy.[9] Their affiliations, their loyalties, their interests, their day-to-day lives—these were all devoted to medicine, their research, the quotidian details of day-to-day operations. The reticence of the documents about much more than technical details is evidence of this silence. People like Wallace Fox, a pioneering TB researcher who led research efforts on domiciliary care and shorter, cheaper treatment regimens via his work in India, Kenya, Hong Kong, and Singapore, and others from the MRC, to say nothing of the long list of WHO personnel who came and went from Kenya, did not seem to concern themselves with matters historians might wish they had. The correspondence, the memos, the medical literature that make up the sources for this chapter and the next—and they are a vast corpus—are for the most part silent on the crumbling empire and the specter of independence. So too are local doctors and medical staff. For Kenyans, of course, independence meant greater opportunities to become doctors, and we begin to see more Kenyans in positions of power in TB research. But it's also true that many Kenyans involved in medical research during the colonial period continued their work unfazed by independence aside from perhaps being pleased to be able to carry out their work with Kenyans in control.[10] Events that we would consider important historically, events that those at the time in other spheres in Kenya and Britain did think important, and perhaps even TB researchers thought noteworthy, were something the actors in this story simply remained silent about.

And that's both fascinated and frustrated me. In India, as we have seen, there was a major, albeit short-lived, homegrown resistance to vaccination that so readily and obviously took the story into the realm of the political and generated substantial commentary. When it came to race and blood and TB in American Indians, as well as people in East Africa and South Africa, what medical people thought about larger social matters was readily discernible from their writing. Their views on race and "primitive people" were not a secret. Medical matters were obviously tangled up in social and political concerns. It's for these reasons that when I began to explore Kenya I was surprised to find that almost no one spoke about anything but TB. Lyle Cummins and Basil Dormer were not just writing about TB: Cummins explicitly commented on racial evolution and modernity; Dormer wrote about the ravages of capitalism and inequality. Wallace Fox and Pierce Kent? Well, they wrote about TB.

Fox and Kent and others, as we will see, knew that the prevalence of TB was tied to social and economic conditions. Indeed, it was those very conditions that much of their work was devoted to overcoming—Fox made it clear, for example, in pioneering research in India, that a hospital stay was not necessary to treat TB. Home care could work. At a time when most thought sick people in the developing world lived in conditions that prohibited them from caring for themselves, this was a powerful and important finding. Developing a treatment regimen that was affordable, readily complied with, and made up of easily accessible, nontoxic drugs was the goal of TB research in East Africa and India. The biomedical challenge was formidable; so, too, many came to realize, were the social and economic challenges—perhaps even more so. But those involved in TB research in the 1950s, 60s, and 70s in Kenya worked through these problems obliquely, never commenting in any explicit way on the sociopolitical structures that might help explain the emergence of drug-resistant TB.

And so the focus here might seem superficially to be on medical bureaucrats and researchers—thus solely on the science of antibiotics. In a way, that's true. For despite the fact that when read carefully and cumulatively, the memos, letters, research protocols, and publications that make up the sources reveal a deep engagement with the nonmedical world, a keen awareness of the social and economic dimensions of the problem, it is also the case that the responsibility for TB control lay with medical people as the disease came increasingly to be seen as a biomedical problem. For an era when many thought of diseases as technical problems this should come as no surprise. The irony should be clear: the biomedical personnel dispatched to tackle TB began to see that TB's life in the social world was just as important, if not more so, than its biomedical profile at a time when biomedicine appeared triumphant and dominant. Yet, of course, biomedical researchers like Wallace Fox and Pierce Kent had very little capacity to change the sociomedical context in which TB flourished. By amplifying their focus on medical research here it's loud and clear that despite their recognition of the social dimensions of TB they were charged with solving it biomedically. Someone like Kent was acutely aware that TB was much more than a technical problem. In Kenya and elsewhere it was not, as Walsh McDermott would have it, a "disease [that] can be decisively altered *without* having to await improvement in the social infrastructure."[11] Despite knowing this, Kent and others had little choice but to approach the problem in this way.

From the moment antibiotics arrived in Kenya they were a source of both hope and concern. There was hope, of course, because now a cure existed. But there was deep concern, too. The concern was drug resistance. By the time antibiotics arrived in Kenya resistance had become a well-known problem plaguing the use of streptomycin in Europe and America.[12] As early as 1952, we find a doctor in rural Kenya refusing to use isoniazid. After reading an article in the *British Medical Journal* that reported very high rates of drug-resistant TB, Dr. D. R. Blomfeld considered the drug too dangerous to use. Blomfeld was prescient, imagining a future—a future he thought "awful to consider"—filled with rampant drug resistance. He was not the only one urging caution. W. S. Haynes, director of the Port Reitz Chest Hospital in Mombasa and the author of the 1948 Kenyan TB survey, thought the MRC's findings in England "so important that we cannot override it here." He was emphatic: "I cannot endorse the policy of using this drug as a large scale outpatient treatment by itself." By the end of 1952 the Medical Department had banned isoniazid from use on an outpatient basis.[13] When A. J. Walker, the director of medical services for Kenya Colony, drew up what he called his "Scheme for the Control of Tuberculosis," drug resistance had become a major concern. He worried that there would never be enough beds for all TB patients. A system of home care was essential. But this then left drug adherence in the hands of patients—and doctors worried about this. A viable system of domiciliary care in which patients reliably took their medicine and stayed out of the hospital became the holy grail of TB treatment. But such a thing did not yet exist in Kenya, and because of this Walker knew that there was a potentially massive problem in the works. The "loose control of domiciliary administration," Walker feared, would guarantee drug resistance, yet so little was still known about how to set up an adequate outpatient system that the quick pace of drug-resistant TB could well outrun the slow gait of progress being made against it.[14]

Walker and others were right to be worried. Antibiotics appeared in Kenya not only well before a system existed for their distribution but also absent adequate training in their basic use. In the years before formal TB treatment programs emerged and drug regimens had yet to be standardized, TB treatment was an ad hoc affair. Without strict drug regimens clinicians established their care on what seemed appropriate based on experiment, common sense, and improvisation.[15] Considering what we know now about drug resistance, one shudders when reading about early antibiotic treatment. In the beginning, doctors in Kenya were flying by the seat of their pants. As a regimen of treatment for TB in Port Reitz Chest Hospital chemotherapy as well as cod liver oil were considered. The course of treatment was casual: "Isoniazid + P.A.S. for say two months, a break of a month and then resumption for another month."[16]

With the warnings of doctors like Blomfeld, Haynes, and Walker going unheeded, and with a lack of infrastructure and a standard of care, drug-resistant TB only grew, so that by the late 1950s and early 60s the problem had become serious. And not only in Kenya. Reports from Kumasi in Ghana and from, as it was then called, Ruanda-Urundi, revealed appallingly high rates of drug-resistant TB—28 percent and 52 percent, respectively, of patients were *presenting* with drug-resistant TB.[17] In a survey in Sudan, 85 percent of patients with a history of previous chemotherapy had resistance to one or more drugs.[18] In Hong Kong the problem of resistance was especially confounding because drugs that worked in East Africa would not work in Hong Kong. No one knew why, but drug resistance had reached alarming proportions.[19] And in South India it was found that "the number of patients excreting resistant strains present a formidable problem. . . . Before very long it may be too late to do anything about it."[20] By the end of the 1950s, Haynes, then the foremost expert on TB in Kenya, considered the problem of drug resistance to be of the "gravest import." "Not only," he wrote, "are the figures much bigger than any have seen reported from anywhere else in the world. But the tendency seems to be for more and more resistance to occur as time goes on." Haynes warned that "if things progress as they are at present, it seems likely that in a short time most of our valuable drugs will be ineffective."[21] Arthur Williams, who had been running small-scale antibiotic trials at Makerere University Medical School in Kampala since the early 1950s, wondered if the time had come to stop putting so much time into figuring out how to treat drug sensitive TB—the base knowledge was there, after all—and instead focus on the "already alarming problems of drug resistant infection."[22] After all, "drug resistance particularly isoniazid resistance is in the forefront" of problems facing those trying to control TB in East Africa.[23]

Finally, and perhaps most concerning, was what Kent turned up in 1958 at the one-year follow-up to his 10 percent sample survey of TB-positive patients in Kenya. The design of his study was simple: he randomly tested 10 percent (or 670 people) of the total annual incidence of TB in Kenya; he found 305 positive cases and began treatment. A year later he went back to those same people to see how they had done. Ninety-five were either dead or had been lost; 69 percent (or 210 people) who had been positive were still alive. For a variety of reasons Kent was only able to collect sputa from 176 of these people for retesting. He began to worry: of those 176 people, 69 were sputum positive on culture one year later; that is, a year of treatment had not cured their TB. And, 62 of those 69 were resistant to isoniazid; 37 of these were *also* resistant to PAS, and a further 7 were in addition resistant to streptomycin. These numbers were not encouraging. We should note in particular that 95 out of the 305 positive cases were either dead or missing. This means that about 25 percent of people who were *known* to have TB were lost sight of and were now—if still alive—spreading partially treated tuberculosis.[24] Add this to the following common scenario described by the principal medical officer in Kenya's densely populated Central Province and it will become clear just how menacing the problem could become: "There are some patients who are under treatment who probably do not have TB, some persist on drugs when a sensitivity test has shown them to be resistant and another combination indicated, and there are many children under treatment for primary TB who do not even have the result of the mantoux test recorded. The doctor has to see that the elementary rules of TB are observed. . . . Thus the TB set up in Nyeri is only just able to cope with the situation and it is clear that if the number of patients continues to increase without an increase in the staff to deal with them, a breaking point will be reached."[25] What the medical officer described was not uncommon: rampant misuse of TB drugs based on poor diagnostics; lots of drug resistance, which of course led to more of the same; and the draining away of precious resources expended on people who did not need them.

The future that Dr. Blomfeld had imagined in 1952 as "awful to consider" had taken only eight years to arrive. Across Kenya drug resistance was a major problem. In 1960 researchers from the MRC reported that they found a "high, unexpected, widely distributed and perhaps unsuspected prevalence of isoniazid and PAS-resistant strains in East Africa . . . that has appeared over a short period of years."[26] P. D'Arcy Hart at the MRC had begun to see that the problem of drug resistance was urgent. Based on the numbers of people presenting with drug-resistant TB—up to 16 percent—this was a problem that if left unchecked would soon render antibiotics all but useless.[27]

Drug resistance had become such a problem in Kenya because antibiotics came to the country before an infrastructure existed to ensure their proper use. What could be done? How could drug-resistant TB be stemmed? The answer was simple: find a short, easily taken drug regimen that combined isoniazid with something else. The consensus was clear: because Kenya's clinical experience with antibiotics had shown that a multidrug regimen, such as isoniazid and PAS or streptomycin, was challenging—irregular drug supply, very long treatment cycle, high default rate, poorly trained medical personnel, no standard treatment, unpleasant side effects, and very expensive—getting a trial up and running to test cheap and effective chemo-therapy drugs was essential. Streptomycin, along with being useless on its own against TB, was expensive and difficult to give—it had to be given by injection and thus required special training and could not be self-administered. A cheaper, easier to use pill would be much better.[28] In Kenya, the high cost of drugs was becoming difficult to bear by as early as 1958, ac-cording to A. J. Walker, the director of medical services, "hence the urgency of the present trials to find cheaper drugs."[29] Shortening the length of treat-ment was also essential. By the late 1950s, out of an estimated fifty thousand cases in the country, there were already eight thousand people in Kenya be-ing treated. But after about six months into the twelve-to-eighteen-month course the default was found to be very high.[30] Shortening treatment, making it cheaper, less toxic, and easy to administer—these were the formidable challenges Kenya faced.

Also important to overcome in these early days was casting aside some old thinking regarding Africans and TB. As we've seen, by the 1950s most TB workers had jettisoned the notion that race and TB were intimate-ly connected. There were some holdouts, to be sure; but thinking of TB as a disease that affected one race more than another, based on *biological not social* differences, was largely a thing of the past. Even so, the emergence of antibiotics brought this issue briefly to the fore again. While clinicians had been using antibiotics with good results, researchers needed to know if Africans would respond to the new drugs because, as Wallace Fox wrote, "It is generally assumed that the effectiveness of chemotherapy in patients with these different racial origins cannot be compared."[31] While the new drugs had been tested in Europeans and shown to be very effective, some doubted that the drugs would have the same effect on Africans.[32] This con-cern was soon put to rest. Because of trials in Uganda, run by Wallace Fox, Paul Hutton, and Arthur Williams at Makerere, as well as less formal stud-ies which were taking place in Southern Rhodesia, for instance, and which were in large part designed to answer the question of African susceptibility to antibiotics, everyone was satisfied that Africans did respond just as fa-vorably as others to chemotherapy.[33]

Whether or not antibiotics simply worked proved to be an easy ques-tion to answer. What came next was not. What was the best way to get anti-biotics where they needed to be? By the mid-1950s researchers from the MRC set for themselves an ambitious goal—Walker's holy grail: developing an effective, home-based, cheap drug therapy.[34] Hutton and Williams had been tackling this question in their work in Uganda when they realized early on that effective chemotherapy might obviate the need for constructing a massive TB infrastructure akin to that in Europe—something that would likely not happen in Africa in any case.[35] By 1956 it was clear a large trial was necessary, and the MRC was up to the challenge. Still basking in the success of its pathbreaking streptomycin trials—the first randomly controlled clinical trials the world had seen—and becoming increasingly important in Britain's postwar, state-sponsored medical research complex, the MRC was both game and uniquely well prepared.[36] The earlier, smaller trials had made clear not only that Africans were susceptible to the new TB drugs but, more important, that the new TB drugs had the potential to *control* the TB problem. Williams, who had been running the trials in Uganda—those first, key trials—and who had been in East Africa investigating TB since the 1930s, realized that the "next trial is going to be of much greater importance than anything we have hitherto tackled. It is going to be on a larger scale, and longer."[37]

The larger trials set out to answer complicated questions. At the heart of these questions was of course the problem of drug resistance, which all admitted could not now be ignored. After the failure of an earlier trial of a sulphone/isoniazid combination to combat isoniazid resistance, the MRC needed to rethink its plans. What would work? Isoniazid was promising but confounding: it was cheap and powerful and easy to give but also needed a companion drug to keep drug resistance from developing. It would not work alone, it seemed. When laying out the trial goals Williams told the Colonial Medical Research Committee that tackling drug resistance was "urgently required" because between 10 percent and 16 percent of patients in their trials to date had been "*presenting*" (emphasis in original) with TB that was resistant to isoniazid.[38] Alongside having to find a cheap and easily administered drug regimen was the need to find one that combated drug resistance at the community level. A cheap drug was no good if it produced TB that was harder to control—in fact, it was worse than no drugs at all. At a 1960 meeting in Nairobi on Africa's TB problem, a group of TB experts reflected on the TB problem across the continent, and to a person they agreed "that any method of treatment which did not result in sputum negativity, was a failure of import both to the individual and to the public health. . . . Mono-drug therapy (INH) resulted in sputum negativity in 40 to 60 per cent of cases: it was considered that the balance might well constitute a public health danger as great as, or even greater than, they would have done had they never been given any treatment."[39] How could no treatment be worse than at least trying some? Because those left uncured were infecting people with drug-resistant strains of TB. A group of doctors in Nigeria echoed these concerns: "Tuberculosis is a public health problem. Any scheme for its treatment must therefore be judged not only by its value to the individuals treated but also by its effect in the community. Failure of treatment is a tragedy for the patient concerned. It is also a waste of scarce resources. From the point of the view of the community, ineffective treatment is worse than none at all, because the patient whose life is prolonged excretes tubercule bacilli for a longer period and his bacilli may now be drug resistant."[40]

To combat this, researchers at the MRC had two options. There might be other companion agents that could temper isoniazid, and there were still questions to be answered about using isoniazid alone—which they needed to answer quickly, "since we believe there are projects afoot to distribute isoniazid liberally in underdeveloped territories."[41] So they decided to learn whether or not thiacetazone would work to hinder isoniazid resistance.[42] Also of the utmost urgency was finding the answers to a set of questions about isoniazid. There was controversy over whether or not very high doses of the drug worked better in cases of isoniazid-resistant TB. It was thought possible that highly resistant strains of TB were not as virulent and thus might be made less infectious when pummeled by very large doses of isoniazid. Different individuals reacted quite differently to isoniazid, and so the hope was that a test could be developed to predetermine who would benefit from isoniazid alone. If such a thing could be made possible, treating large numbers of people, very cheaply, would result.[43] This was thought to be possible because highly resistant strains lacked catalase. The opposite was also questioned: would lower doses of isoniazid work better in drug susceptible TB because of the presence of catalase? As Hart put it, "The controversy centres around whether persons producing a highly resistant strain are less likely to spread the disease to their fellows than those with strains of lower resistance." These might sound like technical details—they are that, but they're more too. Figuring all of this out was of critical importance because of the possibility that higher dosages of isoniazid might actually produce drug resistance. Answering this question, according to Hart, was of "considerable urgency since the WHO is advocating rather indiscriminate use of isoniazid in ordinary dosage in under-developed countries (including Kenya, I believe)."[44] And of course the problem was not at all limited to Africa. Hart considered the question of whether or not to use isoniazid alone or in combination to be the "greatest chemotherapeutic dilemma in the field of tuberculosis in the continent of Asia."[45] Understanding the way isoniazid worked was thus of obvious importance.

The WHO's plans for using isoniazid alone ran up against the sentiments of most in the world of African TB control—they considered using the drug on its own to be a guarantee of drug resistance. But its appeal was understandable: it was cheap and easy to take. And when funds were limited and people clamored for treatment it proved hard to say no. Such was the case in India, where treating people with PAS and isoniazid was considered prohibitively expensive; rather than do nothing, using isoniazid alone was the answer.[46] But some did say no. After the *British Medical Journal* published its results in 1952, many Kenyan doctors, as we've seen, refused to use isoniazid alone, and the Medical Department banned its outpatient use. Others regretted their choice. John Goodall in Nyasaland worried that by giving the drug alone he had done more harm than good.[47] But for the better part of a decade, clinicians in Kenya had to fight against those at the WHO and elsewhere who advocated the use of the drug by itself—something the WHO had been doing since at least 1955 as an alternative to no treatment at all.[48] There is a tragic irony to the WHO's advocacy of isoniazid alone: the conditions under which WHO sanctioned its use—programs unable to marshal the resources to roll out combined therapy—were the very conditions in which isoniazid alone would be the most dangerous. If combination therapy was too much to handle, so too would be the inevitable drug resistance flowering forth from unchecked isoniazid use.

Doctors in Africa knew this and knew too that using the drug alone *was* worse than nothing at all. But then local doctors, it seemed, were no match for prominent people with a sophisticated understanding of TB, such as Johannes Holm, Walsh McDermott, and Hugh Stott, all of whom downplayed the risks of drug resistance from monotherapy. In 1956, during a visit to Kenya, according to the director of medical services, Holm "belittled" Kenyan doctors' fears of drug-resistant TB; Holm considered the risk "more theoretical than practical." He "astonished" the Kenyans when he advocated the continued use of isoniazid alone.[49] Stott echoed McDermott, the American TB expert who had been carrying out research with isoniazid on the Navajo reservation for several years and who had influenced the WHO's position on monotherapy, when he advocated the use of the drug by itself. McDermott, Stott, and the WHO believed that there was more harm in withholding it than there was in the possibility of fomenting drug resistance.[50] Fearing the consequences of using the drug alone was not limited to Kenya. WHO policy met with firm resistance in British Somaliland. There, in 1957, the director of medical services refused to use isoniazid alone, telling the WHO that if forced to do so he and the WHO could no longer work together.[51] Whether or not to give isoniazid alone divided those giving treatment and those making policy, those who were in the field and those who were not. It was a divide that would only grow.

Further, success with isoniazid alone came from trials the conditions of which would be impossible to reproduce. In the case of McDermott—who was one of the first to use isoniazid to treat the disease—his recommendation for using the drug alone came from success with a strictly inpatient and well-monitored group of patients. The conditions under which he used isoniazid alone successfully were wildly different from those found in most of the developing world. To be sure, McDermott and his colleagues carried out their research on the Navajo reservation where the broader social conditions could be said to be akin to those found in East Africa. But considering that the work on the Navajo reservation was inpatient and that the scale was much, much smaller, it was hardly the case that these two places mirrored one another and that one should expect the success of the Navajo work to be re-created anywhere else, much less Kenya. The authors of the Navajo study—McDermott led the team and the research—admitted that single-drug therapy might not be best "for widespread, largely unsupervised use in a population with a high prevalence of active tuberculosis." These were of course the precise conditions found in many places, Kenya among them. Isoniazid might benefit some but would likely do considerable harm in many others. Yet, all this could be tempered by periodical "medical review so that those requiring collapse or excisional therapy can be transported to facilities where they may receive additional treatment." Considered this way, "isoniazid alone represents a simple and surprisingly satisfactory regimen of chemotherapy."[52]

It's hard not to appreciate their optimism, but this way of thinking, much less of practicing, was not exportable. In much of Africa, there were very few or no facilities to transport patients to, to say nothing of the transportation itself. Thus, while McDermott's well-designed study clearly demonstrated, under strictly controlled circumstances, that isoniazid alone could work to cure patients, it had virtually no applicability over the vast majority of the developing world. Pierce Kent pointed out "that some of his [McDermott's] views on tuberculosis are accepted nowhere outside of the United States of America."[53] What had been demonstrated to work in one set of circumstances would not work in another. McDermott's advocacy of isoniazid alone and his influence over others are puzzling, because as soon as he and his co-workers left the hospital and let isoniazid loose the question of compliance and drug resistance rushed to the fore. The possibility of antibiotic resistance via unchecked adherence confronted McDermott just as it did everyone else once outpatient care became the norm. Indeed, he and his team devoted considerable time and effort to devising strategies to combat resistance and poor compliance.[54]

To no one's surprise, when the MRC published its results—results gleaned from work done in India and Kenya—it recommended against using isoniazid alone. The conditions found in both places meant that using isoniazid alone was a bad idea. The need for mass chemotherapy, patients with severe disease, and high rates of primary drug resistance—all of these made the use of isoniazid alone a dangerous idea.[55] But none of this meant that its use was not common all across East Africa—most TB patients and their doctors were not under MRC surveillance, and no one was stopping them from using the drug on its own. Despite the practice "almost certainly" aggravating the problem of primary resistance, it was, like the BCG vaccine, "faute de mieux" across much of the region.[56] When British TB expert H. M. Foreman visited Kenya in 1958 and surveyed the scene, he found that the commonest cause of drug-resistant tuberculosis was the use of isoniazid alone.[57] Yet none of this meant that the WHO wasn't still equivocating over using the drug alone. By the middle of the 1960s, Kent, for one, was fed-up with the WHO and its inability to offer any substantial advice on drug regimens *other* than the misguided recommendation to use isoniazid by itself.[58]

But perhaps things would change. The results from a pilot study showed promise: thiacetazone worked well with isoniazid. A member of the MRC noted that the results were "unexpectedly encouraging" and urged a speedy further trail "if there is a chance that this combined therapy is the answer to the East African problem." The pilot study results were indeed encouraging, but a full trial was called for.[59] And as far as Hart was concerned, trials would continue as long as a mass treatment scheme was absent in Africa and as long as "pre-treatment isoniazid resistance continues to increase yearly as a baffling problem."[60]

The main goal became to "find drug combinations suitable for the mass treatment of tuberculosis in underdeveloped territories." But of course this was not easy: a drug needed to be found that would work well with isoniazid in preventing resistance. It also had to be cheaper and easier to administer than either PAS (which was bulky and expensive and because of its often unpleasant side effects patients might abandon its use) or streptomycin (which needed to be injected). Except for low, but important, levels of toxicity, early results from the larger trial were proving as encouraging as the pilot study: in combination with isoniazid, thiacetazone was keeping drug resistance at bay. Yet, while the results were promising they had been derived from carefully monitored inpatients. Only one half of the equation had been solved; the biological question had been answered: the drugs worked. But the social question—the other half of the equation—was still unanswered. Moving out of the hospital was the next step. The MRC knew that it "is urgently necessary that a careful study of the efficacy of TB1/isoniazid be undertaken also in out-patients." Pressure was building. Well aware of the progress being made, doctors, patients, public health officials, and others did not want to wait before the lengthy process of testing it in outpatients could even begin, much less be completed.[61] They clamored for access to the new combination.

An outpatient trial in Kenya, while challenging, was the next step. The home and the hospital were not alike. The challenges of treating TB on an outpatient basis were formidable; surveillance and compliance were the two most daunting. But then good news came from India: in 1959 Wallace Fox and the MRC showed—in what would become a landmark study—that domiciliary care worked in India. A hospital stay was not necessary to cure people of their TB. The impact of this finding would be hard to overstate: it opened up the possibility that treating TB was possible all across the developing world.[62] Could similar results be achieved with thiacetazone in Kenya? It was time to find out. The trial would be larger than any yet done: three hundred inpatients and three hundred outpatients spread across Kenya, Uganda, and Tanganyika. The scope of the trial, some doctors worried, would push them, their staff, and their facility to the breaking point—it was hard enough keeping up with routine work; adding the burden of the trial might prove too much. The principal medical officer for the Central Province—where, along with Coast Province, TB was highest—was especially leery of taking on more work when even the basics of TB treatment were poorly adhered to. Within a month of his arrival at the hospital in Nyeri he discovered patients without TB being treated for it; those with resistant strains still on their now useless regimen; and children under treatment before a proper diagnosis was made. He wondered how it could be that "In this context it is proposed to launch a MRC trial of out-patients which involves considerably greater supervision than is at present found possible with routine patients." He was frank: Unless he had more help—secretarial assistance, more nurses, another doctor to take care of the routine patients—"we cannot undertake the trials."[63] He also wondered, as few others seemed to have, how the trial would be received by the local African District Councils. Would they accept a change in routine care "in order to be a 'guinea pig' "? Because outpatient trials were much harder to "mask" than inpatient trials, it was inevitable that people would know something was afoot.[64]

"This is depressing" was Arthur Williams's assessment of the early days of the trial. Nothing was working as planned. Too few patients, staff attrition, lack of supplies, local hospitals opting out—not quite "the well oiled machinery" the MRC predicted. Williams hoped things would improve, as "these thiacetazone trials are of key importance for tuberculosis everywhere. They are nowhere being attempted on quite the same scale, and their results are being awaited with no little interest outside Africa as well as here."[65] Setbacks aside, the trial pushed on, and in 1963 the MRC published the results: a cheaper and easier to administer combination had been found.[66] In the end, the trial proved so successful that the Kenyan Ministry of Health and Housing officially replaced PAS/isoniazid with thiacetazone and isoniazid.

Now the real work began: how on earth were they going to get people to take the new combination of drugs? During the outpatient trial the default rate— the number of people who did not take their full course—was discouraging. The drugs worked, but only if people took them—and not enough people were. Figuring out why this was so, and what to do about it, would be far more challenging than developing the drugs in the first place. Ensuring that patients had access to medicine and would stick with treatment for eighteen months—this was something new, and something daunting. It would require a new way of approaching the problem of TB. Unlike BCG, no one resisted antibiotics; no one questioned their efficacy. The converse was generally true: people clamored for them; the effects were miraculous. What was necessary was a way to get them where they needed to be and some way to ensure they were taken properly. As C. Gordon, from the Kibongoto TB Hospital in Tanganyika, wrote regarding the delivery of tuberculosis drugs: "The whole method would involve a departure from the normal system, where the patient comes to the doctor, has medicines prescribed and is presumed to take them."[67]

Normal was not working.

9. The Lost Promise of Antibiotics

Extraordinary progress had been made in understanding how to treat TB. The East African trials proved important. A cheaper and more effective regimen had been found. And research would go on; more breakthroughs would come. For now the MRC and the WHO had had two major victories. The stool they were building now had two legs: they had demonstrated in both East Africa and India that home care could work—a hospital stay was not necessary. And they had found, by the early 1960s, an affordable and efficacious drug combination that the WHO recommended be used across the developing world.[1] The importance of these two achievements cannot be overstated—and they happened fast. It had been only a decade since the WHO had launched the BCG vaccination campaign—the "largest mass action the world has ever known against one single disease."[2] And now, TB could be cured. It went from being a disease that was treated in the hospital with things like cod liver oil and tea to a disease that could be cured at home.

But now, a third leg needed to be in place: transcending the trials and getting the drugs into people's bodies in the real world. The challenge was enormous. The Madras trial was a breakthrough: it showed the world that TB could be attacked outside the confines of a hospital. All the millions without access to hospitals were now able to be treated—and treated with the drugs developed in East Africa. But it's critical to keep in mind that all the patients in the Madras trial were monitored intensely while on treatment; they got what they needed to ensure they stuck with the trial. The trial showed, simply, that domiciliary care could work. Wallace Fox knew that were he to loosen his control over the trial subjects, many might be lost and the study would combust.[3] For this reason, those working in places without a similar level of support—everywhere else, in other words—found that the encouraging results from Madras might actually have little applicability.[4] For the treatment to be effective, patients in home care had to have access to and take their drugs. Without being carefully watched and supported, would they take them? Even in Madras, getting patients to keep taking their drugs for long periods was proving difficult.[5]

Interventions found to be efficacious during a trial were often hard to implement in the field, and home care was no different. Wanting to test the efficacy of home care outside the rigid confines of a trial, the WHO spent a year studying outpatient care in Kenya, only to find that patient compliance was discouragingly low.[6] Within five years of the Madras trial, Johannes Holm concluded that "domiciliary chemotherapy schemes, as applied by many official health authorities today . . . are usually failures."[7] Writing from Ghana in 1960, one British doctor, disillusioned by the clumsy transfer of results from the lab to the clinic, stated that "the outstanding fact emerging from previous clinical research is the manifest failure of chemotherapy to effect control of pulmonary tuberculosis."[8]

The MRC knew this: the relief brought on by the discovery of effective drugs was tempered by profound worry that they would prove worthless in practice. Brandon Lush confessed that the antibiotic trials sponsored by the MRC were "not directly making any real impact on the incidence of tuberculosis in East Africa." His view was sobering. The trials had had indirect value—of what sort he did not say—but "we must not delude ourselves into thinking that the trials by themselves will solve the numerous problem[s] of tuberculosis in East Africa. The trials are essentially confined to treating advanced cases, but it is not possible at present to undertake a proper public health approach to the problem."[9]

The MRC knew also that moving away from testing the efficacy of drug regimens in the lab to "determining the most practical methods of applying them" was the next step. Because so few cases were brought under treatment—most cases went unnoticed, undiagnosed, and thus untreated—"success in defining a 100 per cent effective drug regimen, even one widely and readily applicable, can provide but a limited, indeed nominal, overall effect."[10] Everyone, in fact, knew this. At a 1967 meeting in Nairobi all the major players from the WHO, the MRC, and the Kenyan government lamented the gap between a theoretically possible cure rate of 80–90 percent and the actual rate of less than 50 percent.[11] By the end of the decade not much had changed. Pierce Kent directly compared the results from trials and from the clinics and summed up a decade of sentiment: trials involved selected groups observed under ideal conditions; reproducing their results would be difficult.[12]

What was the solution? Why was it so difficult to get drugs to where they needed to be? And what were the consequences of not doing so? Wallace Fox was one of the era's most astute thinkers on the subject. He knew that solving the biomedical half of the equation did not solve the problem. Few, in fact, were so naive as to think that simply because a successful drug combination had been found it was time to go home. In a thorough, and illuminating, survey of the problem the world over, Fox revealed that getting people to take their drugs was a major problem across the globe. Sometimes it was the fault of the patients: they forgot; they ran out; they sold their drugs. Sometimes it was the doctors' fault: even under supervised administration patients did not always get their proper dosage. What Fox knew was that *people* were at the heart of the problem. Simply possessing the biomedical technology was not enough. He wrote: "The problem of successful prophylaxis or treatment of tuberculosis is not merely a problem of what drug or combination of drugs should be prescribed, and in what dosage or for how long, but whether it is possible to persuade either individual patients or whole communities to cooperate in the long-term self-administration of any medicament."[13]

It was clear to Fox that while patients were at times at fault for not adhering to treatment, there were major problems with drug availability and delivery, the surveillance of patients, the quality of care, the distance patients had to go for treatment—the list goes on. Patients simply not completing their course of treatment was indeed part of the problem. But for patients to do so meant that in every clinic in every rural district and urban center there was an adequate supply of drugs, a competent and helpful staff, and a doctor who knew what he or she was doing. It also meant that patients were able to actually get to the clinics. Rarely were all those things in place. In India, for instance, the National Tuberculosis Institute–affiliated sociologist Stig Anderson knew that the meager drug supply could not match the demand.[14] Expatriate doctors, who often outnumbered local doctors in developing countries, at times ignorantly insisted on following chemotherapy regimes from their own countries rather than what would work where they were. In addition, some doctors, rather than seeing a patient through the entire course of drugs, would stop treatment at the first signs of improvement, mistakenly thinking a cure was in hand.[15]

Yet, despite all this, was it possible to treat TB in Africa on an outpatient basis? Yes and no. Dr. C. G. I. Gordon at the Kibongoto Clinic in the foothills of Mt. Kilimanjaro, in Tanzania, put the lie to any absolute claims to the contrary. On a smaller scale, so, too, did Peter Turner in the Nyeri District of Kenya.[16] But to do so, as Gordon said, meant a "departure from the normal system." It was a system, however, not all could depart from. Gordon could and did. And it was his experience over five years spent building a robust and effective TB treatment program in the late 1950s and early 60s that led him to claim with great confidence that modern methods of TB control could be successfully applied in Africa. Their application needed to be tweaked here and there to accommodate the "mode of life of the African," but there was nothing peculiar about Africans or African conditions that militated against a successful TB program. Gordon took issue especially with those who claimed that poor living conditions made adequate TB care impossible, writing that "the poorest living conditions in Africa are not any worse than the poorest living conditions in parts of the slums of Paris, London or New York and no one has stated in recent years that tuberculosis is untreatable" in those places. Gordon invested his time in "prolonged health education." His work began in the hospital where all patients started their treatment. The initial hospital stay "is of the greatest importance." The patient is at greatest risk, and most infectious, in the first few weeks of treatment. Just as important, "the period in hospital is invaluable as a time when the patient can be 'indoctrinated' in the part he must play in his own cure and in safeguarding the community. This period of health education is perhaps the most important single factor."[17] Kent agreed: an initial hospitalization would be patients' "initiation to a strange new world."[18]

Gordon's investment paid off: it resulted in getting patients to present at clinics when they felt ill—this was an enormous advance over relying on generally inadequate case finding to round up patients. Gordon also fostered community buy-in *before* he began treatment. He held community meetings during which he demonstrated how x-ray machines worked and gave lectures on TB and hygiene. Community participation was essential, he found, if he wanted to ensure compliance with treatment—he essentially got the community to do his surveillance for him. One of the keys to his success was not keeping it a secret. Indeed, he used cured patients as a marketing ploy for his clinic: he gave each of his cured patients—one thousand in 1962 alone— a certificate, ensuring that the "news travelled far and wide."[19] Further, "as a first principle it was laid down that home treatment should be purely an extension of hospital treatment in the home environment and that the patient should be subject to normal hospital discipline." Gordon recruited home-health visitors from the male orderly staff at his hospital; they traveled on foot or by bicycle, covering an area up to twenty square miles. He organized thirty-three simple facilities for outpatient treatment "throughout the area so that all patients could attend weekly at the outpatient centres without undue hardship."[20] He was insistent on this point: "It had been laid down that no patient should be expected to walk more than five miles, so that a very large number of dispensaries were utilised."[21] Patients came once a week to the local dispensary, where they were examined, interviewed, and had their urine screened to ensure they were taking their medicine. Defaulters were, upon first offense, "sternly warned." The second time, "the patient was taken to the local chief for summary admonition."[22]

Did it work? Yes. Gordon randomly selected one hundred patients for a three-year retrospective follow-up. Five had either died or were lost. But ninety-four patients after three years were sputum negative. Gordon never lost sight of more than 5 percent of his patients—as we will see, this was an unusually low number.[23] Yet, for all his success, and despite how sensible his scheme was, it proved almost impossible to replicate. The population Gordon worked with was relatively stable, rural, and lived in the kind of cohesive communities where he was able to effect the level of community buy-in he needed. Yet, that's not really the reason he was successful and others weren't. It's of course part of the reason—the conditions he worked in were more conducive to TB control than those found, say, on the Rand mines in South Africa or in urban India.[24] But Gordon's genius was, after all, his ability to read the local situation and adapt to it. This is not to say it was simple or easily done elsewhere. It is to say, however, that Gordon was among those who knew that curing TB could only be done at the community level with the active participation of patients, their families, their friends, co-workers, and neighbors. Hospital and local dispensary staff were essential; so, too, was the Native Authority.

Getting patients to take their drugs was difficult. Changing the minds of medical people was just as severe a challenge. Getting doctors and other medical personnel to adapt to the new normal—to use a rather anachronistic but apt turn of phrase—called for, according to Anderson, a "complete mental revolution." Focusing on public health at the community level was essential.[25]

All the pieces needed to be in place. TB was truly a social disease. Drugs were a tool. Fox knew this. Yet, as Holm noted, most of these home-care schemes failed. Gordon's work was innovative; it was well planned and well executed. And Gordon had funding. In devising his national plan for home care in the late 1950s Kent knew this would be the crux of the matter: he could draft all the plans he wanted, but if he did not have the money, he would not have the extra staff, equipment, and medicine necessary to make home care work.[26] What Gordon also demonstrated was that a system of sur-veillance was essential; patients' drug intake had to be monitored. This was time-consuming work, but more and more it was becoming clear that without it TB work would fail. Fomenting a "mental revolution" among those treating TB and finding adequate resources to do so would be some of the greatest problems facing TB control programs.

In the early 1960s, Fox knew as much about field research and condi-tions as anyone else in the world. By then he had conducted extensive re-search for the MRC and the WHO in East Africa, South India, Hong Kong, and Great Britain. In 1962, as continuing work in East Africa and India was in full swing, and the results were looking encouraging, Fox reflected on glo-bal TB control. He offered the following sobering observation in a private paper addressed to the MRC's Tropical Medicine Research Board. "Claims for chemotherapy have often tended to be over-optimistic because they have been based on selected groups of patients with drug-sensitive organisms un-der special conditions." In developing countries such conditions were rarely present.[27] Why was this so? Because in TB control, in the early 1960s in the developing world, one problem "stands out above all others. This is whether there is any current control measure which can alter the epidemiological trends of the disease, when applied in communities in the tropics with a high prevalence of tuberculosis, much initial drug resistance, a population that of-ten fails to take oral medicaments regularly and in a context of poor general and nutritional conditions and a minimum of medical and ancilliary person-nel."[28] Effective drugs were well and good, but if the conditions for their application were absent, Fox asserted, they would have no effect at all. He continued his searching critique two years later in another privately circulated paper, this time addressed to the WHO. The "striking progress" made in developed countries in tackling TB between 1954 and 1964 was hardly in evidence in the developing world.[29] Poorly stocked clinics, too few doctors, escalating costs and not enough money, drugs marketed in "dangerously incorrect proportions"—all of these things, and more, plagued TB services in the developing world, Fox wrote.[30] Given these constraints, he warned, clinicians faced "extreme alternatives." Imagine a clinic confronted with two thousand new cases of TB a year. The clinician had a choice: give the best care available (triple-drug chemotherapy, followed by isoniazid plus PAS for six months) to one hundred and expect to cure just about everyone. The remaining nineteen hundred would go untreated. Or, with the same amount of money treat all two thousand patients with isoniazid alone, cross your fingers, and hope for an absolute maximum 70 percent cure rate (but likely far, far lower), leaving the rest untreated and to almost certainly develop drug-resistant infections.[31] What Fox wanted in 1964 was this: "The ideal all-purpose chemotherapeutic regimen that is required is one that is non-toxic, inexpensive, and can be applied successfully in communities with a considerable amount of initial resistance, whether primary or acquired, without the need to know the drug resistance pattern in the individual patient. It would preferably be an intermittent one, effective when given once a week."[32] But he knew he was dreaming. He was describing the ideal treatment regimen; he knew he could not have it, not yet anyway. More than fifty years later, we still don't have it. What Fox imagined has not come to pass.

Antibiotics were let loose in a world unable to ensure their adequate supply or proper use.

If most argued at the time that there was little harm, and potentially great benefit, in using BCG on a mass scale, thoughtful observers argued the opposite when it came to antibiotics. Indiscriminate, large-scale, haphazard use would have dire consequences. If inadequate treatment—for whatever reason—continued to be the norm, the problem of drug resistance in Kenya, and elsewhere, would only become worse. As early as 1961, the WHO reported that approximately 20 percent of TB cases in Kenya were drug resistant.[33]

People like Pierce Kent—hard at work in the field—were becoming more worried as time went by. What concerned Kent most was that he seemed to be shouting into the wind—the cavalier attitude being taken by the director of medical services toward the haphazard TB treatment most patients were receiving galled him. Reports from the field too often had little impact at headquarters. But Kent could not have been more clear. In the starkest possible terms, he wrote to Kenya's chief medical officer in early 1961, "It does not appear to be realised that anti-tuberculosis work with modern drugs necessitates a certain minimum standard of efficiency below which their use becomes not a potential hazard but a definite public health menace—raising, indeed, the question of ethics in their continued use. You are at that stage now in many parts of Kenya, if indeed you have not already passed it in some."[34] Kent's warning was would go largely unheeded.

Kent was not alone. W. S. Haynes joined him in thinking that the government was not taking the problem seriously enough. The problem of drug resistance was clear: Kenya was in trouble. But the Medical Department, according to Haynes, chose to ignore it. The divide between clinicians—like Haynes, Kent, and those staffing the local hospitals and clinics—and the director of medical services was starkly demonstrated in 1961 during a debate over the wording of a Medical Department circular on the colony's general TB practice. Kent and Haynes shuddered when they read the following sentence: "In this circular it is assumed, unless otherwise specifically stated, that the patients' tubercle bacilli are sensitive to the drugs under discussion." Assuming drug susceptibility was the norm, Haynes pointed out, both "sidestepped the issue of drug resistance" and provided an inaccurate description of "the situation obtaining in Kenya at the moment."[35] Further, the circular failed to distinguish between what's known as primary resistance (TB that was already drug resistant when a patient became infected) and acquired drug resistance (TB that converted from being drug susceptible to being drug resistant). Instead, the director of medical services highlighted the number of primary drug-resistant cases (15 percent) and said nothing about the number of cases of acquired drug resistance. Why should this matter? For one, simply leaving out acquired resistance was, as Haynes said, to give a false picture of TB in Kenya. But leaving it out was not solely done by design: no one had any idea how much acquired resistance there was. Further, 15 percent sounded like a reasonably manageable number; ignoring acquired resistance gave the impression, of course, that the remaining 85 percent of cases were drug susceptible. The focus here on primary resistance was important for still another reason. It is an early example of the generally misguided focus on primary drug resistance, a focus that would come to blur the real problem: the development of drug-resistant TB among those receiving inadequate treatment.

Doctors like Kent and Haynes found themselves thwarted time and again by those who made policy but had little understanding of local conditions. From having the director of medical services not take drug resistance seriously to having their concerns about the use of isoniazid alone shunted aside by Holm—Kent and others had grown weary. Consider, too, the astonishing claim—a claim in contrast to all the worry over the problem of drug resistance, even worry expressed by WHO personnel—from the 1960 report by the WHO's Expert Committee on Tuberculosis: "The Committee noted that drug resistance, especially isoniazid resistance, has not proved to be the public health problem originally feared."[36] From where such a claim came is a mystery; it would have been impossible to find anyone in Kenya, and most likely the rest of continent, who would support it.

It's uncertain how much of an impact such a pronouncement had on TB control efforts. Did it give people a pass to ignore drug resistance, to dismiss its threat? It's hard to know, but it's worth keeping in mind that the WHO's Expert Committee and its periodic reports were generally considered guides to the global TB problem. They had considerable impact. What makes the claim especially odd, aside of course from its sheer absurdity, is that the WHO knew about drug resistance in Kenya and knew it was serious and related to patients' ability or inability to take their drugs. When Kenyan doctor James Ang'Awa reported in 1964 that 40 percent of TB patients admitted to the Nairobi Infectious Diseases Hospital were resistant to isoniazid, he derived the figure from WHO-sponsored research begun in 1961, research carried out in response to the growing problem of drug resistance![37] The problem was not limited to Kenya, of course, and the WHO knew well that drug resistance was becoming a problem all across Africa.[38] And Halfdan Mahler, addressing his colleagues in TB control at an international meeting in 1962, implored that "we must not fool ourselves: the resistance problem is already today sufficiently serious to justify considerable expenditure on research for second-line drugs of a cheap and non-toxic nature."[39] None of this was reflected in the WHO's 1960 Expert Committee report.

The gap between what was happening in the field and what was being reported by the WHO continued to grow. As Mahler began to prepare for the eighth meeting of the WHO's Expert Committee on Tuberculosis to be held in 1964, and being especially concerned with the problem of drug resistance, he asked committee members to write him with whatever data they had on the problem of primary and acquired resistance.[40] From India, N. L. Bordia, the adviser-in-tuberculosis to the Directorate-General of Health Services, noted that the only data he was able to provide came as a by-product of clinical work; in most of India TB workers simply did not have the time or resources to do research on the question. The data coming from the MRC studies in the south, he pointed out, could not be transposed onto other parts of the country.[41] This is an important point: the research in India and Kenya, and then only small parts of those big countries, was unique and, really, entirely different from TB research happening almost everywhere else in the developing world—where more or less nothing at all was happening.[42] Thus, Mahler did not learn much from his survey; the responses provided scanty information at best because so little in the way of data was available. Because of this the only conclusion the Expert Committee was able to come to in 1964 was "that adequate information on the present prevalence of primary resistance is still not available."[43] The committee members were similarly reticent when it came to acquired drug resistance: all they had to say was that it "is very complicated," and because accurate data were virtually nonexistent, discerning any sort of trend—was the problem getting worse, better, staying the same?—was impossible.[44]

The Expert Committee was the official voice of the WHO on all matters concerning TB. Its hesitancy regarding the problem of drug resistance was understandable—to a point. It was true that accurate data were not available from many places and that this made it difficult to make any broad statement regarding the problem on a global scale. But considering the field data in hand, or at least available, from both the MRC and the WHO itself in East Africa and South India, to say nothing of the reports from Southern Rhodesia, Ghana, Hong Kong, Nigeria, South Africa, and elsewhere, it seems unfortunate that not more was able to be said about something that people on the local level considered to be an urgent public health problem.

The members of the Expert Committee were not so much loath to rely on local knowledge as they were unaware of it. It's not clear where their data came from exactly, but it's safe to say that Pierce Kent did not have their ear. Very likely they derived their conclusions from large-scale surveys that, while useful, also masked local nuance and, unintentionally, hid from view crucial information. Thus it was ten years later, in 1974 at its ninth meeting, that the Expert Committee on Tuberculosis considered the problem of primary drug resistance—again, those presenting for the first time with active TB resistant to at least one frontline drug—to not be a problem at all. The flood of primary resistance that TB workers once feared had never come to pass. Rates were stabilizing. Indeed, primary drug resistance as a cause for treatment failure, the Expert Committee wrote, was "overrated." No figures are cited, so it's impossible to know what the committee considered an acceptable amount of primary resistance. And that's all that was said about that.[45] But the WHO, and others, had missed something crucial. Primary resistance was only part of the problem. The fixation on it—and then its dismissal as not as bad as previously thought or feared to become—was misguided.

Digging a little deeper into the problem and leaving aside the question of whether primary resistance was "overrated" or not, it's clear that drug resistance, regardless of the Expert Committee's inability to say anything of substance about it, was a problem. It was, first of all, a problem of detection. Who had it? This was a tough question to answer. From a purely bacteriological perspective, it was difficult to get a handle on drug resistance in many places in Africa because sensitivity tests were hard to come by—in Senegal, for instance, doctors had no idea if patients had drug-sensitive or drug-resistant TB because there was no lab.[46] One of the only reliable laboratories was in Nairobi, and it was stretched thin analyzing data from Kenya and the region.[47] But more important, primary resistance was so hard to come to grips with because what was often thought to be primary resistance, it turned out, was not primary resistance at all. Imagine a clinic seeing a patient for the first time. The patient has no record; as far as the clinic knows, he or she has never been treated for TB. If the patient's TB was found to be resistant to antibiotics the natural conclusion would be that this was a case of primary resistance. But that was not necessarily the case.

So what? Why would it matter if a patient had acquired or primary-resistant TB? It's important because the reasons for mistaking one for the other reveal shortcomings, structural deficiencies, and lapses in the treatment of TB. Mistaking one for the other also masks the presence of undetected, freely circulating, infectious cases of drug-resistant TB.

Acquired resistance emerged out of myriad circumstances that all demanded tremendous labor to investigate—labor resources no one possessed.

They all swirl around the difficulties associated with ensuring that patients received and took their drugs. It is here we find the origins of the massive problem we face now: rampant drug-resistant TB brought on by patients' inability to complete their course of drugs. Note: I did not say patients' inability to comply, nor did I claim patients do not adhere to treatment. These are semantic distinctions that matter. Patients' inability to complete tuberculosis treatment, which, not incidentally, could also mean the inability to even begin treatment, is not solely or even principally a problem of patient compliance—that is, individual people simply not taking their drugs. It is a systemic matter involving drug supplies, governments, doctors, home-health-care workers, a clinic's staff, location, and hours, as well transportation availability, and, of course, patients. These days the systemic issue is well recognized as a principal cause of drug-resistant TB, but the disease is still too often a problem laid at the feet of the patient. Few, it seems, have heeded renowned TB expert Lee Reichman's admonishment that "patient compliance is the least of our problems."[48]

It's also a problem that's been under scrutiny for decades; like so much in TB control there's nothing new about it.[49] The terms "compliance" and "adherence" or whatever other term might be deployed are all too confining.[50] What does a national TB program's inability to keep track of patients on treatment have, necessarily, to do with *patient* compliance or adherence? When a program loses a large percentage of its patients, is this a compliance problem or a surveillance problem? Is it a patient's fault when he or she cannot afford the food necessary to ward off the hunger brought on by the drugs?[51]

Whatever we choose to call the problem—and of course that choice matters—it should be clear that while patients play, and have played, an important role, they only do so once an adequate supply of free or very low-cost nontoxic and effective drugs has reached them in a convenient and timely manner at a clinic they have access to, delivered by a well-trained clinician capable and willing to ensure treatment with at least three different medications that patients will have to take consistently for, now six and historically eighteen, months. Keep in mind, too, all of this must happen over and over again millions and millions of times every day. Suggesting that drug-resistant TB is, or has been, caused by lack of patient compliance is incorrect and naive. Discussions of *patient* compliance are fine, but to them must be added a careful and critical look at TB programs. This is of course not a historical concern: treatment default is a massive, global problem only made worse now by the prevalence of HIV/AIDS and multidrug-resistant TB.[52]

Primary resistance was certainly a concern. After all, a patient who came to a clinic having never been treated for TB should, theoretically, have drug-susceptible disease. But patients were not always what they seemed. It's not so much that primary drug resistance was rare in places like Kenya— it was not: it hovered somewhere around 10–15 percent, depending on the time and the place—it's that what was often taken for primary drug resistance was actually acquired resistance in disguise. As I noted earlier, the focus on primary resistance, and then its dismissal in 1974, were unfortunate because what a look at the problem would have revealed was a glimpse into the ways in which acquired resistance was, well, acquired. When the Expert Committee claimed in 1974 that the problem of primary resistance was "overrated," it seemed unaware of what N. W. Horne had pointed out in 1969 in his global survey of drug-resistant TB: it is those with acquired resistance who form the pool of infection where primary resistance "spawns."[53] And if primary resistance was very often in fact acquired resistance, then that pool was even deeper and murkier than anyone knew.

How did primary resistance mask acquired resistance? For one, there were the many, many cases—very hard to track and to stop—of patients appearing at a given clinic denying previous treatment. Patients might present themselves at clinic X saying this was their first visit when in fact they had begun, but not finished, a course of treatment at clinic Y the previous year. When the WHO studied the problem of drug resistance in Kenya in 1961 it found that patients' denial of previous treatment was surprisingly common.[54] Why wouldn't they admit previous treatment? A fresh start. Patients worried that treatment would be withheld were they to admit to previous treatment. And if doctors had little understanding of drug resistance, patients had even less.

Others simply refused to be treated. In Garissa Province in Kenya—a remote area with little infrastructure and even less TB control—it was common for those being treated for TB in the clinic to stop treatment and head home. So common was the practice that the clinic drafted a generic refusal-of-care form; one needed only to fill in the blanks, affix one's thumbprint, and off one went. By signing the form, patients took full responsibility for their failure to complete treatment and were warned of the dangers. For these patients the pull of home was stronger than the threat of drug-resistant TB.[55]

In Kiambu District, just outside Nairobi, some speculated that the Emergency, or Mau-Mau uprising, had created a rural TB epidemic that was impossible to treat because the severe travel restrictions made access to antibiotics all but impossible.[56] Or people might be self-medicating from the abundant sources of illicit and often useless TB drugs available to them. The open market for isoniazid in places like Ibadan, Nigeria, was well known to patients and doctors. In Nigeria and elsewhere this was a market responding to a need: by the late 1950s and all through the 1960s drug shortages plagued TB programs. The same was true in Kenya: by the mid-1950s it had become well known among Kenyans that streptomycin worked to fight TB. Because of this, people demanded it. And what was true in the 1950s and 60s is still true today: all over the developing world not only is isoniazid available in the private market, other TB drugs of suspect origin, efficacy, and safety are too. But governments often did not have enough drugs. And so people bought their own and medicated themselves. At other times *only* those who could pay were given antibiotics. And thus some were getting treatment and some were not, while others were self-medicating. And because of the importation of drugs of little value, some thought they were under treatment when they were not.[57] Or, once they began to feel better, people might share their antibiotics with sick friends or family. Anyone of these scenarios could mean that a patient presenting at a clinic with apparently primary resistance might in fact have acquired resistance.[58]

This was, of course, a problem not limited to Kenya: the high rates of primary resistance reported from elsewhere in Africa were not reliable enough to be counted on as an accurate reflection of primary drug resistance as opposed to acquired resistance.[59] Finally, while patients denying previous treatment or acquiring drugs on the open market surely exacerbated the problem, it was clear, too, that any system of surveillance in place to keep track of those on treatment was not working; clinics routinely lost sight of patients (more on this later).

However it came about, acquired resistance was widespread, but very difficult to measure. It was a problem created by the very conditions people such as Fox and Kent railed against—inadequate treatment and official indifference. "The incidence of acquired resistance," Horne wrote in his 1969

survey of the problem around the globe, "is a serious indictment of therapeutic practice in almost every part of the world."[60]

If we take a moment and examine several surveys of drug-resistant TB in
Kenya, begun in 1964 and followed up at regular intervals into the 1980s,
we'll be able to get a look at the scope of the problem and see that what the
surveys found and did not find were both revealing. What the surveys shed
some light on, of course, was a drug-resistant TB problem, but what they
were unable to uncover was just how serious it was. The inability to gauge
the amount of acquired resistance, and the reasons for failing to do so, were
telling, as they demonstrate that the capacity to assess the problem simply
was not there.

The 1964 prevalence survey determined that 14.7 percent of the TB-
positive population had primary resistance to some drugs. This was high, but
among those who were known to have had previous treatment the numbers
were much, much higher—though admittedly based on fewer patients. For
example, of the thirteen patients who had had chemotherapy for six months
or longer 93 percent had drug-resistant TB. Among those with three months
or more of treatment multidrug resistance was "common." What this means
is that cure rates were very low. Knowing something about cure rates and
about primary drug resistance was important. But what TB workers knew
little about was *acquired* resistance. To be sure, the low cure-rate figures provided some insight—and it was not good. If such a high percentage of the
patients they *found* developed drug resistance after being on chemotherapy,
the thought of how many were out there and not found yet moving about
with infectious, potentially drug-resistant TB was alarming.[61]

The numbers had changed slightly, but the overall picture was the same
ten years later in the 1974 follow-up. About 10 percent of patients had primary drug resistance; again, among those who had had previous chemotherapy the number of patients resistant to antibiotics was substantially greater.
If one were to look at the average the figure would be bad enough: of eighty-
two patients 23 percent were resistant to one or more drugs. But it's when the
numbers are looked at according to length of time on the drugs that things
are even more telling: only two of forty-six patients (or 4 percent) who had
received one month or less of treatment had drug-resistant TB; of the sixteen patients having received six or more months of treatment fourteen (88
percent) were resistant to one or more drugs.[62] Further, we should note that

not only was the percentage of people with drug-resistant TB much higher among those who remained in treatment for six months or longer, there were also far fewer people on treatment.

Two things were happening: most of those remaining on treatment were developing drug-resistant TB, and there were fewer and fewer of them. What this meant was that as people developed drug resistance they left treatment and drifted back into the public with active, drug-resistant disease. And remember: these numbers are based on the people the TB workers found; no one knew how many were out there. Again, the problem was not limited to Kenya. In the early and mid-1960s others reported similar figures in Southern Rhodesia and Hong Kong. And, what's more, just as in Kenya, the development of drug resistance was directly related to length of time on treatment.[63]

The authors of both the 1964 and the 1974 Kenyan surveys made a telling confession—a confession that goes a long way toward explaining how drug-resistant TB became so rampant: they wrote that "no information has been obtained about the number of chronic failure patients within these districts." While this information would of course have been useful, a "more comprehensive survey to obtain information on these aspects would be a formidable undertaking, both organisationally and in terms of the laboratory work-load."[64] The same was true of a survey done in Tanzania around the same time: the TB workers had no idea how many people were lost to treatment.[65] While the MRC had contemplated studying the problem of those who were called chronic infectious patients, the previous survey in Kenya from 1964 said the same: "It provides no information about the size and composition of the pool of chronic failure patients."[66] Even though the matter had not been investigated, the authors of the 1964 survey knew the importance of untreated, infected carriers: they reported that there was a significant difference between those presenting with initial drug resistance who had been exposed to a previously treated individual and those who had not. That is, simply put: if you had contact with someone who had untreated, drug-resistant disease your chances of getting drug-resistant TB were higher than those who had not had contact.[67]

What this of course meant—the point is rather obvious, but it's important—was that most data on TB and the success of drugs came from patients on whom TB workers had data, from patients whom clinics were able to keep track of. They knew almost nothing about those who had vanished.

But as C. G. I. Gordon in Tanzania put it, the "efficiency of home treatment scheme might well be judged by the number of patients who are 'lost.'"[68] Thus, not knowing anything about this group left a large gap. In the Kenyan survey this was an omission by design, and it served to present a not entirely accurate picture of TB control in Kenya. What was left out was as important as what was put in. It was common, of course, to report on the failings of a drug regimen or other technical matters; it was uncommon to report on the limitations of administration. In the case of the Kenyan surveys, data on acquired resistance and lost cases failed to make it into the reports because the data did not exist. The authors knew this and acknowledged the lacuna. It was not an omission designed to mislead. But it misled nonetheless.

In 1963 the sociologists Debabar Banerji and Stig Anderson, working for the WHO in Bangalore, recognized this problem—the problem of not knowing what was left out. In their pathbreaking study of domiciliary care in Bangalore, Banerji and Anderson wrote that "the results of tuberculosis work are often given in terms of a certain proportion only of the patients dealt with. The reader is thereby, whether by design or not, led to too favourable an impression of the over-all value of the work." Their own research on outpatient care was not automatically immune; they, too, had to be self-aware and write in such a way as not to mislead. As they noted, "Even results of this study, dealing with 784 patients diagnosed in a large city clinic, could have been presented in quite rosy terms with no dishonesty other than that inherent in the act of omission."[69] The 1964 and 1974 Kenyan surveys did not intentionally mislead; the results were not particularly encouraging in any case. Yet one does have to read them as much for what's there as for what is not.

It was certainly—obviously—useful to know how effective drugs were. But it also would have been helpful to know more about the population for whom they did not work. Given the number of people on treatment who vanished, the obfuscation over previous treatment, and the availability of illicit drugs it's no wonder no one knew just how much acquired drug resistance existed. And little progress had been made in the ten years between the two surveys in getting people to stick with treatment—only 28 percent and 23 percent, respectively, stuck it out for a full twelve months.[70]

Managing patients in treatment for TB was a challenge. Not being able to account for patients who vanished was understandable. The standard course of treatment took more than a year; drug shortages were common; staffing was thin and ever changing. People also moved around a lot—in Kenya, after the lifting of Emergency-imposed travel restrictions in January 1960 tracking TB patients became even harder in some areas.[71] The problem of errant patients was not a new one; nor would it go away. Doctors in the field in Kenya and elsewhere had been reporting on it for years. Based on reports he had been getting from clinics, Pierce Kent noted in 1957 that they had "lost sight of" around 25 percent of those on treatment, due to staff shortages, resulting in a "steadily increasing number of chronic untreatable (drug resistant) cases."[72] Kent worried about what this meant. "The real significance of the 'lost sight of' cases is, however, the public health aspect of the matter in that the secondary cases to which they give rise must necessarily, in large proportion, be infected with tubercle bacilli which are drug resistant ab initio."[73]

Just to be clear: uncured and infectious patients with drug-resistant TB spread drug-resistant TB, thus compounding the problem. W. S. Haynes was blunt: patients not completing treatment, and vanishing, he wrote, were a "menace."[74] From Ashanti, in Ghana, W. J. Bell reported that 30 percent of patients left treatment by the end of three months; the number doubled before the end of a year of treatment. What did this mean? "Large numbers of partially treated and potentially highly infectious individuals return to their towns feeling temporarily well. . . . It would appear that considerable numbers of partially treated, infectious and already resistant cases of pulmonary tuberculosis are spreading resistant disease throughout the population in Ashanti, and there is reason to believe that the situation is similar in other parts of Ghana."[75]

As the decade progressed, the problem did not get any better. Take a look at Kiambu District, where, in 1968, according to the district medical officer, "despite the published programme, the T.B. Team frequently did not make the scheduled visit to Health Centres, and Dispensaries, and it was found that attendance was poor and little was known of the results of treatment." Not only was the efficacy of treatment unknown, the number not completing treatment was very high. Of the nineteen clinics in the district only one had more patients who could be accounted for than who had been lost. At the Ngenda clinic, for example, twenty-six of forty patients who began treatment were lost sight of. And what's more: these figures were based on patients who had been seen in the previous two years; the files of anyone who had not been seen during the previous two were tossed out. The result:

of the 503 patients brought under treatment in the previous two years 347 were lost. When looked at over ten years the problem takes on a still more ominous dimension. First, the number of patients coming under treatment declined year after year: in 1958, 807 people started treatment; in 1968, the number fell to 204. This decline almost certainly represented a lapse in case finding rather than less TB. Second, and this figure is frankly astonishing: between 1958 and 1968, clinics in Kiambu registered 5,879 patients; they lost sight of 3,473.[76]

It bears repeating what this means: patients lost to treatment were those about whom nothing was known; these were not the people who defaulted but were then found and put back on treatment. These were people with only partially treated tuberculosis—the surest way of developing drug-resistant disease—who had vanished, left to spread TB unbeknownst to anyone.

Case finding is the flip side of compliance. Compliance—and again the term is not entirely adequate—concerns all the myriad ways in which patients do and do not get their drugs into their bodies; case finding is the process by which those patients are found in the first place. It comes in two forms—active and passive—and its success or failure can tell us something about a TB program's profile. Active case finding, which has seldom been used, is the practice of actually looking for TB; it's expensive and time consuming. Passive case finding—detecting cases of TB when a patient presents at a clinic or hospital—is the cheaper, less effective though generally speaking only alternative in places like Kenya. Generally, poor compliance and spotty case finding are two sides of the same coin—if a program is unable to find people with TB, it will also be unable to find them once they've drifted away from treatment.

I noted earlier that in Kiambu the number of people coming under treatment dropped each year between 1958 and 1968 and said that this was likely because of shoddy case finding and not because of a reduction in TB. But what does poor case finding look like? Here's an example: in the summer of 1970 at the Muriania Hospital in the Murang'a District—the site of the Kenyan government's WHO-assisted National Tuberculosis Program pilot project—thirty thousand outpatients came through the hospital's doors for various ailments. Screening for TB revealed fewer than a dozen cases. A statistician from the Ministry of Health rightly wrote that "this is of course unbelievable and indicates a very serious neglect of their part in TB case finding." This sort of harsh judgment was not limited to case finding but was leveled at most aspects of TB control in the pilot program. Staff members weren't doing their jobs, patients weren't being cared for, TB was going undetected almost everywhere. "In general for the District, we notice a return to the bad old system by which patients are not examined at the follow-up periods and where treatment is continued indefinitely for the patients who should be discharged." At many of the dispersed health centers no case finding whatsoever was being done, and in many places patients were being kept on treatment, for no apparent reason, long after they should have stopped—at Makuyu not a single patient had been discharged from treatment since 1968![77]

All this occurred despite what appeared to be a well-thought-out plan to curb TB in the Murang'a District. In fact, the WHO chose Murang'a to be the site of the pilot phase of Kenya's National Tuberculosis Program because it was thought to be a place where local clinics were eager and ready and the medical officer of health was on board; it was a place, too, that had been active in the TB control efforts since the early 1950s when it was known as Fort Hall.[78] Cynics claimed that it was only its proximity to Nairobi that made it appealing. The WHO dismissed this claim as of "merely academic value"—whatever that meant—and declared that there "is no area better or more representative than the Muranga district."[79] This might be so—though many argued it was not—but the fact remained that when the pilot scheme ended in the spring of 1971, after burning through no fewer than seven medical officers of health, the WHO's senior medical officer lamented that the "performance of this test-run area has been rather poor."[80] Problems plagued the program from the start: inadequately trained staff; specialists such as microscopists leaving but not being replaced; lax labeling practices in the lab leading to lost data; dwindling stocks of crucial supplies; and concern over who was in charge—central or local government—among other things, all ensured that the pilot program was doomed.[81]

And yet. The frequent staff changes, the abysmal case finding, the antiquated treatment—all this and more were repeatedly noted. Quarter after quarter the program seemed to be failing; the WHO even started a second test run of the National Tuberculosis Program in Machakos to try and regain some of the footing lost in Murang'a. And yet, when the WHO assessed its time in Kenya in 1973 it had this to say about Murang'a: "The national tuberculosis programme tested in Muranga district was found to be feasible and suited to the health context of Kenya; and it should therefore be expanded to cover the whole country in three to four years time."[82] Two years later it was official: the experience at Murang'a convinced the WHO to expand the National Tuberculosis Program.[83]

It seems, however, that other than the theoretical possibility that the Murang'a pilot program *could* have been successful there was nothing gained from the experience besides the quite useful lesson that Kenya was not ready to run a National Tuberculosis Program. That said, perhaps it was enough for Kenya: when amending the agreement between the WHO and Kenya regarding the WHO's role in Kenya's TB program the parties found that despite some of the problems, such as poor case finding, the "programme model has proved to be well adapted to the sanitary context of the country."[84] What, precisely, was Kenya's "sanitary context"? It's not clear, but one can infer that this meant that the test run in Murang'a was the best anyone could expect.

All this was at odds with the view of W. Koinange Karuga, Pierce Kent's successor as director of the Kenyan Ministry of Health's tuberculosis division. As the program was winding down in the spring of 1971, he reiterated a previous complaint: neither Machakos nor Murang'a was representative of Kenya's TB problem; there was no generic stand-in for the entire country's epidemic. While the two regions were "supposed to reflect what may obtain when the NTP was expanded . . . this was . . . not very convincing." Indeed, the experience at Murang'a should certainly not be used as an argument for expansion. "Many factors," Karuga wrote to the Ministry of Health, "will dilute any conclusions that will be drawn and I do not think the outcome of the report should influence the idea of expansion."[85] While Karuga may or may not have been suggesting that expansion should be stopped, there is no doubt that he did not want Murang'a to be the model.

Patients being lost, cases not being found—these were, of course, problems not limited to Kenya, nor were they going to go away as time went on. A group of French and Algerian TB specialists found that the National Tuberculosis Program in Algeria lost 36 percent of patients in the early 1970s—the vast majority of whom disappeared even before outpatient treatment began, but prior to discharge from the hospital.[86] The problem was rural and urban, but especially acute among those considered nomads—up to 85 percent of whom were lost. Fast-forward to the 1980s. In 1980, in the Mohale'shoek District of Lesotho 96.3 percent of those under treatment defaulted within a few months; the number was much lower in Maseru, the capital—it hovered over several years around 13 percent. But these numbers meant little because they referred only to those patients that clinics could keep track of. A staggering number of people under treatment simply disappeared from view: depending on the year, between 70 percent and 80 percent of patients who began treatment vanished between 1980 and 1983.[87] Nor was this solely a problem of the developing world. In New York City, in the late 1980s, 89 percent of patients on TB treatment at the Harlem Hospital were lost to treatment after discharge.[88] No one knew where they went or if they finished their treatment.

Just after the turn of the century, when yet another TB intervention was being tested—this time isoniazid prophylaxis therapy, of which we will hear more—a research group in Zambia noted that the "main limitation" to their study of the efficacy of isoniazid preventive therapy (IPT) was "loss of patients during follow-up."[89] And the problem is still with us today as a new epidemic—HIV/AIDS—has required that millions of people in the developing world adhere to a lengthy drug regimen. In a study of seventeen antiretroviral therapy (ART) programs in sub-Saharan Africa, and one in India, loss to follow-up ranged from a low of 5 percent to nearly 50 percent; mortality among those lost to treatment but able to be traced went from a low of 12 percent to a high of 87 percent. Among other problems, losing patients to follow-up confounds our understanding of mortality in the AIDS epidemic. Because there is no cure for HIV/AIDS, sticking with ART is critical; stopping is fatal. When the efficacy of ART is gauged in terms of mortality it's of course only possible to report on those able to be followed—whether they're alive or dead. But among those lost, yet able to be traced, it's clear that mortality might be vastly underreported—perhaps by as much as 40 percent![90]

And just as with those who vanished—and vanish still—from TB treatment, we have no idea what's happened to those who have disappeared from ART programs. We can only assume that they are dead.

The problem of "lost sight of" patients was immense, unfathomable. As the surveys of Kenya and Tanzania noted, the problem was so large that even thinking about investigating the chronic failure patients was beyond their ken. And if it was a problem in Kenya, with Africa's most well-developed TB control program and research staff from the WHO and MRC in abundance, imagine the difficulty elsewhere. The patients who vanished became known as "defaulters," labeled noncompliant. But why? And why couldn't clinics keep track of patients? What kept patients from coming back? Figuring out why patients default has been at the heart of TB research for decades. It still is. The tremendous number of patients who vanished from treatment combined with those who did not disappear but stopped taking their drugs or did so only sporadically, but whom the clinics were able to keep tabs on, speaks to the sheer immensity of the problem. As he reflected back on his decades in TB control work, no less a figure than Wallace Fox wrote in 1983 that "world wide, poor patient compliance has been, and remains, the principal cause of treatment failure."[91]

Some thought technological strategies to get patients to take their medicine, from pill clocks to monitoring urine for signs of drug use, might work.[92] Most of these strategies were derived from the notion that compliance with TB treatment was at bottom a patient problem. If clinics could make patients comply then TB control could be achieved. These monitoring devices did not get at the root of the problem; at most they seemed simply to confirm that drugs were or were not being taken—and in at least one case, in a large national survey in Scotland, where these methods of compliance surveillance were put in place they were not checked or monitored with any regularity—that is, people in charge of compliance were not complying![93]

Fox, however, had an expansive view of compliance. To him, compliance went two ways, back and forth between doctors and patients, patients and the health care system in which they were ensconced. Fox's view was shared by almost everyone else in the developing world in the 1950s and 60s and into the 70s and 80s: thoughtful commentators realized that much more was at work than forgetful or lazy patients; they knew too that the problem could not be blamed on cultural differences; nor could it be laid at the feet of those who abandoned their treatment when they began to feel better. All three of these factors were at play, of course. Most commentators realized that what was needed were changes in TB programs: drug delivery and patient monitoring had to be strengthened; staff needed to be shored up; the length of treatment had to be shorter still.

After studying the problem intensively in urban India, Debabar Banerji and Stig Anderson wrote in 1963 that their "essential finding" was that "the straightforward defaulter problem, the classical problem of discontinuation of chemotherapy, is actually a *smaller* problem than the combination of a number of other administrative and organizational problems."[94] In India, Anderson, Banerji and others revisited this theme again and again throughout the 1960s: if India wanted to ensure patient compliance then those in charge of administration and organization of TB services needed to start complying.[95] Similar problems plagued Kenya. When W. Koinange Karuga, for example, toured the Coast Province in 1971 he found that no standard of care was being applied. Patients all over the province were unnecessarily being compelled to travel to the Port Reitz Chest Hospital in Mombasa rather than be cared for locally. Predictably, because this sort of travel was a significant burden default rates were high.[96]

Distance to a clinic, fear of lost wages, whether or not the individual seeking treatment was a mother of small children, age, severity of symptoms, and quality of care—all of these things and more influenced whether or not someone sought out and stuck with treatment. The clinic had to be nearby—no more than three miles or so, especially if you had children in tow or were sick or worked or what have you; patients, it turned out, did not care if their treatment came from a specialized TB clinic or a general hospital, so long as the staff was knowledgeable and competent and the clinic was well stocked; clinics needed to be open after work hours—these were essential.[97]

It seems at times as if in the twenty-first century almost nothing has changed. A major 2007 study of the barriers to treatment completion reads as if written about India or Kenya in the 1960s. The study is a superb rendering of two problems. First, the one it reports on. It's a deeply researched study showing very clearly that TB programs, structural matters, poverty, and so forth, and not simple patient noncompliance, all need to be taken into account to explain treatment failures. But it's also, unintentionally, representative of the perpetual rediscovery of age-old concerns in TB control. This is the second problem it illuminates: there is not much new in the world of TB control; barriers to treatment have been well known for decades.[98] Paul Farmer, in a rousing critique of those who offer culture as a cause of noncompliance, summed up the problem succinctly: "Throughout the world, those least likely to comply are those least likely able to comply."[99]

But what role did patients play? We don't know much about them in Kenya. In contrast to India's National Tuberculosis Institute, in Kenya neither the WHO nor the government nor the MRC had any social scientists on staff. While many doctors and administrators, Pierce Kent of course prominent among them, complained about lack of staffing and money, and here and there occasional commentary could be found concerning why patients might, for example, deny having had previous treatment, almost no one seems to have been concerned with patient attitudes and beliefs. But in the summer of 1969, unsatisfied by the absence of any kind of sociocultural examination of compliance, but humbled by the sheer size of the TB problem, K. Ndeti, the chair of the University of Nairobi's sociology department, headed to Machakos. Ndeti understood the administrative barriers; what he wanted to know was why an individual might not take his or her medicine. What effect, both positive and negative, would the community—both the medical and traditional, as he put it, community—have on one's decision to keep up with care? After spending several months in nineteen clinics, and doing detailed interviews with fifty-nine randomly chosen male and female defaulters, Ndeti offered a series of explanations worth taking a look at.[100]

Patients defaulted for a variety of reasons. For one, they did not always have a clear sense of either their disease or their treatment. One twelve-year-old patient, looked after only by his brother after his parents left seeking new land, was responsible for his own care. He'd not been told how the disease spread; he headed back to school, where no one knew he had TB.[101] And this, Ndeti claimed, was the number one reason an individual might default: poor communication between doctors and patients.

Poor communication might have been the cause of most default, but there were other reasons too that Ndeti spent time puzzling over. He revealed, though he admitted he'd only scratched the surface, that in Machakos an overwhelming number of people believed in what he called "herbal medicine." This left them somewhere between being adamantly opposed to antibiotics to taking herbs and antibiotics in tandem. But when it came to default, even more to blame than a belief in herbal medicine were "traditional concepts of tuberculosis." What this meant was that there were many names for ailments that *could* be TB—symptoms such as coughing, chest pain, and spitting blood were signs of several ailments that all predated the emergence of TB as a separate identifiable illness. Thus, let's say someone had what he or she called *wathe;* it might or might not be TB, but because the individual knew it as *wathe,* a well-known affliction, why go to a clinic to see if he or she had TB?[102] Imagine yourself spending a few weeks wracked by the symptoms of the common cold. Imagine, too, that like most people you know there is no cure; you just have to wait it out. You do not go to a doctor. You drink tea. Unbeknownst to you doctors have found a cure, but they're calling the disease Z-factor. There's not been much in the press about this; what little you've heard makes it sound similar to the common cold, but how could there be a cure for *that?* This might be a crude comparative exercise, but it gets Ndeti's point across: there might well be cultural reasons for not seeking treatment or sticking with treatment, but those reasons have a specificity and depth to them that must be understood and rarely were. It was not simply a matter of lazy or forgetful patients unable to cope with the rational aims of modern medicine.

Poor communication, an overreliance on herbal medicine, and a disconnect in diagnosis all concerned Ndeti, but what he considered a real menace were those he called "witchdoctors." These practitioners both treated and explained TB. According to Ndeti, the witchdoctor "is one of the most advantaged persons in Kenya today. Nobody bothers to probe into his activities or his finances. From the socio-medical point of view he is an impediment to the development of socio-medical services in Kenya."[103] It was this aspect of Ndeti's work, along with the case of two dead defaulters who had been treated by a prominent "witchdoctor," that caught the attention of W. Koinange Karuga. The man with the most influence, and the one allegedly responsible for the two deaths, was John Muia, a well-known herbalist who claimed he could cure TB.

A visit was in order. Karuga put together a delegation that originally included Ndeti (who when it came time could not go) and several others from the health department and set out for Machakos in April 1971. Karuga and his colleagues received a warm welcome from Muia. Dressed in a white lab coat with four nurses in uniform at his side, Muia possessed many of the affectations of Western biomedicine—he even called himself, and was referred to as, Dr. Muia. Karuga knew the delicacy of the situation: Muia had far more influence over patients than Karuga did. In 1971 his patient register revealed that Muia had cured, astonishingly, seventy-four thousand patients of an assortment of ills and that in the four months before the visit he had already seen ten thousand people. Without his cooperation, Karuga knew, TB care and control would be much harder than it already was; with it, it could be much easier. Karuga's fine handling of the situation turned out well: not only did Karuga convince Muia to stop treating TB patients—something he claimed he was reluctant to do anyway because he feared infection—Karuga and Muia also talked about the possibility of using Muia's clinic as a site for distribution of TB medication. As Karuga put it, the "situation here is unorthodox and the solution would likewise have to be unorthodox." He came away from the visit convinced that working against Muia was a dead end and likely worse. The trust established between the two, Karuga thought, needed to be cultivated, not left to rot.[104]

Karuga had learned that Muia was a compassionate, trusted figure who listened to his patients and comforted them when they needed it—something often missing, Karuga lamented, from government clinics. His vast legion of patients clearly believed in *a* system of medicine—it was just the wrong one, according to Ndeti and Karuga. Nonetheless, these were not people unable to comply or unwilling to go to the doctor or who did not pay attention to their bodies—they did these things all the time. Karuga realized that an opportunity had presented itself. This was akin to the realization that C. G. I. Gordon had had more than a decade earlier in Tanzania when he set up his domiciliary care program. Paying attention to what people thought about medicine and how they interacted with it—this was important.

It's not known exactly what came of the visit to Dr. Muia. He may or may not have come to play a role in TB care in the area. The visit did, however, have an impact on Karuga, who realized that flexibility and a keen awareness of the local scene were essential in TB control. Further, within a few years of the visit, and continuing throughout the 1970s, researchers at the East African Tuberculosis Research Center and the MRC, including stalwarts such as Wallace Fox and Hugh Stott, began to look into the use of community leaders in the control of TB, especially case finding. Researchers had come to the unsurprising conclusion that "community Elders were found to have a considerable knowledge of the health of persons living in their locality." In the course of meeting with them, and with little or no prompting, the elders ticked off a list of those with TB. Household heads too, it turned out, knew something of the health of the household. So, why not use them in case finding? The results were mixed, but promising. Household heads did a superb job identifying suspects, but door-to-door interviewing was time consuming and costly. Elders, even though they yielded a "disappointing" number of cases—about one-third—had promise. With a small amount of training and follow-up it appeared that the elders became more adept at identifying suspects.[105]

The recognition that local people possessing intimate knowledge of their community might have a role to play in TB control seems to have been recognized in Kenya only in the early 1970s.

Work on the problem of course continued. Intermittent and short-course chemotherapy—and their eventual merger—showed great promise. Working from the premise for now that directly observing patients taking

their drugs was the best way to ensure compliance, but knowing that the resources simply were not there to do this every day with every patient in
every developing country—think of the labor involved!—the reasoning behind intermittent therapy was obvious: less frequent intake of drugs meant
less frequent monitoring. Intermittent chemotherapy, those working on the
problem in Kenya hoped, would solve the problem of patient noncompliance.[106] But intermittent therapy, even once a drug regimen was found that
was considered as reliable as standard daily chemotherapy, still faced the
same problems: the controlled conditions of the trial were not the same as
those in the field.[107] Getting patients to take their drugs, even if they had to
do so only twice per week, would still be difficult.

What if the duration of treatment could be curtailed? Imagine a drug
regimen that was shorter and in which drugs only needed to be taken a few
times a week? Trials to sort out the efficacy of short-course chemotherapy,
which became a very real possibility with the development of the fast-acting
drugs pyrazinamide and rifampin in the late 1960s, were under way by the
early 1970s in East Africa, Singapore, Madras, and Hong Kong.[108] By the
middle of the decade short-course chemotherapy had been shown to be effective. It was the last major breakthrough in TB treatment.[109]

Chemotherapy that worked, was easier to take, and relied on cheaper
drugs, plus a shorter, intermittent schedule—once these breakthroughs came
to pass, innovation in TB treatment ground to a halt. These milestones in the
treatment of TB were all achieved within a generation—from roughly 1950
to 1975. Nonetheless the problems remained the same: there was still no way
to ensure that drugs got into patients' bodies. Each of these breakthroughs
was instrumental in creating a useable and effective TB treatment regimen.
They were technological triumphs. And up to a point they were only that:
successful innovations that *could* cure tuberculosis.

During a period in which global public health practitioners and policy makers were supposedly either lulled into complacency by the promise and allure
of medical technology or confidently claiming that disease could now be de-
feated, we see here those on the ground, doing the work, showing the opposite: TB control is and will remain very difficult.

In the decades following World War II experts hatched plan after plan
to improve the lives of the less fortunate in the developing world. Sometimes
these plans went awry; they were at times overambitious and poorly planned.

But in the world of TB control these were not years characterized by over-optimistic bloviating. For every hubristic claim, for every time someone or some committee glossed over the TB problem, many, many more worried and complained and mostly carried on. In 1967, ten years after warning against optimism and a decade into an unprecedented period of research success in demonstrating efficacious methods for TB control, Johannes Holm, by then the director of the International Union Against Tuberculosis, had not really changed his view. He wrote in frustration to the director general of the WHO: "At a time when we have the means and the knowledge to control tuberculosis and we know that if the technical policies and general recommendations of the WHO are followed, an effective tuberculosis programme can be implemented without high costs, it is distressing to see that so little progress is made to bring tuberculosis under control in Africa. The poor countries of Africa need help from outside first of all in form of equipment and supply, and evidently more than the WHO and other U.N. agencies can provide."[110] Sadly, Holm's assessment, in perhaps slightly different form at the margins, would be echoed over and over again in the coming decades.

The MRC broke it down starkly: in East Africa alone there were an estimated three hundred thousand cases of TB; sixty thousand new cases were added each year. Twenty thousand people were on treatment; half were cured. These were not figures anyone was cheering about.[111]

A vaccine to prevent TB and drugs to kill it: these were what everyone in TB control pursued—and still pursue. But too much—the disease itself, the people manufacturing and the people taking the drugs and the vaccine—complicated their efficacy. TB workers recognized the extraordinarily difficult work involved in applying modern technology, in the form of antibiotics and the BCG vaccine, to a problem as complicated as TB. Some may have been more pessimistic than others, but no one thought it would be easy.

In 1964, in a major survey of TB in tropical Africa, the WHO concluded that "unfortunately no information is available to show whether this situation is a fairly stable one or whether there are marked tendencies towards improvement or deterioration."[112] Despite years of work this kind of assessment was common. The disease was studied and studied; clinical trials launched and run; much money spent—and still those most intimately familiar with TB work lamented that the disease was not under control, nor did they even know if their efforts at control were doing any good, and the medical technology available was far from perfect.

In Kenya, more was done to combat and study TB than in any other country on the continent. And yet, more than two decades into a period of sustained and robust research and fieldwork the director of the Tuberculosis Investigation Centre confessed in 1978 that "unfortunately there is little information available to show whether the situation has been a fairly stable one or whether there [is a] marked tendency towards improvement."[113] Two years later, in 1980, the MRC sadly came to same conclusion regarding TB in the developing world as a whole, saying that "there is no evidence that its incidence is declining nor that it will necessarily decline in the near future without the introduction of better methods of control specific to such countries."[114]

It would only get harder. By the mid-1970s, as we've seen, the biomedical technology and know-how to cure TB were well known. But putting it all to work remained an enormous challenge. In Hong Kong, for instance, a tremendous amount of labor had gone into controlling TB in the 1960s. Real gains were made. Yet after a decade of hard work TB still killed more people than all other infectious diseases combined.[115] The work on antibiotic treatment pioneered in East Africa and India in the 1950s, 60s, and 70s changed TB control forever. But as a group of TB experts convened in 1982 by the WHO and the International Union Against Tuberculosis lamented, the major beneficiaries of all this research had not been the countries where it was needed most. Instead, affluent countries with adequate facilities, plenty of resources, and of course much less TB had been the real beneficiaries.[116] Developing countries were living laboratories but clinically moribund.

And then came the biggest challenge of all. Reports began to trickle in from across eastern and central Africa—TB rates were on the rise. What was going on? In 1987, a doctor from the Kigoma region of Tanzania reported that "a disturbing factor in the incidence of tuberculosis became more clear this year."[117]

PART THREE

Failure, 1975 to the Present

10. The Making of the HIV/TB Pandemic

It is possible that AIDS reflects and magnifies diseases that are
endemic to a particular locality.
—Gnana Sunderam et al., 1986

The combination of both diseases could be at the root of a horrifying
hecatomb in the years to come.
—J. Prignot and J. Sonnet, 1987

As the [AIDS] epidemic continues to unfold, the greatest opportunist
may prove to be *M. tuberculosis*.
—Richard Chaisson, 1989

We are facing one of the greatest public-health disasters since the
bubonic plague.
—J. L. Stanford, J. M. Grange, and A. Pozniak, 1991

For adults infected with HIV in developing countries, the primary
illness and cause of death is now HIV-associated tuberculosis.
—U.S. Agency for International Development, 1993

The combined epidemics of HIV and tuberculosis (TB) present a
public health challenge unlike any other faced this century.
—WHO/IUATLD Joint Statement on HIV and TB, 1994

Take a look at the epigraphs. They tell the story of the early recognition
of and increasing alarm over the HIV/TB coepidemic. Yet when one considers all the attention paid to HIV/TB by the end of the 1980s—attention

manifest in meetings, research publications, editorials, and funding poured into projects—it is maddening to read statements like the following, from a 2008 WHO report on isoniazid preventive therapy, intensive case finding, and infection control (known as the "Three *I*'s"). The report noted that "it has become increasingly clear that HIV and tuberculosis co-infection (TB/HIV) is a major public health threat to people living with HIV that directly jeopardizes the success of ART scale-up."[1] Of course, by the time this was written it had been abundantly clear for two decades that HIV/TB coinfection was "a major public health threat."

The WHO's 2008 statement is distressingly similar to many other things one reads about HIV/TB written in recent years. A 2013 editorial in the *Huffington Post* written by Michael Sidibé, the director of UNAIDS, is typical. His editorial, a call to arms full of absolutely true and tragic figures about the staggering toll HIV and TB are taking in Swaziland, could have been written about Zambia in 1990.[2] Writing to commemorate World AIDS Day in December 2013, Cheri Vincent, the chief of the infectious disease division at U.S. Agency for International Development, praised the progress made in fighting AIDS. But she had to remind the global community to not forget TB.[3] In 2010, a veteran of the epidemic, Anthony Harries, of the International Union Against Tuberculosis and Lung Disease, and his colleagues rightly asked, "When will we act?" The global response to the "onslaught [of HIV/TB], particularly in the killing fields of east and southern Africa, has been," Harries and his colleagues claimed with considerable and warranted fury, "timid, slow, and uncoordinated. If this situation had been a war—more deaths from AIDS have been recorded than there were military deaths in World War II—our efforts would have been ridiculed as half-hearted and ineffectual."[4] Wondering when we will act is understandable considering not only the scope of the problem but also that this question has been asked repeatedly. Many have been asking similar questions for some time now—Harries even asked one himself more than twenty years ago![5]

Long before Harries published his 2010 plea, impatience regarding action on the HIV/TB epidemic had set in. More than two decades earlier, in October 1989, a group of experts gathered in the Geneva headquarters of the WHO to try to hammer out a set of guidelines for how national TB programs might operate in the face of HIV. At the end of their report the authors wrote that the "actions recommended in this report should be taken as soon as possible to avoid further lost opportunities and to increase the possibility that the 'TB/HIV' problem will finally be addressed successfully."[6] That was in 1989.

Six years later the WHO was still revving its engine. When a different group of experts met in 1995 they determined that "the first objective is to implement studies addressing the research priorities. The Global Tuberculosis Programme is in a position directly to make a start on some of the priorities."[7] From hoping to "finally" do something about HIV/TB in 1989 to resolving to "make a start" on figuring out what the research priorities were in 1995—this form of regression was all too common. And, sadly, in the decades since, we have come only marginally closer to "finally" addressing the problem of HIV/TB. Writing in the *Lancet* in 1991 a trio of British and Zimbabwean TB specialists warned that "despite the WHO's Alma Ata declaration of Health for All by the Year 2000, sub-Saharan Africa will be lucky if the tuberculosis problem is not far worse in that year than it is today."[8] They were right.

Kevin De Cock, then of the London School of Tropical Medicine and Hygiene, wrote in 1994 that what was needed to tackle the co-epidemic was better coordination of HIV and TB services; international will and financial support; and the deployment of the most advanced forms of diagnosis and treatment.[9] Some of the details have changed—or better put: things have gotten much worse as many more people are coinfected and multidrug-resistant and extensively drug-resistant forms of TB have emerged as urgent problems—but De Cock's decades-old article mirrors many written today that call for the same things. Indeed, the "Three *I*'s"—intensive case finding, isoniazid preventive therapy, and infection control—have all, perhaps at times in slightly different forms, been advocated for more than twenty years.[10] The use of IPT (isoniazid preventive therapy) in developing countries, as we will see, has been a subject of debate for much, much longer.

Now, a depressing repetition of recommendations has set in.[11] Top TB and HIV experts know this, too. Paul Nunn and Kevin De Cock, from the WHO, and Alasdair Reid from UNAIDS, began their 2007 survey of the field in the following way: "One might have expected, some 23 years after the first reports of HIV-associated tuberculosis (TB), that there would be close coordination in policy making on HIV/TB matters internationally and that control programs would be working closely together at the country level. In fact, neither the TB nor the HIV community, in our view, has responded adequately to the problems posed by the interaction of TB and HIV infection."[12]

For a quarter century or more TB and HIV have been the two halves of a deadly, deadly partnership. A new disease breathed life into an old and intractable one. And now TB is the leading cause of death among people with HIV, and has been for decades; it eclipses all other risk factors for the reactivation of latent TB and progression to active disease.[13] In Africa as a whole TB has gone from an incidence rate of 146 per one hundred thousand in 1990 to 345 per one hundred thousand in 2003.[14] One group estimated that HIV is responsible for a 6 percent annual increase in TB case rates in sub-Saharan Africa.[15] And figures for places like the township of Khayelitsha, outside Cape Town, are much higher: in 2005 incidence was 1,283 per one hundred thousand, and 76 percent of patients with TB were coinfected with HIV.[16] In 2007, because of HIV, the world saw 1.3 million new cases of TB; half a million died.[17] Because HIV leaves the body incapable of fighting infection its impact on tuberculosis has been absolutely staggering.

HIV/AIDS, since it announced its arrival in 1981, has changed the face of the earth forever. The demographic, economic, epidemiological, and cultural impacts of the disease are immense. The history of AIDS is only just now being understood and written. The scope of its impact means that no single history is ever likely to be written; at a minimum we're a long way away from such a chronicle. For now, we can tell parts of the story. Here, I'll explore elements of the new plague's deadly partnership with an old scourge.

Thanks to epidemiologists, molecular biologists, and others we now know where and when HIV first emerged—central Africa in the early part of the twentieth century. We know now that colonization, urbanization, and migration cleared the path for the disease to blaze its way across the continent and out into the world beyond.[18] Now no place is free of its effects. What we've also known for a quarter century or more is that tuberculosis and HIV have formed a deadly relationship, merging in some places, like much of sub-Saharan Africa, into a coepidemic (see figure 4). How did this happen?

It's a story of remarkable historical amnesia. The synergies between HIV and TB were discovered decades ago. HIV's devastating effect on TB was recognized early and often. Taking the problem seriously, the WHO began to respond. But just as momentum was increasing, as we will see in the next chapter, all the energy required to keep it going vanished as priorities shifted. And for a decade, HIV/TB was virtually ignored. So, too, was multidrug-resistant tuberculosis. It's clear that in the early to mid-1990s the

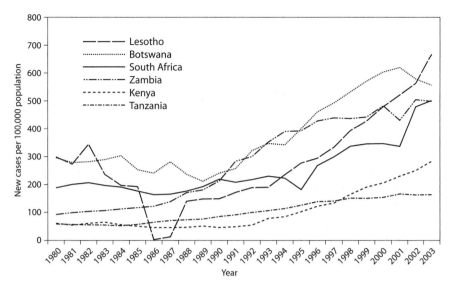

Figure 4. TB in the era of HIV in eastern and southern Africa. (From Elizabeth L. Corbett, Barbara Marston, Gavin J. Churchyard, and Kevin M. De Cock, "Tuberculosis in Sub-Saharan Africa: Opportunities, Challenges, and Change in the Era of Antiretroviral Treatment," *The Lancet* 367, no. 9514 [2006]: 926–937, copyright 2006, reprinted with permission from Elsevier.)

staggering increase in TB, fueled by HIV, put the disease back on the global health agenda, from which it had dropped off by the end of the 1970s. But in a tragically ironic twist, HIV, the very thing that made TB a global emergency—a declaration the WHO made in 1993—was left out of global TB control policies until well into the twenty-first century. Convinced that a cost-effective solution had been found to the TB problem, the WHO, national TB programs, and the World Bank—a new and powerful player in global health—focused singularly on what came to be called DOTS (directly observed therapy short course). DOTS, however, did not take into account HIV, nor did it have any provisions for multidrug-resistant tuberculosis. As a result, HIV/TB and MDR-TB were allowed to careen out of control.

By the end of the 1970s there was reason for cautious, very cautious, optimism. Theoretically, TB could be controlled. Short-course chemotherapy was a major breakthrough; if it could be implemented it might actually help to turn the tide. But TB programs were fragile. And then the unexpected arrived. Thinking back on this time, Annick Rouillon, of the International Union Against Tuberculosis and Lung Disease, wrote in 1991,

> In the long history of tuberculosis in man, despair follows hope,
> triumphs and tragedies succeed each other. We have made no ex-
> ception to the rule. . . . Having duly waited for certainty before
> proposing conclusions, we had no sooner started to feel joyful at
> the great significance of the new system of delivery of Tuberculosis
> measures in poor countries of the developing world than we start-
> ed, once more, to be extremely worried. This time, it was the ob-
> servation of an increasing number of unexplained deaths. By
> 1986–87 we had begun to note that some patients, young patients,
> were dying who were reported initially as new smear positive cas-
> es, seemed to have followed a proper treatment regularly and
> whose sputum had converted to negative. Dr. Styblo and his col-
> leagues in Africa checked for various possible errors in diagnosis
> or in recording, or pitfalls in the Programme. But, of course, THAT
> WAS HIV![19]

When Rouillon wrote these lines Africa and the world were ten years into
the epidemic, and HIV/AIDS was well on its way to putting a stop to any
progress that had been made in controlling TB. By the time Tanzania reported its first case of AIDS in 1981 African TB programs were barely containing
tuberculosis. Arata Kochi, the chief medical officer of the WHO's TB Unit,
declared at the end of the 1980s that the "AIDS epidemic is having a devastating effect on tuberculosis control."[20] Raymond Bretton, a French doctor
who had been working in the Ivory Coast for more than two decades, told
the *New York Times* in 1990 that "this is a terrible thing. I thought I had succeeded in fighting tuberculosis, but now it's all back to zero."[21] Bretton considered the two together their own new disease.[22] The following year, after a
visit to the Ivory Coast, where he found staggering numbers of TB patients
who were also HIV positive—25 percent in 1988 and 45 percent in 1990—
Dr. Zhi-Yi Hu of the WHO's Global Program on AIDS wrote that "tuberculosis can be considered the most frequent HIV-related opportunistic
infection in Africa."[23] A French researcher in the Congo likened HIV/TB to
a time bomb silently ticking away.[24] And that bomb, Peter Eriki, the WHO
representative in Brazzaville, said in 1992, "has led to an increase in tuberculosis morbidity reducing or tending to *wipe out* progress made so far."[25]

By the early 1990s the devastation that unchecked AIDS was having on
TB was obvious; evidence had been mounting since the early 1980s. Major
medical journals like the *Journal of the American Medical Association* and the

Archives of Internal Medicine published pieces in 1983 that made clear the connection between the two diseases.[26] Jonathan Mann, who would go on to run the WHO's Global Program on AIDS, suspected TB would play an important role in the AIDS epidemic and started collecting data on TB among those with HIV in 1985 while working in what was then called Zaire.[27] That year alone Mann found that 40 percent of a sample of 231 hospitalized TB patients in Kinshasa were HIV positive.[28] The following year, in Lusaka, Zambia doctors reported high rates of TB associated with HIV.[29] These reports and others began to appear alongside calls for taking TB seriously in the face of HIV; they became relatively common by the late 1980s and early 90s. And these were not lone voices chiming in from the margins of the medical world. Articles appeared in all the major publications—*Journal of the American Medical Association*, *New England Journal of Medicine*, the *Lancet*, the *British Medical Journal*, and many others. Some even argued, as early as 1986, that TB might be predictive of the presence of AIDS—that is, an uptick in TB meant AIDS was lurking.[30] In 1987 two authors characterized the presence of TB among AIDS patients as already "staggering," noting that controlling HIV infections "is now essential to tuberculosis control."[31] By the late 1980s, Paul Farmer found, rural Haitians considered the two diseases intimately linked—TB went from being AIDS's "little brother" to its "big brother" from the mid- to late 1980s.[32] And finally, R. L. Colebunders and his colleagues wrote from central Africa in 1989 that coinfection was becoming so common that TB patients could be used as "sentinel populations to detect HIV-related illnesses in selected regions."[33] By the mid-1990s the leaders of South Africa's National TB program realized that "HIV related TB is likely to be the single greatest challenge to TB control in the country."[34]

When the experts from the WHO's TB division and its Global Program on AIDS met in 1990 to discuss how preventive antibiotic therapy—which we will hear more about in the next chapter and which can be administered to HIV-positive people not yet infected with TB—might alleviate some of the TB burden threatening to overwhelm Africa, they explained the problem well: "Before the HIV epidemic, developing countries achieved at best an annual decline of some 3–5% in tuberculosis, as evidenced by notifications and surveillance of the annual risk of infection. The present increase therefore represents a tremendous setback in control efforts. In addition to the direct consequences regarding the case-load, it is very likely that the increased incidence of pulmonary tuberculosis will entail a similar increase in the risk of infection which, in turn, will result in an increase in tuberculosis in the entire population in future years."[35] Just to be clear, what they were worried about is that HIV can, and often does, cause inactive TB to become active. HIV's relentless attack on the immune system can render one unable to fight TB, and thus inactive disease can become active. And because TB is highly contagious it spreads easily from person to person. With the rise of HIV-activated TB, that meant more cases of TB, which meant a rise in infections. Workers in the field were worried too: a group of Zimbabwean researchers noted in 1989 that TB "is the only complication of HIV which could prove a significant public health hazard to the [HIV-] uninfected population."[36] This is precisely what has happened. Of course, the problem was not limited to Africa—Haiti and Thailand were hard hit; so too was Brazil in the early days.[37] The Pan American Health Organization, WHO's affiliate in Latin America, drew up guidelines for dealing with the coepidemic in 1992.[38] But Africa was, and is, suffering the worst.

In 1990, in a draft of the WHO's "Guidelines for National Tuberculosis Control Programmes in View of the HIV Epidemic" the authors noted that in "numerous areas of the world, an epidemic of tuberculosis is occurring as a result of the HIV epidemic." Tanzania had, by the end of the 1980s, begun registering a 7 percent annual increase in TB cases; in other places in Africa the annual increases by the end of the decade ranged from 2.6 percent to 30.9 percent.[39] To put more specificity to those figures look at Zambia, where TB cases had been more or less stable from the mid-1960s through the early 1980s. Then, they exploded: in 1988 there were 12,876 new cases of TB; in 1980 there had been 5,342. By 1993 there were more than twenty-three thousand new cases.[40] What had been an endemic disease had, very quickly, turned into an epidemic and had become Zambia's leading cause of adult death.[41] Researchers in Uganda, where HIV rates were among the highest in Africa in the late 1980s and early 1990s, cited "alarming figures" when it came to TB: between 1991 and 1992, TB cases jumped from fifteen thousand to more than twenty thousand. Because of HIV, excess TB cases, they worried, might approach fifty thousand per year.[42] At the four hospitals where HIV/TB coinfection was being tracked, between 46 percent and 64 percent of TB patients aged twenty to forty were HIV positive.[43] Uganda was not alone: the U.S. Agency for International Development estimated in 1993 that because of HIV/AIDS Kenya would add between twenty-four thousand and fifty-three thousand new cases of TB each year.[44] As a group of Kenyan researchers noted that same year, in the understated style of medical journals, "The pattern of tuberculosis in Kenya seems to be changing."[45] The Global Program on AIDS was blunt: because of AIDS, in Africa "since 1986 . . . an almost exponential increase in reported tuberculosis cases has occurred."[46]

And on and on without end. Reports of HIV's almost incalculable effect on TB were abundant in the mainstream medical press and the files of the WHO. The combination of TB and HIV was a problem impossible to ignore.

That the convergence of an uncontrolled TB epidemic and a newly emerging disease—HIV/AIDS—presented the world with a formidable challenge was already well known nearly three decades ago. The situation was dire, and anyone paying even the slightest attention knew it. The WHO knew it. Urgency, and even panic at times, colored discussions. The experts were watching a tragedy unfold. It's hard to imagine the helplessness some felt. Thirty years earlier antibiotics and optimism first made their way into East Africa, India, and other parts of the developing world. An incurable disease became curable. Now the gains made—however tenuous—were on the verge of being erased. When a group of TB and HIV experts got together in 1990 to discuss chemoprophylaxis for TB in the HIV-positive population they could not have been clearer about just how bad things were: "Throughout the consultation, the participants expressed a sense of urgency because of the increasingly disastrous situation with respect to dual infections and a feeling of frustration resulting from difficulties in starting the studies that are needed if disaster is to be averted."[47] Disaster: it's not often one encounters that kind of word when reading the generally antiseptic meeting minutes coming out of the WHO. Yet this was the climate, the consensus, at the time: impending doom.

It's impossible to imagine that there was anyone working in TB or HIV/AIDS who would have denied the critical importance of tackling the two diseases simultaneously. In 1988 the WHO and the International Union Against Tuberculosis and Lung Disease stated that the incidence of coinfection "obviously calls for coordination of the tuberculosis and AIDS programmes at the national level."[48] The two diseases were merging into a coepidemic, especially in Africa but elsewhere as well. This was well known; HIV/TB was not ignored. Those involved did more than simply cite figures and decry the coming crisis. They began to devise control strategies.

The WHO considered HIV/TB a research priority by the late 1980s.[49] In 1988, worried that a combined epidemic of TB and HIV could become a grave public health problem, researchers at Projet SIDA in Zaire were working on research protocols to learn about such things as the risks people with both HIV and TB posed to family members and other household contacts.[50] Research can of course take time to bear fruit, but knowing that fast action was needed, Arata Kochi, then in charge of TB at the WHO, wanted to get moving. Writing Jonathan Mann, Kochi said: "There is an urgent need to develop 'tentative guidelines' based on available information and by taking into account the operation reality of developing countries." There was simply too much TB in Africa, Kochi wrote, to wait "until the research produces the findings which will be used for the guidelines."[51] In the Ivory Coast, a project run by the WHO and the U.S. Centers for Disease Control and Prevention was hoping to answer essential questions about the relation between HIV and TB—did standard antituberculosis treatment work in HIV-positive people? Was TB in HIV-positive people more infectious?[52] That was in 1989. By the next year the WHO and its partners launched eight major field research projects with seven more scheduled to begin in 1991.[53] The sheer volume of work published in leading medical journals in the late 1980s and early 1990s on the relationship between AIDS and TB makes it clear that the coepidemic was not ignored. Publishing the results of robust research projects on HIV/TB was so common, in fact, that Richard Chaisson, who had been involved in HIV/TB research since the beginning, wondered in 1995 if an article he had submitted to *JAMA* would see publication in such a high-profile journal because of the "recent spate" of articles on HIV/TB.[54]

HIV/TB was on the map. An urgent problem was being addressed.

But the challenges would be formidable. To begin with, by the time AIDS emerged TB had been ignored for a decade or more. Innovation in TB treatment had in fact ended in the mid-1970s with the development of short-course chemotherapy.[55] TB was no longer, and had not been for some time, the focus of what the WHO called in 1953 "the largest mass action the world has ever known against one single disease."[56] By the early 1990s it was in fact the opposite: a neglected disease.[57] At the end of 1993 the U.S. Agency for International Development, for example, cut its entire overseas TB budget, thus slashing the WHO's already tiny TB funds by a third.[58] Donors and governments, the WHO complained, did not think the TB epidemic "sufficiently serious."[59] A group of TB experts gathered in Geneva in 1995 was blunt in its assessment: "Consistently, the world community has failed even to implement those effective and well tried measures against tuberculosis that have existed for almost 40 years."[60]

That HIV/AIDS appeared at a time when TB research, and general interest in it, was at its nadir is a tragic coincidence. After nearly three decades of sustained work in TB control, by the mid-1980s very few were paying the disease any attention—a WHO/International Union Against Tuberculosis report noted in 1982 that many in the developed world worked under the false assumption that TB was no longer a problem. Funding plummeted.[61] The WHO had drastically cut its TB budget, and the British Medical Research Council—the leader in TB research in the developing world from the 1950s to the 1980s—shut down its TB unit in 1986 when Wallace Fox retired. The network of labs it created in Africa lay dormant.[62] Further, despite all the work done on TB control—the rollout of the mass BCG vaccination campaign, the development of effective and inexpensive antibiotic regimens, outpatient care, and short-course chemotherapy—Johannes Holm, the former director of both the WHO's TB Unit and the International Union Against Tuberculosis, declared in 1984—just as HIV/AIDS was going to explode in Africa—that these efforts had little appreciable epidemiological benefit.[63] Karel Styblo, of the Union, lamented at the meeting in Geneva in October 1989 that "it is regrettable that in at least the last decade, tuberculosis has been ignored by much of the international health community." This was especially appalling, according to Styblo, because the "magnitude of the tuberculosis problem in developing countries is staggering."

And then came HIV. Styblo, usually calm and restrained in his scientific papers, was clearly alarmed. He went on to note at the meeting that "there is no doubt that *balance between tubercle bacillus and man in the absence of man-made interference* (i.e. case finding and treatment) *which had existed in the pre-HIV era, was disturbed by HIV, an event observed for the first time in the last 100 years*" (emphasis in original). Styblo warned that the "impact of HIV infection on the epidemiological situation of tuberculosis is so large that—under certain conditions—the tools available at present for tuberculosis control will fail to restrain the increase not only in the incidence of tuberculosis disease but also in the transmission of tuberculosis infection, due to HIV infection."[64]

TB, a neglected disease that few cared about and some thought was no longer a threat, was actually on the verge of becoming uncontrollable. Amid great concern and facing a daunting challenge, the experts gathered in Geneva in 1989 looked hard for a ray of light in the darkness. They hoped that "the association of tuberculosis and HIV infection may increase public awareness of the seriousness of the world tuberculosis problem. If this increased awareness is translated into concern, funding, and action tuberculosis programs throughout the world will be strengthened and significant reductions will be achieved in morbidity and mortality."[65]

This is what the world had come to: TB had become so neglected that it was hoped that one devastating disease—AIDS—would help bring fresh awareness to another. That's in fact what happened. The WHO, and the global health community generally, began to take renewed interest in TB in part as a result of the increase in HIV-related TB. The WHO even went so far as to officially label the TB epidemic a global emergency in 1993.[66]

But it might have been too late. National TB programs—once WHO's great hope for TB control in Africa, and, as we've seen in the case of Kenya, not terribly successful—were in a shambles. Even Tanzania, home to East Africa's most successful TB program and with the continent's most enviable short-course chemotherapy program—rolled out nationwide in 1986—was in trouble. By the summer of 1990 the program in Dar es Salaam was on the "verge of collapse."[67] At least one prominent critic, D. R. Nagpaul, former director of India's national TB program, complained that not enough money had been put into national TB programs and that in many places all the talk about integration of health services had been just that, talk. The result was little or no integration, on top of a dismantled national tuberculosis program.[68] On the eve of Kenya's AIDS tidal wave, W. Koinange Karuga, formerly in charge of Kenya's TB program and now director of medical services, lamented in 1986 that TB, despite no other disease having had so much attention lavished upon it, was still a major problem. The poorly handled shift from a vertical program of TB control to one decentralized to the local communities under the well-intentioned guise of "Primary Health Care" resulted in a loss of momentum, a confused set of priorities, and inconsistency. The program poised to become—in fact, *designed to be*—the poster child for African TB control was not working.[69]

Kenya's problems were not unique—TB programs continent-wide were in dire straits. The WHO rather obviously noted in 1994 that "currently low TB cure rates and weak TB systems will require urgent and substantial strengthening before co-infection with HIV becomes more prevalent."

What "poor programmes" did well, sadly, was "keep infectious people alive longer and thus increase TB transmission."[70]

Look at Zambia. By 1990 Zambia's TB program, according to one WHO observer, was extremely weak, yet at the end of the 1980s, a decade when TB admissions more than doubled in some parts of the country, TB was Zambia's number one hospital death.[71] Early, somewhat tentative data showed that in 1987 40 percent to nearly 60 percent of AIDS patients also had TB.[72] In 1992, 72 percent of all new TB cases also tested positive for HIV.[73] And all this in a country that had virtually no money: massive budget deficits in the 1970s, due to the collapse of the copper economy, led to borrowing from the World Bank and the International Monetary Fund, which, when Zambia was unable to pay back its loans, led to severe structural adjustments in the 1980s, which in turn translated to drastic reductions in spending on health.[74] Despite generous funding from the WHO to study the impact of HIV/TB in children, shortfalls in the country's paltry TB budget meant there was no money to follow up patients in the study. Default rates were very high. And worse than that, a steady supply of drugs could not be counted on—both pyrazinimide and isoniazid ran out on more than one occasion.[75] Added to this, tragically, was the fact that the cheap and effective and widely available drug thiacetazone—the antibiotic that TB specialists in Kenya had spent so much time on in the 1960s—could not be used in HIV-positive patients. It was too toxic; its use could lead to a fatal skin rash.[76] And thus a *new* regimen had to be devised. Because of all this, Zambia, the TB specialist for the Ministry of Health warned in 1992, "is on the verge of an emergency with respect to TB control."[77]

Others wondered about the continent as a whole—was Africa lost, experts wondered at a WHO meeting in 1990. Was there simply no way of dealing with the HIV/TB coepidemic?[78]

Active TB was widespread, and TB infection was near universal; southern Africa had the highest incidence of TB in the world in the pre-AIDS era.[79] Thus, by the mid–1980s, just as HIV/AIDS was boiling to the surface in Africa, TB control efforts were greatly diminished but the disease had not gone anywhere; globally eight to ten million new cases emerged per year, and three million people died.[80] As we've seen, this was well known among those paying attention. And it was not that they simply noted a rise in TB; the early work on TB and HIV in Africa recognized that TB, even without

HIV, was still a major killer in Africa despite the availability, for decades, of effective and affordable chemotherapy.[81]

The coincidental decline in TB research and control efforts in the face of a still massive TB epidemic in Africa as HIV/AIDS was emerging is only part of the problem. HIV/AIDS, while by no means ignored entirely, was neglected in Africa in the early years of the epidemic. It took the world time to notice. In 1985 Halfdan Mahler, the director general of the WHO, downplayed the significance of HIV/AIDS, noting that "AIDS is not spreading like a bush fire in Africa. It is malaria and other diseases that are killing millions of children everyday." To him, focusing on AIDS took precious resources away from more important diseases—and it's worth noting TB was not one of them.[82] Mahler needed to be convinced that AIDS, especially in Africa, was the problem some thought it was. Initially, the African epidemic did not receive the same level of scrutiny from the biomedical and epidemiological communities as did the European and American epidemics—epidemics initially confined to intravenous drug users and gay men. The experience in the West was not easily transferred to Africa, where the epidemic was very different.[83] And despite the attention Africa did eventually receive from the WHO's Global Program on AIDS between 1986 and 1990—which saw some successes, such as stemming the epidemic in Senegal and Uganda, for instance, and which Mahler eventually supported enthusiastically under the direction of Jonathan Mann—by the mid–1990s there were no signs AIDS was slowing down.[84]

HIV/TB got out of control not only because TB had been neglected and the WHO was slow on the uptake when it came to African HIV. The co-epidemic also thrived because the WHO, as many noted at the time, was in crisis, and the world at large was not paying much attention to AIDS in the developing world.[85] When UNAIDS published its book-length history of the global response to the epidemic in 2008 it began by noting that coordinated, global efforts to fight the disease did not come for fifteen years after the first case—"15 years during which the world's leaders, in all sectors of society, had displayed a staggering indifference to the growing challenge of this new epidemic."[86] By the late 1980s the WHO was losing influence and had very little money. At the end of the decade financial crisis forced drastic cuts in key programs, including for TB.[87] But the WHO was facing the twentieth century's worst pandemic. At a time when the WHO was in a less than optimal position to lead many still looked to it for leadership because there was no one else around. The late 1980s through the late 1990s was the most confusing and incoherent time in global health in more than a generation, but it was also a time when coherence and consistency were needed more than ever. For what we now know was a brief time—1987 to 1990—the WHO's Global Program on AIDS (GPA) was the undisputed leader in the field, taking on HIV/AIDS like no one else. During that time, even while the WHO budget overall was shrinking, the GPA was blessed with what were called "extra-budgetary funds"—funds earmarked by donors for programs of their choosing.[88] As a result, the GPA was not short on money. But beginning in 1990 when Jonathan Mann resigned—a period characterized by Gary Slutkin, an early GPA employee and TB specialist, as one of "great turmoil and confusion"—things started to decline. Within three months of Mann's departure, along with his key staff, Slutkin maintains, contact with African countries was virtually lost. Two years later the entire African country staff was gone.[89]

Shortly thereafter the GPA's new leader, Michael Merson, began the process of dismantling the GPA. Many in the global health community—or, rather, in the global health bureaucracy—began to think that GPA had accrued too much power and was having a hard time working with other U.N. agencies. Duplication of efforts was becoming more and more common. A unified agency was necessary to fight the global pandemic. And "thus began," as the authors of the official history of UNAIDS put it, "the tortuous process that would result in the establishment of UNAIDS."[90] That process lasted four years, until 1996; it would be another two years before UNAIDS was able to command the global stage. And so it was that between roughly 1990, when Mann resigned, and 1998, when UNAIDS was firmly established, the fight against HIV/AIDS was left without a clear leader.[91] While interest in TB had experienced an upsurge due to its connection to HIV/AIDS, attention to the coepidemic lost focus.

The set of circumstances noted above—the global indifference to TB that had set in by the end of the 1970s; the appearance of a new disease meeting an old and intractable one; the initial neglect of HIV/AIDS in Africa; the incoherence and lack of leadership in global AIDS policy—are at the root of the problem. Looking back in such a way, it seems almost inevitable that TB would become HIV's number one coconspirator in Africa.

What could be done?

11. Prevention, Cure, and the Search for the Cheapest Solution

Once HIV had arrived, once its power was felt, the association between TB and HIV made sense—of course the two would merge and feed off one another. The natural history of TB, TB experts like John Murray noted early on, made it HIV's perfect companion. Considering the high rate of TB infection already present on the continent, Murray very simply declared in 1990, the "explosion of tuberculosis in Africa . . . is predictable."[1] But still, the speed and force of the new coepidemic took most by surprise. No one was prepared. The TB programs that might have been able to manage the problem—national programs like Kenya's—were not up to the task, and even well-run ones, like Tanzania's, appeared to be no match for HIV/TB. Thus, by the early 1990s, the world found itself caught off guard and faced with a problem the likes of which no one had ever seen. What could be done? The WHO showed some initial interest, but momentum was hard to maintain. After the initial alarm, the first urgent calls for action, the recognition that a tragedy was unfolding, a period—a crucial period—of quiet neglect set in. There were, of course, those committed to HIV/TB, but work on the problem became marginalized as other priorities emerged. As TB had become a neglected disease by the late 1970s and early 1980s, HIV/TB was by the mid-1990s, if not neglected, then certainly shoved out of the spotlight.

To the picture of the general neglect of TB, the slow response to AIDS in the developing world, and the waning influence of the WHO another element must be added. Just as the WHO's hold on the global health agenda began to weaken, and perhaps even because of it, the World Bank's began to strengthen. The bank's interest in health had been growing steadily from the late 1960s. In 1979 the bank created a new department—the Health, Nutrition, and Population Department. What thrust it into the world of TB control was work in the late 1980s—which began to be published in various forms in the early 1990s—on the cost effectiveness of TB treatment. Cost effectiveness is not the same thing as cheap, though they are related. Health care economists and policy makers who latched onto cost effectiveness did not compare the raw cost of an intervention; they calculated its potential benefits relative to its cost. Was a given intervention, in other words, a good investment?

Cost had been considered in the past. In Kenya, as we've seen, reducing the cost of TB treatment was a principal goal of both the British Medical Research Council (MRC) and the WHO. But something changed. By the late 1980s health had become intimately connected with economic development—a healthy population was a more productive one, and thus "investing" in health became important. Of course, health and development did not suddenly entwine themselves in the 1980s. Indeed, it is arguable that the potential connection between good health and economic growth has always been one of the principal drivers of the global health agenda.[2] What was different as the twentieth century drew to a close was that at a time when the WHO was falling out of favor in the international community, and thus losing funding from donors fed up with its supposed bureaucratic lethargy and waste, the World Bank, with untold resources in its control, stepped into the void. By the beginning of the 1990s the bank's loans for health care projects surpassed the WHO's entire budget.[3]

The bank had certainly not been keeping this a secret. But it was not until 1993, when it published its *World Development Report, 1993: Investing in Health,* that many began to take notice. Widely regarded as a watershed moment, the publication of *Investing in Health* signaled the beginning of a new era. Bill Gates credits the report, among other things, with sparking his interest in global health—an interest that has now grown into the world's largest philanthropy, the Bill and Melinda Gates Foundation.[4] What most captured people's attention was what the bank called a DALY (disability-adjusted life year)—the amount of potential productive life lost to illness. Once DALY entered the lingua franca the question then became: how many DALYs could be saved by which interventions, and how much would they cost? Would a given intervention salvage enough of a person's productive life to be a wise investment? Was an intervention, in the final, and it must be noted most important, analysis, cost effective?

Seeing health care in this way was novel; it also had an elementary appeal that many found hard to resist. Who would not want programs to be cost effective? It seemed to make so much sense that it became hard to see things any other way. It began to seem obvious, even natural: if something was not cost effective, it cost too much and could not be done. And once an intervention was found not to be cost effective its chances of survival were slim. The infiltration of this way of thinking into the world of global health was a triumph of neoliberalism. By contrast, when the MRC developed thiacetazone in Kenya in the 1960s as a way to reduce the cost of TB care and cure more patients, its development was not predicated on its being a cost-effective investment in neoliberal terms. The goal in Kenya was to cure TB; reducing the cost of doing so was absolutely essential. But the commitment to curing TB was the primary goal; that did not waver. What had changed by the 1990s was that wanting to cure TB, per se, was not the goal. Cost effectiveness dictated the diseases eligible for treatment or prevention. The diseases themselves were not necessarily the priority; their cost effectiveness was. For a disease to be a wise candidate for control it had to be a cost-effective investment: the return on the monetary outlay required to control it needed to be part of the equation. That return was, generally, the amount of productive life saved were an individual spared a given affliction. This kind of calculus emerged out of disparate sources—the well-known rise of neoliberalism, frustrations of the first world with the profligacy of the third, fears that developing nations were driving the agenda of global economics (most evident in the backlash over the United Nations' "New Economic Order"), and the perception that resources were diminishing and priorities needed to be set.[5]

In the world of global health the turn to cost effectiveness, which had its very public debut in *Investing in Health,* can be traced to debates in the late 1970s over the WHO's move toward primary health care and its "Health for All by the Year 2000" campaign. Social justice and equity, alongside a growing frustration with overly technical, vertically oriented interventions, guided the WHO's director general, Halfdan Mahler, to move the world toward primary health care. Mahler's enthusiasm for integrated care over specialized, targeted approaches was already evident by the late 1960s when he had developed his interest in folding TB programs into countries' more general health services. When he became director general in 1973 he devoted his considerable energy, and deployed his legendary charm and powers of persuasion, to primary health care. China and its "barefoot doctors," as well other developing countries the world over in Africa, South America, and South Asia, had been successfully experimenting with primary health care. UNICEF and the WHO began to take notice. With the old strictures of public health crumbling, Mahler sensed a "revolution" blooming in the dust. As he told the World Health Assembly in 1975, "We could . . . become the *avant garde* of an international conscience for social development."[6]

Mahler announced his revolutionary agenda at the now famous International Conference on Primary Health Care in Alma-Ata, in what was then the Soviet Union, in 1978. Attended by three thousand delegates from all over the world, it was a massive global affair. The declaration that emerged out of the conference was a denouncement of medical elitism, the neglect of the rural poor, top-down health campaigns, and useless, expensive technology. Instead, the declaration was a rousing call for community involvement, "appropriate technology," the construction of rural health centers, and the central place of basic health care in economic well-being. The World Health Assembly approved the declaration the following year.[7] Under Mahler's leadership it appeared that the global health community was on the cusp of real change. It was indeed—just not in the way Mahler envisioned.

Within a year everything had changed. Quickly following the Alma-Ata conference was another meeting. "Health and Population in Development," convened in 1979 by the Rockefeller Foundation at the Bellagio Conference Center in Italy and organized by the heads of the World Bank, USAID, the Ford Foundation, and the Canadian International Development and Research Center, offered an alternative approach. The meeting had been inspired by the work of two health economists, Julia Walsh and Kenneth Warren, especially their paper "Selective Primary Health Care, an Interim Strategy for Disease Control in Developing Countries." While the goals of primary health care and "Health for All by the Year 2000" were admirable, Walsh and Warren, as well as the attendees, considered them unrealistic and vague. Instead, Walsh and Warren offered specifics. They classified diseases as either high, medium, or low priority. Their ranking was based explicitly on the cost effectiveness of a given intervention. TB, for example, was a medium priority even though it was "highly prevalent" and caused "high mortality." Why? Because it was difficult to control and thus not cost effective.[8]

The Walsh and Warren paper and the conference set in motion what we now know was the beginning of the end of primary health care. It also signaled the arrival of cost effectiveness and the growing dominance of neo-liberalism in setting the global health agenda. Primary health care in the spirit of Alma-Ata was never put in place. It *was* too vague; it was not clear to many just what it entailed. Cost-effective, technical, measurable solutions to health problems—like childhood immunizations, for instance—became the order of the day.[9] Thus, while the concept of a DALY—the formal mechanism by which cost effectiveness could be calculated—had its international debut in 1993, thinking in terms of cost effectiveness had been around for more than a decade by then. The World Bank, for its part, had been calculating cost effectiveness for at least half that time.

And, as it happened, TB led the way. Beginning in the late 1970s, with AIDS not yet on the horizon, the International Union Against Tuberculosis teamed up with the Tanzanian government to tackle TB. Karel Styblo, a brilliant M.D. and epidemiologist and one of the few people still doing research on TB, led the effort. Styblo's success in Tanzania revealed that even in a poor, developing country TB control could work. One of the key insights was that standard course chemotherapy—which lasted anywhere from twelve to eighteen months—was not working. Too many people defaulted; too few were cured. It simply took too long. Styblo began to pilot short-course chemotherapy; when the pilot programs proved successful he rolled it out countrywide in 1986. Early evidence suggested it was working: reducing the regimen to six months increased cure rates. This was a breakthrough: short-course chemotherapy had been shown to be efficacious in trials but not yet in field conditions in a developing country. A few elements needed to be in place: a vigorous, government-supported TB program capable of case finding and ensuring compliance and a ready supply of drugs. Considering the results Styblo was achieving—cure rates of up to 90 percent!—and with AIDS just barely registering, he predicted that "tuberculosis would cease to be a public health problem" by the year 2000.[10] One can only read such a prediction now with unease and regret.

Because it was efficient, cheap, and effective Styblo's work caught the interest of those interested in the cost-effectiveness of programs in the developing world. Styblo joined forces with Christopher Murray, a Harvard M.D. and an economist, and Annick Rouillon, the president of the International Union Against Tuberculosis and Lung Disease ("Lung Disease" was added to the union's title in 1986), under the auspices of a World Bank project, the Health Sector Priorities Review. In 1990, three years before the publication of *Investing in Health,* they wrote a paper—the influence of which cannot be overstated—that claimed: "Taken together the studies on the cost-effectiveness of both standard 12-month and short-course chemotherapy show that tuberculosis chemotherapy is an excellent invest- ment relative to virtually any health intervention."[11] Their claim was further buttressed by research on case finding and treatment with short-course chemotherapy from programs supported by the International Union run- ning on what was by then called the Styblo method in Malawi and Mozambique as well as Tanzania. Again, TB treatment with short-course chemotherapy was found to be cost effective.[12] Three years later, when *Investing in Health* appeared, it had been determined that TB caused more DALYs than any oth- er disease. Because the cost of drugs was so low and the burden was so high TB treatment became the single most cost-effective intervention on the plan- et. The investment reaped returns many times over. *Investing in Health* de- clared that TB treatment must be part of the "essential clinical package" of any country with a TB epidemic.[13] TB, long a neglected disease, was now considered too serious and too cost effective to ignore. One has to wonder, for a moment anyway, had TB been found not to be cost effective, would neglect have continued apace?

With the success of short-course chemotherapy in the developing world the World Bank decided to go big: it aimed to transform China's TB program. With a $50 million loan China implemented a new TB program in 1991. When the first report came from the program it appeared to be success- ful: case detection and cure rates were up.[14]

Had there been a breakthrough?

Tuberculosis had, in a very short time, gone from being a neglected disease to becoming once again the focus of considerable international attention. The details will come later in the chapter, but for now suffice it to say that the focus of the World Bank and the WHO in the 1990s on TB via what came to be called DOTS (directly observed therapy short course) rivals the antibiotic revolution of the 1950s and 60s; and, at least in ambition if not execution, it was the equal of the BCG campaign—perhaps in more ways than one.

But what was to be done about HIV/TB? Was there any way to control the coepidemic? Treating TB, of course, was an option—and would become an increasingly appealing one. But with TB programs for now in disarray many began to focus on prevention. Was it possible to forestall at least some new infections? Theoretically, yes. Isoniazid preventive therapy (IPT), also called chemoprophylaxis, might just work. The idea was, and is, simple: give HIV-positive people infected with the TB bacillus, but without active TB, a course of prophylactic isoniazid to prevent the onset of active TB. In 1992, the top TB people at the WHO declared that "in view of the high risk of tuberculosis in dually-infected persons, prevention of tuberculosis in such persons is clearly a high priority. Administration of preventive chemotherapy to HIV/tuberculosis co-infected persons has therefore been considered as one of the most critical interventions to limit the increase in clinical tuberculosis that is expected from the pool of HIV/tuberculosis co-infected individuals."[15]

It sounded simple. It turned out to diabolically complicated.

IPT has a long history spanning some six decades. Its theoretical possibilities have always fascinated researchers. It's occasionally been seen as a solution to the TB problem. Suppressing the onset of TB, rather than treating it after it arrives, has an obvious appeal. Before HIV/AIDS, IPT had been tested repeatedly in a variety of settings around the globe. The U.S. Public Health Service began trials in 1955.[16] That same year American Indian reservations became, once again, a hive of activity.[17] Basil Dormer—Lyle Cummins's South African nemesis in the debate over virgin soil theory—began using IPT with great success in high-risk infants in Durban in the late 1950s and advocated its much wider use.[18] Early in the next decade, the WHO identified "the problem of the efficacy of large-scale chemoprophylaxis" as one of the four "urgent" priories in TB research.[19] And simultaneous with the MRC's chemotherapy studies, the WHO also carried out IPT trials in Kenya and Tunisia. Based on the work in Kenya, which had been designed to see if chemoprophylaxis could work among household contacts of those with active TB, the WHO determined in 1964 that preventive therapy worked.[20]

One of the most fascinating trials, of which little is known, was run by the chief medical officer of Gold Fields, a mining company in South Africa.

Substituting isoniazid with Neotizide, P. Smit began work in 1962. He eventually administered his tonic to forty-one thousand miners. Smit spiked the miners' *marewu*—a maize-based mildly alcoholic beverage virtually all miners drank—with Neotizide. Remarkably, by the end of 1967 Smit reported marked reductions in TB, especially compared to mines where workers were not drinking Neotizide-enhanced *marewu*. Realizing his method did not ensure that all miners were getting prophylaxis at all times, and that some might be getting more than others, Smit let his results speak for themselves: the large-scale distribution of Neotizide-laced *marewu* was reducing TB on the mines. Using a nontoxic dose of Neotizide, Smit came up with an unconventional method for reducing TB—a method the statistician for the South African Chamber of Mines claimed was working. After Smit published his results in 1968, however, his work on TB appears to have stopped. In a discussion of Smit's Neotizide trial held by members of the Mine Medical Officers Association there was concern over long-term efficacy of the intervention as well as maintaining its use with a highly mobile population—there was up to 90 percent turnover year to year in the labor force. It seems once Smit's trial was over the program ceased.[21]

By the end of 1960 trials had been run all over the world. And for the most part IPT worked: it reduced the onset of active TB.[22]

Among all the IPT trials two stand out. The first is the oft-cited, but never emulated, work done in Alaska. Led by George Comstock, the Alaska work began between 1957 and 1959 and follow-up continued throughout the 1970s.[23] The trials were tightly controlled studies of IPT's effect on an entire community, not just obviously high-risk portions of the population. And it worked: it appeared to demonstrably reduce TB.

There are a number of important features of the Alaskan work. Before the advent of the IPT program TB rates were staggering: a 1949–1951 tuberculin survey revealed that the annual infection rate among Alaskan natives was 24.6 percent. But by 1957 it had dropped to 8 percent—still among the highest on the planet, but an extraordinary reduction. Once the IPT trial was under way, almost certainly in part as a result of IPT, the annual infection rate dropped again, to around 1 percent. Thus it was clear by 1961 that the infection rate was, according to Comstock, "quite low."[24]

While the drop from 1957 to 1960 was remarkable it was not entirely attributable to IPT. IPT was added to an already very robust program. By the time IPT began, a very well-organized system of emergency TB control had been in place since 1954. The program included a doubling of hospital beds as well as a reduction of time spent in the hospital. There was also an innovative and vigorous program of ambulatory chemotherapy. When IPT began, the annual rates of infection and incidence were falling precipitously.[25] One key question in all IPT work concerns its long-term effect—will IPT stave off TB over time? Because TB was already so rapidly in decline this question could not be adequately answered in Alaska. As Comstock wrote, "In large measure, the observation period is still too short because the risk of developing tuberculosis decreased sharply with time for all the populations participating in the Public Health Service cooperative trials and, as a consequence, fewer cases are available for analysis each successive year."[26]

The trials were done in two phases—one in 1958–59 and the other in 1963–64. The second phase, carried out in and around the town of Bethel, turned up a problem that would plague researchers from then on—recruitment and follow-up. Overall the trial was successful, but a few elements are noteworthy. First, the trial failed in the town of Bethel itself. Few people from town volunteered for the trial, and no door-to-door publicity and recruitment campaign was carried out as it was in the smaller villages. Further, the town's "constantly shifting" population made following cases especially tough. In the smaller villages, enrollment was more successful but still disappointing. As cases declined, fewer and fewer people lived in the shadow of TB. The disease was becoming a memory; fewer people were inclined to seek preventive treatment. All of this, the authors of the initial report on the trial noted, meant that "the threat of tuberculosis has ceased to be strong motivation for community action."[27]

By 1970, TB had fallen even more dramatically. By that year the incidence rated had dropped, from 1,842 per 100,000 in 1952, to 141 per 100,000. Most of these cases showed signs of previous disease indicating that new infections were few. There were no deaths from TB in 1970.[28] It was in the context of steadily declining annual rates of infection that the IPT trials were carried out.

The Comstock trials have rightly been hailed as pathbreaking. They have become well known as one of only two successful community-wide IPT trials. The other trial in which an entire population was given IPT was among a broadly similar population in Greenland. When the results were published in 1966, the authors considered the trial successful in reducing TB, but they pointed out several things of note, each of which would be concerns in the years to come. First, distributing IPT to an entire community was a significant strain on resources. Second, the efficacy trailed off over the six years of follow-up. Third, the authors recommended that IPT should not be given to an entire community; it should only be given to at-risk groups, because too many people received IPT in vain.[29]

Despite their success neither of these trials inspired similar work. Unlike mass prophylactic campaigns against sleeping sickness in the decade and a half after World War II, in which more than ten million pentamidine injections were administered to healthy, but at-risk, people in the French, Belgian, and Portuguese colonies in Africa, mass IPT never caught on.[30] As early as 1960, despite it having been "definitely . . . established as effective," IPT in Africa faced "insurmountable" obstacles.[31] In contrast to a single shot of pentamidine, chemoprophylaxis with isoniazid was an extended affair that demanded far more logistical organization than a mass needle campaign. And while the WHO declared in 1963 that determining whether or not chemoprophylaxis was an "urgent" research priority, the following year—without ever actually testing its efficacy—the WHO's Expert Committee on Tuberculosis discouraged its use on a large scale, arguing that the cost, the logistical difficulties, the likelihood of defaulting, and other concerns all made it unfeasible.[32] When the Expert Committee met again and issued its next report in 1974, it considered the use of isoniazid preventive therapy to be "irrational."[33] In 1982, citing fears that its implementation might take resources away from curative treatment—this would become a common refrain in the future—the WHO and the International Union Against Tuberculosis declared that "in practice [IPT] has virtually no role in developing countries."[34] IPT appeared to be dead.

But then HIV changed everything. Within less than a decade IPT went from having "virtually no role" in TB control to become, again, one of the WHO's research priorities. With remarkable speed IPT raced to the top of the agenda. It became vitally important to know if IPT would work among HIV-positive people.[35] And, just as important, could IPT work on the scale necessary to control the HIV/TB epidemic in places where the coinfection was exploding? If it worked, its benefits were obvious. As Jonathan Mann, the first director of WHO's Global Program on AIDS, wrote in a 1989 memo, "Delaying or preventing TB may be the single most important thing that can be done in developing countries for prolonging the survival of HIV infected persons."[36] By 1989 the WHO and the International Union Against Tuberculosis and Lung Disease had decided that testing the efficacy of IPT was an urgent priority.[37] The following year an editorial in the *Lancet* urged the international community to get to work quickly on efficacy and feasibility studies—after all, IPT might be something that could have a real effect on the dual epidemic.[38]

Momentum was gaining. That same year the WHO convened a group of TB and HIV experts who recommended that "WHO should vigorously promote studies of tuberculosis chemoprophylaxis in HIV infected persons as a major priority for research."[39] Almost immediately, and with great gusto, the WHO sponsored IPT trials in places as diverse as Haiti, Zambia, Uganda, and Thailand. When researchers from the London School of Tropical Medicine and Hygiene launched the Zambia trial they called IPT the "only current available intervention method . . . likely to reduce the occurrence of HIV-associated tuberculosis."[40] The WHO's TB leadership, including Arata Kochi, considered IPT "one of the most critical interventions to limit the increase in clinical tuberculosis that is expected from the pool of HIV/tuberculosis connected individuals."[41] IPT was back in the spotlight. What was once considered "irrational" had become an essential weapon in the war against HIV-related TB.

Just as in Kenya in the 1960s when antibiotic research was in high gear, two essential questions needed to be answered. Would IPT work, and if so would it do so when transferred from a trial to the field? First came efficacy. Nothing could be done until this question was answered—an early iteration of the Zambian trial could not even get WHO approval because the researchers wanted to consider compliance and cost alongside efficacy. Until it was known whether IPT would even work cost and compliance simply did not matter.[42] Once the WHO decided to try to answer those two questions work quickly got under way.

But then it was slow going. Getting a trial up and running anywhere resources were in short supply was hard work. Adding HIV/AIDS to the mix made it even harder. For example, in Uganda it proved difficult to recruit people for the study. While the researchers identified nearly two thousand HIV-positive people eligible for the study, only 12 percent of them volunteered to be tested for TB and potentially join the study. Why? Because no provision had been made to ensure anonymity at Kampala's AIDS Information Center—people who had tested positive for HIV had to wait in the public corridor of the center before being tested for TB. There was no private space, and thus it would be easy to tell who had tested positive for HIV as they awaited TB testing.[43] The same was true in Zambia: people worried that others would learn they were taking medicine and assume they had HIV, a disease to which there was great stigma attached.[44]

Other problems emerged as well. The WHO eventually approved the Zambian trial, and it was scheduled to get off the ground in August 1992. Drugs that were supposed to arrive in July actually arrived in October—and cost substantially more than originally budgeted for; many patients presenting for inclusion in the study did so with abnormal chest x-rays, leaving them ineligible.[45] Recruitment into the study was difficult for another reason as well: futility. In Zambia, as in other places, testing for HIV was both limited and a hard sell: everyone knew nothing could be done. Researchers hoped IPT might change this, that at least controlling TB might lure people into the trial. Because the country's TB program was quite weak and resources were hard to come by, enthusiasm for a TB prevention program was hard to muster. But as one WHO observer grimly put it, "Support for such a prevention programme was not entirely rejected."[46]

The trials, despite all the difficulties, nonetheless proceeded. And remember: these initial studies studied only efficacy, not feasibility. At this stage, the operational challenges noted above were not important. Did IPT work? Results began to appear in the early to mid–1990s, and they confirmed what had been known about IPT in the pre-HIV era: it reduced the incidence of TB.[47] By the middle of the decade it was clear IPT worked in trial conditions. The results were so clear that further trials would be unethical. While IPT's place in the world was by no means secure—whether or not it *would* work still needed to be answered—its role in easing the burden of TB among people living with HIV was promising. The possibilities were such that three prominent researchers confidently claimed in the *Lancet* in 1995 that "for the HIV infected individual in Africa or Asia, preventive therapy for tuberculosis may represent the single most useful intervention for prolongation of healthy life."[48]

IPT was ascendant. A therapy which had been around for decades, but which had never been deployed on a large scale, now looked poised to become a lifesaver for millions.

Once efficacy had been established—IPT will work among HIV-positive people—feasibility became the next challenge—would it work, and would it be cost effective, in real-world settings? This, of course, was not a new problem. IPT no doubt reduced the incidence of active TB in HIV-positive people; the science was not in dispute. The question had *always* centered on whether or not it *would* work. Indeed, more than two decades earlier, in her 1970 review of IPT in the pre-HIV era, Shirley Ferebee—an expert on chemoprophylaxis at the U.S. Public Health Service—wrote that "isoniazid treatment of infection is biologically so good now that sociological research on how to conduct successful programs is imperative." For Ferebee, figuring out how to get the drugs to where they needed to be and then into people's bodies was much harder than figuring out what happened once they got there. As she noted, "It must be admitted that scientific study of social factors is far more difficult than study of the interaction between drug, bacilli and host." And a large part of the problem was the research community itself. The problem of getting patients to stick with their treatment, of motivating them to do so, was "so large and diffuse that it must be broken into many small piece for a series of studies, a course unattractive to most investigators who hope that each step toward understanding will be a giant step." In a priceless instance of understatement, Ferebee further noted that "humans make difficult subjects for research because their opportunities for deviating from a prearranged protocol are infinitely more varied than those of laboratory animals." Researchers failed, it seems, to understand this. And according to Ferebee, the difficulties in figuring out what did and did not motivate patients "[lay] with the investigator," who insisted on testing multiple things at once rather than methodically investigating approaches one by one.

Ferebee's point was simple: scientists rarely took the same time and care to investigate social factors that they did biological ones. By 1970 the scientific basis for IPT had been settled. And because of that, she argued, "Surely the most important task ahead is social research to determine the efficient and economical ways to bring treatment to those who can benefit."[49] Or, in the terms used in the 1990s: did IPT in the era of HIV/AIDS work, as they say, "under program conditions"? Was it feasible and cost effective? In the real world the results appeared to be mixed. Regarding the Zambian trial, Australian HIV expert David Cooper had his doubts. He worried that "even if the study has a positive benefit of TB prophylaxis, the analysis of the cohort so far suggests that such a strategy will be difficult to implement in an African context."[50]

What was the problem? Just as in TB treatment, so too in IPT: compliance became a major, perhaps the dominant, obstacle. Hugh Stott warned about this in 1959 when Kenya and the WHO began their IPT study.[51] It has remained a problem ever since. When Ferebee surveyed the world scene in 1970 it turned out that adherence—along with cost, of course—was an enormous problem in rolling out IPT more often.

The challenges thrown up by poor compliance and adherence in the early days of HIV-era IPT trials were daunting. After struggling to get people to come back to the clinics after their initial visit—many were lost to follow-up—Dr. Alwyn Mwinga decided to ask her Zambian patients why they skipped their appointments. The answer was rather simple: Lusaka's sprawl combined with its expensive and inefficient public transportation meant that study participants had to spend precious time and money to get to the clinic. As Mwinga put it: "Given that the majority of the patients in the study are not acutely ill, it is easy to see how attendance at the clinic may not be high in their list of priorities on which to spend scanty resources." When researchers explained to subjects the value of the research it turned out that they well understood the importance of the work. But this was not enough. According to Mwinga: "In a situation where there is a high rate of inflation with an ever increasing cost of living and growing unemployment an intellectual understanding will not make up for a deficit in the pocket!" The solution: pay the patients. How much? A dollar and some soft drinks each time they came to the clinic.[52] Still, even with money to pay for transportation and diligent efforts by project staff to keep track of patients, around 30 percent simply disappeared.[53]

Understanding patients has always been difficult. No one who has given the matter any thought disputes this. Yet, despite the critical importance of so-called patient behavior—how many times does one need to read that poor compliance is at the heart of TB control's failure to be convinced of this?—it still seemed to be the case that by the mid–1990s those working in TB control needed to be reminded again. Ferebee would surely have agreed, but likewise been frustrated, had she been at the 1995 WHO meeting, twenty-five years after her article appeared, at which it was discussed how "in the past, tuberculosis control programmes have generally not been successful in using findings from the social and behavioural sciences, and yet patient behaviour underlies all our control strategies."[54] Despite this statement not being true at all regarding the pathbreaking work done in India in the 1950s and

60s on the importance of social factors in controlling TB, it was a fair characterization of the general state of affairs: almost nothing had changed since Ferebee implored researchers to get working on the social barriers to implementing IPT.

As researchers discovered, patients behaved in unpredictable ways, and circumstances changed. For example, in Zambia they began to notice that some patients who had been lost started to show up as time went by. Why? They were sick. At the six-month follow-up point a patient might feel fine and decide to skip out on the trial; at eighteen months he or she might have AIDS and active TB. What's more, the cost of living rose dramatically in Zambia in the early 1990s, and in 1992 the country instituted a fee-for-service model rather than the free care once offered. Sick patients with no money returned to the trial seeking care. Grim circumstances served as incentive to get back to the clinic. Other patients were lost because they were, by design, impossible to find. Because of the powerful stigma attached to HIV/AIDS in Zambia, some patients recruited into the study gave false addresses, not wanting to be found.[55] Contrast this with experience of researchers in northern Thailand, where "one of the unexpected outcomes of the IPT is that the symptomatic HIV positive patients are going to hospitals requesting the INH [isoniazid] preventive therapy."[56] In Haiti, knowing people would avoid an HIV testing center, researchers working on chemoprophylaxis combated this problem by advertising their study as a TB control project.[57] In Zambia, add the problem of false addresses to the high cost and inconvenience of traveling Lusaka's labyrinth and it becomes clear why so many patients were lost sight of. In Uganda, where two separate studies were under way—one on efficacy and another on feasibility—the problems were similar. Patients found the distances they needed to travel for follow-up to be burdensome; others had sick relatives to care for; some came for their appointments only to find that the clinic had no drugs; still others did not want to be seen going into the clinic—they feared the stigma of TB. Some were simply too busy.[58] If this litany does not sound familiar, it should—these are precisely the same problems TB workers had been dealing with since the advent of antibiotics in 1950s.

As mundane and quotidian as these might sound, they are the things that in studies of its feasibility and cost effectiveness doomed IPT. Instead of identifying the barriers, embarking on a research strategy to try to figure out how to improve adherence, and then devoting the resources to implement such a program, it was easier to simply give up. The nuances of people's lives were not teased out in the scientific literature. Rather, a convenient shorthand—the "African context"—was deployed. And in that context IPT would not work. The feasibility study from Uganda was published in *AIDS* in 1995. It was not encouraging. Not enough data, too many barriers, too many patients lost—all these meant, at a minimum, that more work was needed on feasibility.[59]

When the difficulties of carrying out IPT treatment in Africa were encountered, but well before they were fully understood or any attempts were made to overcome them, enthusiasm for IPT began to wane. But it was not only the challenges of IPT that caused the initially strong support to atrophy. These were desperate days. The early 1990s were a period of rapid change, a period of what could appear to be a helter-skelter scramble for solutions. Resources were limited, as those working in the world of HIV and TB control were reminded again and again. The World Bank took on the dominant role in global public health just as it confronted the effects of compelling countries to whom the bank, and the International Monetary Fund, had lent money to undergo structural adjustment—effects that included pitifully diminished health programs. Having run out of money, Zambia's TB program was in such dire straits that an untold number of patients died for want of antibiotics.[60] Furthermore, frustration had set in; not enough progress was being made in the burgeoning coepidemic. The WHO lamented at an HIV/TB meeting in 1995 that the "present research agenda is stuck."[61]

Cost-effective solutions were absolutely essential. And just as IPT research was getting off the ground in the early 1990s one such solution might have been found.

12. Prevention versus Cure

The Neglect of HIV/TB and
Multidrug-Resistant TB

In 1994, as isoniazid prophylaxis therapy stumbled, the World Health Organization announced a new direction. Making its debut in the "Framework for Effective Tuberculosis Control," the "revised strategy adopted by WHO is simple: All countries with a TB problem must provide standardized short-course chemotherapy (SCC) to, at least, all sputum smear positive TB patients." The revised strategy did not include IPT. Rather, in boldface, the WHO declared, "Cure is the best prevention."[1] Soon to be packaged as DOTS (directly observed therapy short course), the new strategy was, for a decade, hailed as the final solution. The simple act of watching patients take their medicine, it was hoped, would ensure success. But what of HIV, which, after all, many at the time thought was responsible for the upsurge of TB in the first place? In addition, what of the countless numbers of cases of TB in the HIV-positive population that would go undetected and untreated because of the many people with HIV who have a smear *negative* sputum test? DOTS policy did not concern itself with HIV. Both HIV and the emerging multidrug-resistant TB disaster (MDR-TB is defined as TB that is resistant to the two frontline drugs rifampin and isoniazid) were noted as afterthoughts: once the new framework was in place, "systems to monitor HIV seroprevalence and drug resistance in TB should be added."[2] They never were. Thirteen years later a group of prominent researchers from the Centers for Disease Control and Prevention in Atlanta as well as institutions in Kenya and Zambia called the merging of HIV and multidrug-resistant TB the "perfect storm."[3]

Up to a point, DOTS was a novel intervention. Or at least that was the way it was marketed. A key component of the strategy Karel Styblo and the International Union Against Tuberculosis pioneered in the late 1970s and early 1980s was the direct observation of patients taking their drugs. Ensuring that drug regimens were adhered to, especially in the first, intensive two months of treatment was crucial. While directly observing patients has come to be the heart of the program, DOTS is actually made up of several elements. For DOTS to work there must be top-level political commitment; funding has to be adequate and regular; drugs and diagnostics must be readily available at all times even in the most out-of-the-way places; staff need to be properly trained; and, finally, the health system must be capable of ensuring that treatment is adhered to. When all these are in place—which of course they rarely are in the developing world—you've got DOTS. From the moment it first appeared on the global health agenda in 1994 until the early years of the new millennium DOTS was *the* TB intervention. With the World Bank making support of TB programs contingent on the adoption of the new the program the gospel of DOTS spread far and wide, and did so very quickly. Five years after its emergence, 120 countries had, at least nominally, adopted DOTS. To secure funding, for example, India, already home to a well-established though not necessarily effective TB program, developed a DOTS program that sparked considerable controversy over the ethics and necessity of directly observed therapy.[4]

Stunning assertions flowed forth: the WHO claimed in a 1996 publication that "where the health system is working even moderately well, the DOTS strategy is extraordinarily effective, typically achieving cure rates over 90%."[5] But where in sub-Saharan Africa were there TB programs reliably implementing all five strategies? In many places, of course, the health system was *not* working "even moderately well." With the advent of AIDS even Tanzania's program, as we've seen, was on the verge of collapse. At a discussion on DOTS in the late 1990s, focused on the question "Is DOTS the health breakthrough of the 1990s?" Jaap Broekmans of the Royal Netherlands Tuberculosis Association—a major supporter of various national TB programs—pointed out to the assembled, in what can only be described as obvious and understated, that "weak political commitment, poor programme management and insufficient capability to carry out directly observed treat-ment are important factors."[6] Indeed, one could argue that these were *the* limiting factors and without them DOTS would fail. Even so, and despite considerable debate in the scientific and academic communities over DOTS, the WHO hailed DOTS as perhaps *the* breakthrough in TB control.[7] It was marketable, simple to understand, and required no new technologies.[8] It's easy to see why DOTS became so attractive an option: it offered the hope of solving one of the most intractable problems in TB control: compliance. In these respects and others it was the antithesis to IPT, which appeared com-plicated, required embarking on a new path if not a new technology, and, in comparison to DOTS, could not be less marketable—chemoprophylaxis and isoniazid preventive therapy are nothing if not a mouthful.

At first glance DOTS makes sense: watching to make sure patients take their medicine sounds like a good idea; so, too, does having government support, a regular supply of drugs, and so forth. And DOTS can work, but apparently not as well in Africa as anywhere else in the world.[9] But it's clear, too, from several studies, that treatment outcomes in these cases don't appear to be better under DOTS than they are without it. Programs vary from place to place, and infection rates remain high. It's not the magic bullet it was touted to be; a universal solution has not been found.[10] By 2005, a dec-ade after its formal adoption, DOTS was theoretically available to 89 percent of the world's population. Yet only 27 percent of cases were actually enrolled in DOTS programs.[11] And in places with established MDR-TB, DOTS can be more harmful than helpful. How could this be? In a place where resistance already exists to first-line drugs like isoniazid and rifampin, a DOTS program will revert to, for example, a short course of pyrazinamide and ethambutol at doses insufficient to treat active TB but in doses large enough to boost resist-ance. Further, if a patient's TB was not cured DOTS also called for retreat-ment with rifampin and isoniazid, whether there was resistance or not. Paul Farmer calls this the "amplifier effect," and it's a cruel irony of the DOTS program: the unintended worsening of the MDR-TB problem.[12]

What's more, the central component of DOTS is really a rebranding of an old and well-known intervention—Wallace Fox pioneered the use of directly observed therapy in the 1950s, even paying patients to take their medicine. Like so much in TB control, what appeared new was not. Further, the dominance and dogma of DOTS has tended to overshadow all other in-terventions. And it was adopted by the WHO with virtually no research to back it up.[13] By the end of the 1990s even Christopher Murray, upon whose work, among others, the WHO relied to promote the global expansion of DOTS, began to wonder if DOTS was enough. It had been slow to catch on, and other interventions, like IPT, might also be called for in the face of HIV/TB.[14]

This thumbnail sketch of DOTS might seem an unduly negative assessment; it's not quite meant that way. In theory DOTS makes sense. Who could argue with its basic premises? The problem is not with DOTS, per se, or with the several places where it has worked, or with its theoretical possibilities. DOTS was a response to what was clearly a severe, intractable, and urgent problem—a response that appeared to be an affordable way to combat a formidable foe. Well-meaning people devoted considerable energy to its implementation. My concern is with none of that, really, but rather with the way in which it was adhered to rigidly for a decade without clear evidence to back it up or a recognition that it might not work in all places at all times or, often enough, not given the resources it needed to ensure its success. Finally, it took little to no account of HIV/TB or MDR-TB—even Arata Kochi, the former director of TB programs at the WHO and one of the architects of DOTS, admitted this. In a 2006 interview, he lamented: "One thing I didn't do well is develop an additional strategy in addition to DOTS for HIV/TB. That is my regret."[15] There are echoes here of the BCG vaccination years: hope and faith meant DOTS did not come under intense scrutiny until years after it was rolled out. Its successes were used as evidence of its universal appeal, while its failures were considered anomalies. What seems to have happened is that a series of commonsense, and, it must be said, well-known strategies, were repackaged under a new name, DOTS, that when introduced to the world were touted as the final solution to the TB problem. A great discovery had been made, according to some. But what DOTS really is, in many respects, is the collation of several different strategies into a new package that has as its centerpiece—even if unintentionally—the direct observation of patients while they take their medicine. This feature of the DOTS approach is of course an effort at addressing an age-old problem: compliance. And in that respect it's nothing new at all. What DOTS did well, initially at least, was draw new attention to TB. What some feared it would do—siphon off resources from other promising interventions or stymie research—is difficult to prove.[16] That there was a fixation on and rigid adherence to DOTS from 1994 to roughly 2004 is undeniable.

It's also clear it did nothing to address either the HIV/TB epidemic or the problem of multidrug-resistant TB.

DOTS was introduced around the world with little or no initial research to support its efficacy—unlike for IPT, no trials were run, for example. The early studies that demonstrated the efficacy of directly observed therapy, and influenced its adoption, were retrospective and did not control for the effects of other components of a TB program.[17] And despite it being potentially cost effective it still actually *cost* a lot of money—New York City's effort to use directly observed therapy to combat the HIV-fueled upsurge in TB in the early 1990s cost in excess of a billion dollars.[18] When DOTS was first implemented it took little or no account of HIV, and it did nothing for those with multidrug-resistant TB. For example, in South Africa DOTS did initially strengthen the country's TB program, but any potential gains made by curing people were overshadowed by the massive increase in cases brought on by an uncontrolled HIV epidemic.[19] DOTS is, according to one study, "failing to control TB" in the HIV-positive population.[20] Even in well-run programs in South Africa's mining industry, where DOTS is adhered to, TB case rates have increased fourfold since 1990 because of the extraordinary increase in HIV—from 1 percent of the workforce to 30 percent in the 1990s.[21]

DOTS can work; DOTS has worked. It has helped to contribute to a reduction in the global TB prevalence in some places, but not in Africa, where HIV/TB wreaks the most havoc.[22] On a massive scale in China, over ten years, the World Bank–sponsored Endemic Disease Control project rolled out the world's largest program. It worked—and seems to have continued doing do, as the twenty-year review of China's commitment to DOTS has shown.[23] The country achieved cure rates of more than 85 percent. But that's not the whole picture. Case detection barely climbed above 50 percent—DOTS has been most effective in reducing TB in known cases, not in finding new ones. Further, in some areas of China actual direct observation of treatment reaches no more than 5 percent of those on treatment, and many have considered the policy unnecessary and ineffective; patient interviews indicated that actual completion rates were lower than reported; and up to 22 percent of patients had run out of drugs in the previous week or simply not taken their antibiotics. The official policy—all patients must be directly observed—was only occasionally carried out.[24] China has the world's largest number of TB cases, estimated at 11 percent of the global total. The experience in China encouraged the WHO to launch DOTS worldwide. But was it a good example for the world? Key to China's seeming success were two things: robust political and financial support at the local and national levels and a well-organized TB program in which information, supplies, and other resources flowed freely between all levels.[25] In other words, the conditions under which DOTS was rolled out were ideal for its success.

Directly observed therapy has worked in other places, too. With funding from the WHO and the South African Medical Research Council, David Wilkinson and his colleagues have shown, over a number of years and under trying circumstances, that DOTS can work in rural KwaZulu-Natal, South Africa. Wilkinson's program relied on community health workers and voluntary laypeople to deliver drugs and watch patients take them. By harnessing the resources locally available—willing and able community members, including traditional healers, long the bane of modern biomedicine, and shopkeepers—Wilkinson has been able to demonstrate that community-based care is sustainable and cost effective.[26] He also knows DOTS is not new.[27] But even in rural KwaZulu-Natal it does not help with patients who simply vanish—a significant problem in a place where people are constantly on the move in search of work.[28]

While DOTS can and has worked, it is not necessary in all circumstances for effective TB treatment, nor is it especially effective at reducing a large burden of TB when only a small number of practitioners adopt it. For example, several small-scale homegrown programs in Nepal and India, which also rely on community health workers, but which don't use directly observed therapy and are not part of a national program but are run by nongovernmental organizations, have been successful. By contrast, on a much larger scale, all Indian Ministry of Health TB facilities are, the WHO said in 2009, supporting DOTS. The vast majority of people being treated for TB in India, however, are not seen in government clinics. They are under the care of one of the country's eight million private-sector prescribers. These doctors are easier to access and do not adhere to DOTS, because either they don't know about it, the proper drug regimen is hard to come by, or they're uninterested in enforcing what many consider the system's inflexibility. Whatever the precise reason—and again this is not an indictment of theoretical possibilities of DOTS or meant to call into question its successes—DOTS is not reaching most Indian patients.[29] In Rio de Janeiro, one study found, standard treatment, and not directly observed therapy, was both cheaper and more cost effective.[30] In Pakistan DOTS was counterproductive: forcing people to report to a clinic for observation resulted in some abandoning treatment, as it was costly and inconvenient to get to clinics. DOTS might have been more cost effective for a program, but at least in Pakistan it was clearly not cost effective for patients.[31]

When looked at on a global scale it's become clear that DOTS is *not necessarily* any better than standard short-course chemotherapy.[32] It's also not clear how effective it is in the long term, as very little work has been done studying the problem.[33] Finally, while encouraging results have come out of some small-scale programs, like one in Nigeria that achieved 100 percent compliance, scaling it up would, those running the study admit, cost a tremendous amount of money[34]—so much in fact that its cost effectiveness might wane.

The secret ingredient in successful TB programs is not directly observed therapy.

Several things have been unfortunate about DOTS. To begin with, it was promoted, and then rolled out, as a novel and extremely effective form of TB control when it was actually neither. It was not novel and it was not known to be effective in all places at all times. It's become clear as more and more programs have been studied that DOTS in the real world faces real-world problems. Further, because DOTS during its heyday had been promoted as a one-size-fits-all approach, little or no thought went into how it might be received in the myriad local situations into which it would be introduced. There seems simply to have been an abundance of faith that its commonsense appeal would prevail. It's not at all surprising, then, to read that there has been an astonishing array of responses to DOTS; that, it turns out, not all programs are well run; that in some places where DOTS is nominally in place it's not so in practice; that drug supplies are not always reliable or patients always well treated. All of which adds up to the not very remarkable conclusion that DOTS is not universally applicable and that there must be flexibility dependent on local circumstances.[35]

Perhaps most important of all is that it took many in the global health bureaucracy a long time to learn that DOTS is not the universal panacea it was thought, or hoped, to be. And in the meantime, the dogma of DOTS prevented, in some cases, attention to other pressing problems. Of course, as we have seen and will explore more below, this was the case with HIV/TB. But it was also true when it came to MDR-TB—something, according to one official at the Centers for Disease Control and Prevention, the DOTS policy "obstinately neglected" until 2006.[36] In Peru, for example, the strict adherence to DOTS because of faith in the gospel of cost effectiveness completely ignored and in some ways made worse the problem of MDR-TB. Because DOTS was considered by so many to be cost effective, and, dare I say, a magic bullet, veering away from it to treat the admittedly more expensive MDR cases was a very tough sell. Many believed, with no more than faith in DOTS, that simply sticking with the program would take care of MDR-TB.[37] Because treating multidrug-resistant TB was *more* expensive than treating drug-susceptible disease, it was considered *too* expensive.[38] Ostensibly objective, rational cost-effective analysis had been reduced to its essence: a hierarchy based on what was cheapest, not what was most effective.

But faith is powerful. It can blind one to alternative ways of seeing the world. As with BCG before it, that's what happened with DOTS. Did the possibility of preventing TB stand a chance?

For a few years the WHO moved at a furious pace to learn whether or not IPT would stem the tide of TB in those with HIV. But the commitment to IPT proved short-lived. During the height of research, political and administrative support for IPT was, publicly, lukewarm at best. While IPT studies were well under way, and the WHO was seemingly committed to chemoprophylaxis, the TB program, the Global Program on AIDS, and the International Union Against Tuberculosis and Lung Disease crafted and published a joint statement on IPT in 1993. It read like an endorsement, if only a weak one, but was really a death sentence. It's also a remarkable example of linguistic acrobatics. They wanted to have it both ways: for and against IPT. The first point in the summary of recommendations is the following: "There is sufficient information to support the recommendation of isoniazid preventive therapy for tuberculosis infections." Hovering above that sentence was a footnote that read: "However, isoniazid preventive therapy is not recommended for implementation as one of the components of the tuberculosis control strategy in programme settings worldwide."[39] A better example of waffling would be hard to find. Two recommendations about the same therapy that advocate different things. Yet the authors did add more teeth to the statement when they wrote the following: "Programme implementation of preventive therapy would only be considered in areas where tuberculosis programmes are achieving the global targets established by WHO (i.e., successfully treating 85% of detected smear positive cases and detecting 70% of existing new smear positive cases) and where voluntary testing and counselling for HIV infection is available. This will also require close collaboration between National AIDS and Tuberculosis Control Programmes."[40] Which is to say: nowhere in Africa. Thus began the beginning of the end.

In the context of cost effectiveness, IPT never really had a chance. When Murray, Styblo, and Rouillon's research appeared alongside the World Bank's *Investing in Health* and demonstrated that *treatment* was the answer, it was the beginning of the end for *prevention*. Even though the TB leadership at WHO predicted, as recently as 1992, that preventive therapy would be more cost effective than treatment, there appeared to be no turning back.[41] Chemoprophylaxis might have a place in TB control, among high-risk groups like those with HIV—still apparently just a risk group and not a massive portion of the population—but as a research group including Murray and Styblo wrote in 1994, "Case finding and chemotherapy for smear-positive pulmonary tuberculosis is the mainstay of control strategies."[42] Styblo, never a fan, had come out against IPT several years earlier: despite claiming that "there is no doubt that adequate chemoprophylaxis could significantly decrease the occurrence of tuberculosis caused by HIV infection," Styblo cited IPT's cost, logistical difficulties, and worries over patient compliance as reasons for not even trying it.[43]

Cost effectiveness was a crucial consideration. Knowing which was cheaper—treating people with active TB or paying to prevent it—was of course important, especially so when it appeared that the world would only be willing to bear the burden of the cheapest intervention. Once cost effectiveness became the benchmark by which all control efforts had to be evaluated—and again I am not naively suggesting cost is not important; of course it is—it appears to have become the case that only *the one* most cost-effective control measure would be pursued. There did not seem to be room for both DOTS and IPT. DOTS was considered to be more cost effective, so DOTS it was.[44] Considering, as a group of researchers in Zambia put it, that "neither tuberculosis programmes nor AIDS control programmes can afford the interventions that are needed in this unequal world," deciding which cost less was vitally important. For their part, the Zambian researchers thought that chemoprophylaxis would be the cheaper intervention—the expense of treating and caring for people with active TB would be, on balance, more costly than screening for eligible IPT candidates. Finding "innovative ways" to start people on chemoprophylaxis was important, as IPT was "one of the few positive things that can be done for the millions of people already infected with HIV that may have an impact not only on the quality and quantity of the life of an individual patient but also on the spread of tuberculosis within the community."[45]

When IPT was abandoned and DOTS was embraced those millions of people were cast aside.

Of course, it was not as if the WHO or the World Bank, or anyone else, said to the world: it's either DOTS or IPT; you can't have both. But that's what happened. DOTS was found to be cost effective, though its efficacy was not well understood, and so it gained supremacy. IPT, though without being thoroughly studied, was found not to be cost effective. But what this precisely meant was unclear. To many, IPT appeared to be more costly than DOTS—but then according to the World Bank's influential *Investing in Health* so did every other intervention for every other disease. So, in relation to what was IPT not cost effective—the cheapest intervention on the planet? The most expensive? Of course, putting things in terms of cost effectiveness is a form of ranking. But it's crude. And by that I do not mean crude as in imprecise or unrefined, awaiting a fine-tuning; I mean crude as in primitive and blunt.

While related, DOTS and IPT are not simply two alternatives to the same problem. They should never have been examined side by side as if they were. Yet, at a 1995 WHO meeting on the HIV/TB epidemic—the same one noted above, where it was said that the research agenda was "stuck"— Murray effectively did just that. He reported that modeling had suggested that IPT "is a very cost effective intervention in HIV-infected individuals." He then went on to say in the same sentence that "short-course chemotherapy is about four times more cost effective."[46] It is certainly possible that those at the meeting could and did tease this all apart. Still, it's hard to see how most would have heard Murray saying two separate things: first, that IPT is a cost-effective intervention for its intended benefit—preventing TB in those who are HIV-positive; and second, that short-course chemotherapy is a cost-effective intervention for its intended target—treating those with active TB. Rather, it's more likely that most left the meeting thinking nothing more than that treatment was the most cost-effective TB intervention; that IPT was four times as expensive; and that therefore to control TB, treatment was the way to go. Yet what those advocating IPT would likely have pointed out was that by not preventing TB in HIV-positive individuals the number of TB cases increased and thus the costs of treatment increased—to say nothing of the lives lost. Indeed, that's just the argument made by Murray's Harvard colleague Jody Heymann two years before. In a rousing essay in favor of IPT Heymann made the case that it is the more cost-effective intervention, especially when one factored in, as she did, the crushing number of new TB cases brought on by HIV. Preventing new cases would save far more money than would letting TB become active only to be treated. Preventing TB would not only benefit those individuals receiving prophylaxis, it would also, of course, mean that they would not infect others. Heymann did not suggest, not at all, abandoning treatment; what she argued was that accepting the value of treatment should not forestall the use of IPT. Further, prevention, over time, would reduce the costs of treatment not because treatment itself would be cheaper but because there would eventually be far fewer people who needed it.[47]

The argument fell on deaf ears.

Rejecting IPT was based explicitly on the perception of its place in the cost-effectiveness rankings. But it was also shunted aside because of its theoretical potential to siphon resources away from more cost-effective treatment programs. When the WHO and UNAIDS revisited the question of IPT in 1998 they made all this quite clear. IPT had much going for it: "There can no longer be any doubt that treatment with isoniazid of PPD-positive individuals living in a setting with a high prevalence of TB will reduce the risk of developing active TB in the short term to around 40% of what it would have been without treatment." Even without a skin test IPT was still looking good: on the basis of studies, "it is therefore possible to state that treatment with isoniazid in HIV-positive individuals, in whom a PPD skin test cannot be performed, living in a setting with a high prevalence of TB will reduce the risk of developing active TB in the short term to around 60% of what it would have been without such treatment." The report even allowed that "IPT may provide a cost-effective intervention for those known to be HIV-positive."[48]

Yet IPT was still found wanting. For example, IPT might have been cost effective for HIV-positive individuals, but the problem was that the vast majority of people did not know their status. And testing people for HIV simply to learn their eligibility for IPT—why it was assumed this was the primary reason for testing is unstated—was itself, the unexamined claim went, not cost effective. Because of this IPT should be reserved for those who know their status or in places where there is "sufficient" demand for testing. The policy statement concluded quite sensibly that IPT should be "promoted as an intervention for those living with HIV." Yet in the same sentence the statement went on to say that it should not be promoted "as a primary strategy to control the public health burden of tuberculosis."[49] Of course the policy statement does not say so, and there is room to see things otherwise, but as with Murray's statement above this has the effect of suggesting that IPT and treatment are addressing the same problem. In addition, by claiming that IPT would not reduce the public health burden of TB but would help those who are HIV-positive, the statement intimates that HIV-related TB is not part of the public health burden of TB. At a minimum, it suggests that reducing TB in the HIV-positive population will not help the more burdensome problem of the general TB epidemic.

Further, the WHO and UNAIDS worried that IPT would "drain" resources from "already overstretched TB services." To ensure that this did not happen the priority for TB programs had to remain the "detection and treatment of active cases, as formulated in the DOTS strategy." What might happen were IPT to appear? It might lead to "less effective detection and treatment of active cases," which would result in ongoing transmission and thus negate the effects of IPT.[50]

Rejecting IPT was based on an abundance of mights.

Lest it seem that I am offering the merely plausible interpretation of the position of the WHO and UNAIDS—which in effect was a consensus statement from the global health leadership—to be that IPT and DOTS were in direct competition with one another in the battle to control TB, let me make clear that I am reporting the explicit position of the WHO and UNAIDS: DOTS and IPT were considered potential solutions to the same problem. "The evidence shows that PT is not an alternative to the DOTS strategy for controlling TB, even in areas with a high prevalence of HIV." A clearer statement cannot be found—though it was followed by this jarring lament: "However, many opportunities for providing PT to people living with HIV have been missed and this has led to many cases of TB that could have been prevented."[51] Without an endorsement or funding from any of the players—the WHO, the World Bank, IUATLD, UNAIDS—was it any wonder that "many opportunities" to use IPT and thus prevent TB had been squandered? It's a surprising statement because of who delivered it: the very entity that was in fact ensuring that many more opportunities would be lost.

DOTS killed IPT. Once DOTS emerged it rather easily toppled IPT from its precarious position. As a program, DOTS was invincible. The early success of DOTS in places like China alongside the inconclusive IPT feasibility studies—studies that were not allowed to play out—from the mid-1990s; the WHO, UNAIDS, and the International Union Against Tuberculosis and Lung Disease recommending against it in all but the most ideal circumstances; the claims about its expense; and, most important, putting the two in competition with one another in the battle over resources— all these added up to the death of IPT at the hands of DOTS. That IPT and DOTS are related, though crucially different, interventions seems not to have mattered. It was either/or: treat or prevent. Richard Chaisson, an early and persistent champion of IPT, recalls being publicly attacked as "immoral" at the annual meeting of the International Union in 1993. His crime: he advocated IPT. Doing so at the time was seen by many as the same thing as advocating against treatment.[52] Jim Yong Kim and his colleagues at Partners in Health had the same charge leveled against them: it was morally suspect to advocate treating MDR-TB, seen as a hopeless cause in poor countries, because it would take valuable resources away from patients suffering from drug-susceptible TB—TB treated by strict adherence to DOTS.[53] A choice had to be made, and the world chose DOTS.

The point here is *not* to make the case that IPT is better than DOTS. Aside from my not having the expertise to say such a thing, it would, by the pitting the two against each other, also contradict a claim made above. My aim is to offer a historical argument. What I am suggesting happened was that at a chaotic time in the world of TB control, when the WHO perceived the planet to be in the throes of global emergency, something had to be done, and done quickly. Pressured to choose only one intervention, one based on its cost effectiveness, the WHO chose DOTS. IPT was subjected to intense scrutiny—as it should have been. DOTS, on the other hand, was rolled out far and wide very quickly without nearly the same level of examination and was presumed to be *the* solution for all places at all times. IPT's critics needed only to point out its *potential* flaws for it to fail; DOTS's critics were shouting into the wind. Murray, Styblo, and Rouillon's World Bank–sponsored work, which picked up on that done by Styblo in Tanzania, work sponsored by the International Union (of which Rouillon was president) became like gospel. All true believers followed it. Unlike DOTS, IPT was not tied to a particular faith. But, as with BCG in an earlier time, faith won out. By the mid-1990s, in the midst of several ongoing IPT trials and surrounded by mounting evidence that it worked, DOTS was triumphant.[54]

But then consider the following. In 2012 a group of prominent TB experts reviewed global strategies to control the disease in the preceding decade and a half. They discussed the ups and downs, reported on case rates, mortality, and so forth. Among the litany, they lamented that IPT was "an inconsistently implemented global policy." Others complained that only between 2 percent and 2.5 percent of eligible cases received it.[55] Considering all that came before—the low priority assigned to IPT, the skepticism surrounding its feasibility, the dominance of DOTS—this is not terribly surprising. With few crusading on its behalf it was of course used sporadically. What's surprising is the lament itself. Something had changed. As we've seen, IPT had been championed in the early 1960s and the early 1990s. Was it now, again, a priority? By the end of the 1990s IPT was, if not dead, on life support. Then, in a remarkable reversal, IPT came back. Money and AIDS were responsible.

One of the first to breathe new life into IPT was Christopher Murray. In 1998, he and Joshua Salomon published an important paper in *Proceedings of the National Academy of Sciences*. It began with a question. Was it time to think beyond DOTS? The work in Malawi, Mozambique, Tanzania, and China which showed that 80–90 percent of cases could be cured under DOTS was not being borne out worldwide—only 11 percent of cases, the WHO reported, were being cared for in DOTS programs. And so Murray and Salomon considered that "given the pace of uptake of DOTS, the heavy emphasis of WHO on smear-positive pulmonary cases only, and the magnitude of the remaining problem, it is worth examining whether considerable gains against tuberculosis can be achieved through promotion of DOTS alone."[56] They modeled several different scenarios that, given a variety of variables, might play out between 1998 and 2030. If only DOTS were used, they projected that there would be 171 million new cases and sixty million deaths from TB—this was the best-case scenario. At worst there would 249 million new cases and ninety million deaths. Murray and Salomon concluded that DOTS, effective as it could be, simply was not enough. Too few cases were being found, for one. They did not at all advocate abandoning DOTS; they recommended supplementing it with other effective interventions. Like IPT.

Regarding IPT, Murray and Salomon made two unconventional points: first, unlike UNAIDS and WHO, they argued that identifying HIV-positive people through voluntary testing and starting them on IPT would forestall, between 1998 and 2030, nearly forty-three million new cases and prevent just under seventeen million deaths. And this would be achieved by screening only 10 percent of the HIV-positive population each year. Recall that UNAIDS and the WHO in their policy statement did not think voluntary testing would capture enough people to make IPT worth it. Murray and Salomon argued that it would. Even more unconventional was their suggestion that high rates of compliance with IPT were not absolutely necessary. As they wrote, "Even with modest completion rates, a mass preventive therapy campaign could alter significantly the course of the tuberculosis epidemic."[57] If followed, this would make feasibility an entirely different matter. Coming from Murray and Salomon, who by the late 1990s were veterans in the war on TB, this kind of unconventional thinking could not be ignored. But they were not naive. They knew this would cost a lot, take tremendous energy, and require the commitment of the global community.

Murray and Salomon were by then among a growing number who, by the end of the 1990s, supported IPT. In fact, enough work had been done that two meta-analyses—papers that examine the conclusions of a group of studies—came out in the *British Medical Journal* and *AIDS* within a year of one another. These two prominently placed reviews reported that IPT was effective.[58]

But efficacy was one thing; cost was another. For years, as we've seen, IPT was assumed to not be cost effective. This turned out to be just that: an assumption. Little to no work had actually been done on the question. That, too, began to change. Added to Murray and Salomon's argument that DOTS was not enough, especially when it came to the HIV/TB coepidemic—something, recall, that DOTS did nothing about—was emerging research on IPT's cost effectiveness. While the 1995 feasibility study from Uganda did not bolster IPT's case, work coming out of South Africa and Zambia, and unpublished data from Thailand, began to show that IPT might be cost effective.[59] Then, a year after Murray and Salomon's salvo, came another influential paper. The title of Jensa Bell, David Rose, and Henry Sacks's paper was itself a declaration: "Tuberculosis Preventive Therapy for HIV-Infected People in Sub-Saharan Africa Is Cost-Effective." The authors began from the premise that IPT worked, as it had been known to since Shirley Ferebee's 1970 paper, but aimed to show that it also made economic sense. In addition to simply comparing the costs of treatment with those of IPT, the study discussed the expenses associated with secondary cases—those cases of TB that would emerge if IPT were not implemented—and social costs—the expenses and lost wages patients would incur were they to develop active TB. When all these were considered together the paper came to a firm conclusion—a conclusion that did not force a face-off between DOTS and IPT but added it to the armamentarium: "The addition of TB preventive therapy to the case-finding and treatment strategy currently in use in sub-Saharan Africa will result in saving money."[60]

Just as in the late 1980s and early 1990s when HIV brought TB new attention, it did so again in the early twenty-first century. The initial burst of interest had its origins in fear; the second in an equal measure of hope and despair. When the two were first linked, most commentators paying any attention feared a catastrophe; they were of course correct. And this fear sparked a brief but intense interest in dealing with HIV/TB—money flowed from the WHO into national programs to tackle the two, and research on IPT was a priority. Then came the dominance of DOTS. Attention to HIV/TB faded for nearly a decade.[61] The opposite was the case for HIV/AIDS. From the moment it was discovered AIDS was the focus of intense scientific attention and, crucially, activist agitation. Both scientists and activists—sometimes they were one and the same—relentlessly pursued a cure, a vaccine, a treatment. As a result, a series of regular scientific breakthroughs were made, and the disease went from being a death sentence to becoming a chronic, treatable affliction. This is not to say that its devastating effects disappeared; obviously they have not. And access to life-saving drugs has been unequal, sometimes staggeringly so. Still, by the early twenty-first century the face of AIDS had changed: no longer was antiretroviral therapy (ART) thought to be too costly and too complicated for those most in need; drug costs have plummeted; more are now in treatment than ever before; and funding has remained far more abundant than it has for TB.[62] There was some hope that the menace could be contained, but there was despair too—despair because many believed HIV's most reliable companion was slowing progress down. Something had to be done about TB—compared to AIDS, a disease attracting only a fraction of the world's attention.

This began to change on the eve of the global rollout of ART when activist organizations like the Treatment Action Group—a prime mover in the global effort to reduce the cost of ART, which made the rollout possible to begin with—saw that TB had no champion and took up the cause.[63] The scale-up of ART came at a time of increasing interest in HIV/AIDS. The WHO's "3x5 Initiative"—an effort to get three million people onto ART by the end of 2005; the Global Fund for AIDS, Tuberculosis, and Malaria, formed in 2001; and the U.S.-based President's Emergency Plan for AIDS Relief (PEPFAR), announced in 2003, all worked to facilitate the rollout of ART around the world. These efforts theoretically assured access to many previously doing, and thus dying, without ART. Those with HIV could now live longer lives—but not if they had TB. All of this also meant that preventing TB might now make more sense.

This is of course a grim admission. If what it took to implement IPT was the fact that HIV-positive people were now living longer, and had greater access to ART, then it suggests that when this was not the case improving their lives and stopping the spread of TB was not enough.[64] When discussing the early days of IPT Richard Chaisson said that this was indeed the case: on top of the arguments about cost was a sense of futility. Some wondered: why bother; these people are going to die anyway.[65] The wider availability of ART by around 2005 provided some incentive to refocus attention on HIV/TB.

Momentum was gaining. With the realization that without an adequate means of controlling TB much of the effort put into ART in sub-Saharan Africa would be lost, the WHO set about figuring out what could be done. In 2003 a group of HIV and TB experts met in Geneva, among them Mark Harrington of the Treatment Action Group, by then very active in promoting the cause of TB. Coming out of that meeting was the WHO's "Interim Policy on Collaborative TB/HIV Activities." The policy, announced in 2004, had three legs: establish the mechanisms for collaboration; decrease the burden of tuberculosis in people living with HIV/AIDS; and decrease the burden of HIV in tuberculosis patients. Decreasing TB among those living with HIV/AIDS would be accomplished by intensifying case finding and bolstering infection control in hospitals, clinics, and other hotbeds of infection. Perhaps surprisingly, given its history, isoniazid preventive therapy too was considered essential.[66]

HIV/TB was now, rather suddenly considering all that had come before, front and center on the global health agenda. If there was any doubt, it was dispelled in the summer of 2004 when Nelson Mandela took the stage at the Fifteenth Annual International AIDS Conference in Thailand and announced a grant of nearly $45 million from the Bill and Melinda Gates Foundation to support work on HIV/TB in Africa. Mandela stated, "The world has made defeating AIDS a priority, but tuberculosis remains ignored. Today we are calling on the world to recognize that we can't fight AIDS unless we do much more to fight TB as well."[67] This was a call, of course, that others had been making for years.

By the end of the decade, isoniazid preventive therapy—now considered cost effective and essential for those living with HIV and at risk for TB—alongside intensified case finding and infection control, had become an integral part of the WHO's so-called Three *I*s initiative for fighting HIV/TB. The Three *I*s initiative, announced in 2008, emerged because "it has become increasingly clear that HIV and tuberculosis co-infection (TB/HIV) is a major public health threat to people living with HIV that directly jeopardizes the success of ART scale-up."[68] Of course, by the time this was written it had been abundantly clear for more than two decades that HIV/TB coinfection was "a major public health threat." This kind of rediscovery was all too common. If any in the world of TB control missed the new interest in IPT the top leadership in WHO's STOP TB department and UNAIDS published an editorial in the *International Journal of Tuberculosis and Lung Disease* urging action. With no irony and seemingly no historical consciousness the editorial lamented the fact that IPT had been, because of skepticism, "relegated to the back burner." But those days were over.[69] And with evidence mounting that, when used in combination, IPT and even more powerful highly active antiretroviral treatment (HAART) significantly reduced mortality from TB, the case for preventive therapy simply got stronger.[70]

IPT was back. Remarkably resilient, IPT had now lived at least three lives: born in the 1950s, it was a WHO priority by the early 1960s but then fatally labeled "irrational" in the early 1980s; revived in the late 1980s because of HIV only to be dispatched back to the grave in the mid-1990s; and then again resurrected in the early twenty-first century. Its appeal seems hard to resist.

But it's not perfect. Far from it. Despite IPT now being official policy, its rollout has been slow; most patients eligible for preventive therapy are not getting it.[71] In South Africa and elsewhere, doctors have been resistant to prescribing IPT—they're unclear on the guidelines, not sure of its benefits, and find it difficult to always accurately rule out active TB.[72] And research questions remain. Two of the most important are under active investigation: Can it work on a large scale in community with a massive HIV/TB burden where the risk of infection or reactivation are high? And what's the most effective duration of treatment? The first question was the focus of the large and ambitious Thibela study of IPT among miners in South Africa. Beginning in 2006 the Aurum Institute of South Africa embarked on the largest community-wide IPT trial to date, the aim of which was "to have a large and rapid impact on TB incidence and prevalence." Confronted with an intractable TB epidemic among miners in South Africa—among whom rates of TB are between three thousand and seven thousand per one hundred thousand—Aurum decided that a novel approach to IPT was necessary. Reasoning that the whole community was at risk of developing TB, Aurum decided to treat the entire population, in a cluster-randomized fashion, rather than a targeted subset. While novel in the era of HIV/AIDS, community-wide IPT, as previously noted, has been done before. The Aurum trial was explicitly modeled after the Alaskan work.[73]

But was the Alaskan trial an appropriate model for the Thibela study? Were the conditions in the two places similar enough to warrant even the possibility, much less the expectation, that Thibela could replicate George Comstock's success in Alaska? There were several significant differences between Alaska and the Thibela study areas; foremost among them was that in Alaska, by the time the study began, there was already a declining rate of new infections. This is a set of circumstances very different from those that were present in the Thibela study area, where the infection rate was staggeringly high and showed no signs of decline. Of course, there was also no HIV/AIDS in Alaska. The Thibela study failed to show a community-wide impact; immediately after patients ended their nine-month course of IPT its protective effect was lost. One possible reason for this is that the risk of infection with active TB is so high both in the tight confines of the mines and the miners' living quarters, combined with high rates of HIV and silicosis, that one might simply be unable to ward off infection without perpetual protection.[74] It's possible, in other words, that under such high-risk conditions continuous IPT might be best.

In fact, the duration of efficacy has been a long-standing question. It's become all the more so since 2011, when the WHO endorsed a six-month regimen—and after the results of the Thibela study one imagines the question will gain even more attention. Following the WHO's six-month guidelines, South Africa immediately embarked on a national IPT program and overnight doubled the number of people on the planet receiving IPT.[75] The scale-up of IPT in South Africa was impressive and very rapid. In addition to only being a six-month regimen, it started without first doing a tuberculin skin test.[76] Without one having to first do a skin test—screening for active TB is done by other means—the logistical barriers to IPT have been greatly reduced. But as Stephen Lawn and Robin Wood point out, "While eliminating the need for TST assessment simplifies IPT implementation, the downside is that the intervention no longer targets the minority of patients who stand to gain benefit. Thus, large numbers of patients are treated needlessly, undermining cost-effectiveness."[77] Lawn and Wood's caution against indiscriminate IPT is virtually the same as that offered by the authors of the Greenland study nearly fifty years ago—too many people needlessly treated, resulting in a waste of limited resources.[78]

It is in this context that ongoing research in Botswana, and elsewhere, is so important. Botswana, like South Africa, follows WHO guidelines and provides six months of IPT without first doing a skin test. To test the efficacy of such a regimen, in Botswana a group began a six-month course of IPT; after six months one arm received a placebo for thirty additional months, while the other arm continued on IPT for thirty more months. The protective benefit of IPT in the six-month arm was lost two hundred days after the six-month course ended; the arm continuing IPT showed considerably better results.[79] This work, along with the results from the Thibela study, seems to be making it clear that for IPT to be effective patients must remain in treatment much longer than initially thought—perhaps for at least three years but possibly a lifetime, depending on their risk of infection. Length of treatment, the risk of reinfection, the possibility that isoniazid might not actually be the best preventive agent, the epidemiology of HIV/TB in a given area, concerns that using isoniazid as a preventive agent might promote drug resistance—all of these factors must be understood.[80] It remains to be seen just how effective IPT will be in places like South Africa and Botswana. So far, there and everywhere else, it's progressing slowly. There are of course no long-term data yet available.[81]

While most of the focus here has been on isoniazid prophylaxis therapy, multidrug-resistant TB suffered a similar, though not identical, fate. Like

HIV/TB, drug-resistant TB has been rediscovered. As we saw earlier when looking at Kenya, it has been around for decades; multidrug-resistant TB was simply the natural extension of an old problem that was then willfully ignored. What also connects IPT specifically and HIV/TB generally with MDR-TB is that they were neglected in favor of treating drug-susceptible TB at a time when it appeared that a stark choice had to be made. The cost effectiveness of DOTS lured people into thinking the only thing that could be done was the supposedly most cost-effective intervention. But it's clear cost effectiveness is a moving target: when drug companies lowered the prices of second-line TB drugs, for example, it was suddenly cost effective to treat MDR-TB. Decades ago now when cost effectiveness was first applied to tuberculosis it appeared to offer a rational, objective measure for how best to combat the disease. But by applying cost-effective analysis, those in global health leadership operated as if the elements that went into the analysis were neutral and stable facts, not human inventions. The examples of MDR-TB and IPT make clear this is not the case. Cost effectiveness also forced people to think that what had been deemed cost effective was the best and only intervention. That is, DOTS might be cost effective, but did this mean it was the best and only intervention for the myriad ways in which TB operates in the real world? Of course not.

As with IPT, multidrug-resistant TB was ignored, and now it's not. But Paul Farmer and Salmann Keshavjee, two leaders in the effort to expand treatment for MDR-TB, have called the scale-up of treatment for MDR-TB "abysmal."[82] It's true that a tectonic shift in thinking about MDR-TB took place in the late 1990s: many in global health began to appreciate that it could be treated in poor settings. Arguments about it not being cost effective to treat MDR-TB—arguments based on limited data, as well as dramatically overinflated drug costs—began to crumble under the weight of evidence.[83] Thanks to the pioneering work by Partners in Health in Peru of actually treating and curing multidrug-resistant TB, the notion that it was a hopeless cause was challenged. Médicins Sans Frontières, Partners in Health, and others worked to bring drug costs down; they plummeted by up to 95 percent. Suddenly, treating MDR-TB was cost effective.[84] But while a major change in thinking has taken place, and MDR-TB, like IPT, is no longer a victim to spurious arguments against it based on the claim that it's not cost effective, a commensurate commitment to action has not taken place. When compared to HIV, which thanks to efforts like PEPFAR has seen extraordinary increases in treatment, MDR-TB seems still to have been virtually ignored—perhaps an emergency plan for TB, just as for HIV/AIDS, is what's needed.[85] Salmaan Keshavjee, the former chair of the WHO's Green Light Committee for lowering drug costs and increasing access, recently called his own program "phenomenally unsuccessful."[86]

The combined neglect of both the HIV/TB pandemic and multidrug-resistant TB has been one of the greatest public health tragedies of the last generation. The neglect of HIV/TB is made all the more tragic because by the mid-1980s many saw it coming; toward the end of that first decade of the pandemic the WHO actually tried to do something about it. Those efforts were then abandoned. Drug-resistant TB has been a problem even longer and consequently been neglected for a much greater time. It's taken an awfully long time, but it does now seem to be the case that neither MDR-TB nor HIV/TB can be ignored. What that means remains to be seen.

Conclusion

As we historians get closer and closer to the present we get nervous because we inch closer and closer to no longer being historians. As one approaches the present it becomes harder and harder to come to an end. Narrative structure in historical writing demands a conclusion, an endpoint to which all that came before has been moving. We are not accustomed to simply finding a place to sign off, content that the story will go on. Our stories end.

Not so here. For the recent past suggests that any neat ending that I might want to impose on this story will not last. The story of TB control in the era of HIV moves at such a pace that it's hard to keep up—once an endpoint might appear to have been reached, things change. It's also maddening. The urgency, for example, with which IPT is called for now sounds so familiar. So, too, with drug-resistant TB; it seems almost nothing is new. As I have gotten closer and closer to the present, this book has at times veered away from history and become a reflection on the current moment. That is so because we live in the time in which this book takes place and in the world created by the events recounted here. Everything in the preceding pages is a way to explain how we've arrived at this moment. That makes writing a conventional conclusion a challenge. The story is not over. The book is at times as much about the present as about the past. There are times, too, when I think we might have reached a point where, if it can be said to ever do so, history is repeating itself. Writing the story of HIV/TB first made me think this way. The confluence of HIV and TB was discovered once and then discovered again. Then, as I wrote more and more I began to think I could say the same for drug-resistant TB: much of the way drug-resistant TB is written about today—its causes, consequences, challenges—sounds a lot like what was written about Kenya in the 1960s. And it's not because people lack imagination; it's that the contours of the problem, its topography, were mapped decades ago. We've been exploring the same terrain ever since.

There is danger in not paying attention to history. In the case of HIV/TB the consequences have been inefficient, perhaps even tragic repetition as the problem has been discovered, forgotten, and then discovered again. Arguing in favor of racial explanations for susceptibility to TB, when it's based on historical pedigree, relies on a profound misreading of evidence from the past as well as ignores the fact that a previous generation of researchers abandoned the search for a racial explanation when it became clear that the poster children for such a phenomenon—American Indians, black South Africans, and so on—could not actually be said to be racially predisposed to TB. By critically examining the ways in which discursive categories have been constructed we might be able to move beyond them. Trotting out American Indians as the population that best exemplifies the salience of virgin soil should be stopped. Just as American Indians became a category stripped of all historical context in attempts to make a biomedical argument, so too did "Africans" become, in the early years of research on AIDS, a category: hypersexualized, nonmonogamous, spreaders of AIDS. Influenced by earlier discourses on African sexuality vis-à-vis syphilis in the colonial era, early AIDS researchers focused intensely on sexuality to the exclusion of other possible areas of research.[1] Drug-resistant tuberculosis is not a new problem. It's a very old one brought on by circumstances that have barely, if at all, changed. There is variation in the details, certainly, but the broad contours of the problem have been well known since the early 1960s when, in the case examined here, a rampant drug-resistant TB problem emerged in Kenya and elsewhere. The only thing that's really different is that the problem has gotten worse. Even after repeated failures, after success in one place could not be replicated in another, faith in the efficacy of the BCG vaccine won out over skepticism, resulting in the largest failed medical intervention in world history and quite possibly the forestalling of research into a more viable alternative. That kind of faith was present, too, in the rush to declare DOTS the solution to the world's TB problem. BCG *might* have forestalled research into other vaccines; DOTS *did* stymie other interventions. It ignored HIV and multidrug-resistant TB.

But what to make of this? What is the value in now knowing this history? In part to learn to be humble: people to whom problems they are just encountering seem new and fresh might do well to consider they might not be the first responders. It's also worth keeping in mind that history does not march progressively onward; we are not always getting better. The history of TB control is arguably an example of regression. Knowing all this is also important because it can be valuable to take a long-term perspective with the hope that by doing so it might be possible to discern patterns or to see where the possibility for change might have become stuck or to see things that might have worked and have since been abandoned or left to atrophy. But analyzing the past can take time—time many don't have. Almost fifty years ago, when assessing the WHO's TB work in Kenya, Kurt Toman—who would go on to write what's now become a classic in TB literature known by its vernacular name *Toman's Tuberculosis*—wished he had been able to spend more time looking at the history of TB control in the country. He suspected that a look at the origins of the program could help explain the present. He began his "private and strictly confidential" 1966 report with the following: "To get a full understanding of the present situation of Kenya-4 [the name of the WHO's project] it would have been probably best to study the project from its beginning seven and a half years ago. Many of the existing problems could have been traced back to the earlier stages of the project." Alas, time forced Toman to move on. "After the initial attempt the writer had to give up the idea to analyze and evaluate the past although it has a definite bearing on the certain present difficulties. But that would have been a too comprehensive and time-consuming affair."[2] One can only wonder what Toman might have determined about the past's influence on the present; he gave the matter not a shred more thought.

Seeing the past's particular impact on the present of course has value. But it might also be worth thinking about whether or not having a historical consciousness more generally could be an aid in forestalling rediscovery.[3] It would be more powerful to think historically about TB at all times— realizing that TB is a problem *of history*—rather than using history to bolster or undermine a given approach.[4] For example, when the Aurum Institute modeled its community chemoprophylaxis program in the South African mines on the work done by George Comstock in Alaska, it was not thinking historically about the problem of TB but using history to support its approach. Similarly, in contemporary debates over what's called "treatment as prevention" in the world of HIV/AIDS control both those who advocate the approach and those who don't deploy history to aid their arguments. History, in these cases, is used strategically. It's often simplified. What's necessary is more work like Randall Packard's on malaria—work that shows, over a long period of time and in many different places, what has and has not worked to control the disease, in an effort to demonstrate that short-term technological solutions are not the answer.[5] Thinking historically can mean a method of approaching the study of the past that argues for reaching beyond merely memorizing facts; it's often connected with teaching students how to work with historical materials the way a historian would—to take context and contingency into account, for instance.[6] This is, of course, a valuable pursuit; historians do it all the time. But I'm not really interested in having public health people or doctors and so forth act like historians and do historical research. They have enough to do. Nor am I suggesting that historians be tasked with telling the history of a given intervention or what have you—though that too can be important. What I mean when I say that TB is a problem of history and that those involved in TB control should think of it as such is that everything about the disease as we now know it has been determined by history. We are living within that history. While the notion of a useable past is appealing and might even, in this case, be applicable, history is not simply something from which to draw lessons; to be used as pedigree for a particular approach—"Well, it worked in the past"; or as a warning against repeating old blunders—"We've been down that road before." Almost everything discussed in this book is not in any sense over or even past.

The history of TB control in the twentieth century and into the twenty-first, as we've seen, is one of major breakthroughs and significant setbacks. The focus here has been on the setbacks, to be sure, but I hope not at the expense of completely tossing out the breakthroughs and thereby ignoring the extraordinary work people have done and are doing. As I have researched and written this book, aside from doing conventional historical research, I have talked to many people about TB control; read as much as I can from the current literature; and during two trips to South Africa spent time observing the challenges doctors and patients and others face attempting to control the disease in extremely trying circumstances. Gavin Churchyard at Aurum in Johannesburg and Tony Moll at the Church of Scotland Hospital in Tugela

Ferry—to name just two prominent people among many others working on TB and HIV in South Africa—taught me more about the hard work of controlling the pandemic than I would have otherwise been able to learn. I became powerfully aware of the difficulties and awed by those who spend their days, their lives, combating this insidious disease. Even so, much of this book might be seen as an affront to that work—and a particularly offensive one, as it comes from an outsider not embroiled in the day-to-day challenges of controlling the disease. It is of course not meant to be so.

Yet, does such an indictment as that offered in this book demand a culprit? Perhaps, but I don't think there is one. For this reason, I have tended to not focus on individuals, choosing instead to focus on structures and, in any given case, the series of decisions that have been made within the confines of those structures. Those structures might be: a way of thinking about race that determined action; the confines of cost effectiveness; the trap of compliance repeatedly snaring people into believing that controlling TB hinges on patient behavior; the well-meaning, though lumbering, behavior of a global bureaucracy; and the willful blindness to readily apparent failures. It's the rare individual who has had a discernible impact on any of these things— and generally if they did (save perhaps Lyle Cummins) I am more generally favorable toward them than not. My point is that I have been much more interested in exploring how TB control has not worked rather than in casting aspersions on—or creating heroes of—those operating within a set of structures not of their own making. Wallace Fox—whom I greatly admire for his technical and clinical acumen as much as for his ahead-of-his-time observations on the perils of being seduced by the allure of antibiotics—effected great change. But in the end, even his work could not transcend the world in which he operated. In 1986, when he retired, the Medical Research Council's TB unit was shut down; no longer would the British government, increasingly conservative, fund the unit's work. The closure of the TB unit coincided with the shift toward cost-effectiveness; it came, too, at a time of global complacency toward TB. And it happened at the dawn of the African HIV/ TB tragedy. All of which is to say that even Wallace Fox—by any measure an important, perhaps even singular, figure in the history of TB control— worked in a world that placed great restraints on what was possible.

So, finally, what does a historian have to offer? Observing that those working in TB control do so in a world that constrains the limits of the possible is not terribly satisfying. Tell that to someone working in a township clinic in Johannesburg, or anywhere else, really, and his or her likely response will be "Tell me something I don't know." What a historian can offer is the evidence needed to show, over a long period of time, just what those constraints have been, in order that it might be possible to transcend them rather than nurture them.

Notes

INTRODUCTION

1. C. J. Murray and J. A. Salomon, "Modeling the Impact of Global Tuberculosis Control Strategies," *Proceedings of the National Academy of Science* 95, no. 23 (1998): 13881–13886.

2. For the most recent summary of TB's development and its place in human consciousness see Helen Bynum, *Spitting Blood: The History of Tuberculosis* (New York: Oxford University Press, 2012).

3. For the six components of the strategy see http://www.who.int/tb/strategy/en/.

4. Agnes Binagwaho, Paul E. Farmer, Sabin Nsanzimana, Corine Karema, Michel Gasana, Jean de Dieu Ngirabega, Fidele Ngabo, et al., "Rwanda 20 Years On: Investing in Life," *Lancet* 383, no. 9940 (July 2014): 371–375.

5. Ross Upshur, Jerome Singh, and Nathan Ford, "Apocalypse or Redemption: Responding to Extensively Drug-Resistant Tuberculosis," *Bulletin of the World Health Organization* 87 (2009): 481–483, 483. Noting that improper treatment of TB creates drug resistance and that this is a human, not natural, creation has been done by many others. See, for example, Michael Iseman, "Tailoring a Time-Bomb: Inadvertent Genetic Engineering," *American Review of Respiratory Disease* 132, no. 4 (1985): 735–736.

6. On doing this kind of medical history see the thoughtful essay by Allan M. Brandt, "From Analysis to Advocacy: Crossing Boundaries as a Historian of Health Policy," in *Locating Medical History: The Stories and Their Meanings*, edited by Frank Huisman and John Harley Warner (Baltimore: Johns Hopkins University Press, 2004), 460–484. I am also sympathetic to Richard Horton's plea—Horton is the editor of the *Lancet*—for medical historians to reengage themselves with current problems in health, medicine, and disease. Richard Horton, "Offline: The Moribund Body of Medical History," *Lancet* 384, no. 9940 (26 July 2014): 292.

7. This phenomenon is not exclusive to TB. For the World Bank's and others' "discovery" of British colonial-era agricultural development schemes decades after their initial introduction see Joseph Morgan Hodge, *Triumph of the Expert: Agrarian Doctrines of Development and the Legacies of British Colonialism* (Athens: Ohio University Press, 2007), 270–271.

8. Helen Epstein, *The Invisible Cure: Africa, the West, and the Fight against AIDS* (New York: Farrar, Straus and Giroux, 2007), 209.

9. Poliomyelitis, Fact Sheet No. 114, World Health Organization, March 2014. http://www.who.int/mediacentre/factsheets/fs114/en/.

10. Quoted in E. Cochrane, "Tuberculosis in the Tropics, Part I," *Tropical Diseases Bulletin* 34, no. 10 (1937): 743–773, 743.

11. S. Lyle Cummins, *Report on Tuberculosis in Burma* (Rangoon: Superintendent of Government Printing and Stationery, Burma, 1939), 29.

12. "Tuberculosis amongst the African Population of Nairobi," no date but filed with papers from 1956, RN/11/14, Kenya National Archives (hereafter KNA).

13. Margaret Humphreys, "No Safe Place: Disease and Panic in American History," *American Literary History* 14, no. 4 (2002): 845–857.

14. Iñaki Comas, Mireia Coscolla, Tao Luo, Sonia Borrell, Kathryn E. Holt, Midori Kato-Maeda, Julian Parkhill, et al., "Out-of-Africa Migration and Neolithic Coexpansion of Mycobacterium Tuberculosis with Modern Humans," *Nature Genetics* 45, no. 10 (2013): 1176–1182. There are many books on the neolithic expansion. A fairly recent one, written by a renowned archeologist, is Ian Morris, *Why the West Rules—for Now: The Patterns of History, and What They Reveal about the Future* (New York: Farrar, Straus and Giroux, 2011).

15. Much of this general description of TB relies on Helen Bynum's excellent *Spitting Blood*. Bynum notes that the "key words for mycobacteria are longevity, resilience, and ubiquity." Bynum, *Spitting Blood*, 4; on grave sites, see pp. 6–7.

16. See Bynum, *Spitting Blood*, for the most up-to-date survey of the literature on TB.

17. Simon Szreter, "Rethinking McKeown: The Relationship between Public Health and Social Change," *American Journal of Public Health* 92, no. 5 (2002): 722–725; J. M. Grange, M. Gandy, P. Farmer, and A. Zumla, "Historical Declines in Tuberculosis: Nature, Nurture and the Biosocial Model," *International Journal of Tuberculosis and Lung Disease* 5, no. 3 (2001): 208–212.

CHAPTER 1. THE RISE OF RACE

1. Portions of the material on American Indians have been published in Christian W. McMillen, " 'The Red Man and the White Plague': Rethinking Race, Tuberculosis, and American Indians," *Bulletin of the History of Medicine* 82, no. 3 (2008): 608–645.

2. Sebastien Gagneaux and Peter M. Small, "Global Phylogeography of Mycobacterium Tuberculosis and Implications for Tuberculosis Product Development," *Lancet Infectious Diseases* 7, no. 5 (2007): 328–337.

3. Noel H. Smith, R. Glyn Hewinson, Kristin Kremer, Roland Brosch, and Stephen V. Gordon, "Myths and Misconceptions: The Origin and Evolution of Mycobacterium Tuberculosis," *Nature Reviews Microbiology* 7 (2009): 537–544.

4. For insights into these questions see J. M. Grande, M. Gandy, P. Farmer, and A. Zumla, "Historical Declines in Tuberculosis: Nature, Nurture, and the Biosocial Model," *International Journal of Tuberculosis and Lung Disease* 5, no. 3 (2001): 208–212.

5. E. Schurr, "Is Susceptibility to Tuberculosis Acquired or Inherited?" *Journal of Internal Medicine* 261, no. 2 (2007): 106–111, 106.

6. Gagneaux and Small, "Global Phylogeography of Mycobacterium Tuberculosis and Implications for Tuberculosis Product Development."

7. Julio Delgado et al., "Ethnic-Specific Genetic Associations with Pulmonary Tuberculosis," *Journal of Infectious Disease* 186, no. 10 (2002): 1463–1468.

8. Marc Lipsitch and Alexandra O. Sousa, "Historical Intensity of Natural Selection for Resistance to Tuberculosis," *Genetics* 161, no. 4 (2002): 1599–1607.

9. William W. Stead, "The Origin and Erratic Global Spread of Tuberculosis: How the Past Explains the Present and Is the Key to the Future," *Clinics in Chest Medicine* 18, no. 1 (1997): 70; see also Stead et al., "Racial Differences in Susceptibility to Infection by Mycobacterium Tuberculosis," *New England Journal of Medicine* 322, no. 7 (1990): 422–427; Stead, "Genetics and Resistance to Tuberculosis: Could Resistance Be Enhanced by Genetic Engineering?" *Annals of Internal Medicine* 116 (1992): 937–941. Stead's oft-cited *NEJM* article is deeply problematic for one simple reason: his finding that blacks were more susceptible to TB than whites did not take into account at all previous exposure to various risk factors for TB; he thought of the white and black subjects of his study as blank slates with no past. See Christian Lienhardt, "From Exposure to Disease: The Role of Environmental Factors in Susceptibility to and Development of Tuberculosis," *Epidemiologic Reviews* 23, no. 2 (2001): 288–301, 296.

10. Adrian Hill, "The Genomics and Genetics of Human Infectious Disease Susceptibility," *Annual Review of Human Genomics and Genetics* 2 (2001): 273–400, 273; on TB see Igor Kramnik, "Genetic Dissection of Host Resistance to Mycobacterium Tuberculosis: The ssti Locus and the Ipr1 Gene," in Bruce Beutler, ed., "Immunology, Phenotype First: How Mutations Have Established New Principles and Pathways in Immunology," *Current Topics in Microbiology and Immunology* 321 (2008): 123–148; for a recent overview of natural resistance to HIV see Jon Cohen, "HIV Natural Resistance Field Finally Overcomes Resistance," *Science* 326, no. 5959 (11 December 2009): 1476–1477; Herbert W. Virgin and Bruce D. Walker, "Immunology and the Elusive AIDS Vaccine," *Nature* 464 (11 March 2010): 224–231.

11. "The Control of Tuberculosis in Kenya Colony," by A. J. Walker, medical officer, Colonial Medical Service, 1941–, Nairobi, April 1949. National Association for the Prevention of Tuberculosis Essay Competition Winner, 1949, Radcliffe Science Library, Oxford.

12. S. Lyle Cummins, "Tuberculosis in Primitive Tribes and Its Bearing on the Tuberculosis of Civilized Communities," *International Journal of Public Health* 1 (1920): 138–171, 137.

13. For Winnebago see W. J. Stephenson, agency physician, Annual Report of the Commissioner of Indian Affairs, 1897 (hereafter: year and ARCIA); William G. Coe, Sanitary Report, Yakama Reservation, ARCIA, 1887, 306; for children succumbing to the "usual inherited tubercular troubles" see Ann Egan, "Report of Superintendent of Klamath School," 30 June, ARCIA, 1903, 290; see also Report of Charles C. Logan, Navajo Agency physician, who wrote that the principal disease among the Navajos was TB, due to heredity and the way they lived. ARCIA, 1904, 142; James S. Perkins wrote in "Tuberculosis—Its Cause and Prevention" that children "inherit the tuberculous diathesis, which predisposes them to tuberculous infection." ARCIA, 1902, 422.

14. ARCIA, 1904, 34, 35.

15. Woods Hutchinson, "Varieties of Tuberculosis According to Race and Social Condition," *New York Medical Journal* 86 (1907): 625; from the same year on lacking "resistive vitality" see no author, "Suggestions in Tuberculosis," *Medical News* 87, no. 8 (1905): 365; on Indians, evolution, susceptibility, and TB see "Bacteria as Empire Builders," in G. Archdall Reid, *The Principles of Heredity, with Some Applications* (New York: Sutton, 1905), 182–188; see also p. 150 where he declares Indians the most susceptible.

For a similar set of ideas in circulation in Canada at the same time see Megan Sproule-Jones, "Crusading for the Forgotten: Dr. Peter Bryce, Public Health, and Prairie Native Residential Schools," *Canadian Bulletin of Medical History* 13 (1996): 212–213.

16. Carroll quoted in Isaac W. Brewer, "Tuberculosis among the Indians of Arizona and New Mexico," *New York Medical Journal* 87 (1908): 982. Brewer wrote to doctors and superintendents at a number of reservations and asked them their thoughts on TB. For races, including Indians, being susceptible to TB see also Karl Von Rouck, "General and Specific Resistance to Tuberculosis Infection," *American Journal of Medical Sciences* 137, no. 3 (1909): 695; for Indians being "unselected" for TB see no author, "Tuberculosis among Natives of Alaska," *Journal of Heredity* 8, no. 4 (1917): 177.

17. Francis E. Leupp, "Fighting the Scourge among the Indians," *Transactions of the Sixth International Congress on Tuberculosis*, vol. 3 (Philadelphia: William F. Fell, 1908), 574.

18. Associate Committee on Tuberculosis Research quoted in Maureen Lux, "Perfect Subjects: Race, Tuberculosis, and the Qu'Appelle BCG Vaccine Trial," *Canadian Bulletin of Medical History* 15 (1998): 282.

19. Brian Dippie, *The Vanishing Indian: White Attitudes and U.S. Indian Policy* (Lawrence: University Press of Kansas, 1982).

20. James R. Walker, "Tuberculosis among the Oglala Sioux Indians," *American Journal of Medical Sciences* 132, no. 4 (1906): 600.

21. Laffer to CIA, 1 December 1910, CCF 98384-10-700, Warm Springs, reel 23, in Central Classified Files, 1907–1939, Series C: Indian Health and Disease, part 1, Reports on Medical and Nursing Activities (Lexis-Nexis, 2005) (hereafter IHD, part 1).

22. *Tuberculosis among the North American Indians: Report of a Committee of the National Tuberculosis Association* (Sen. Comm. Print, 67th Cong., 4th Sess., 1923), 4.

23. Colony and Protectorate of Kenya, Annual Medical Report, 1926, 31.

24. Charles Wilcocks, "Notes on Tuberculosis in Dar-es-Salaam," *Kenya and East African Medical Journal* 5 (1928): 206.

25. League of Nations Health Organisation, *Interim Report on Tuberculosis and Sleeping Sickness in Equatorial Africa* (Geneva, 1923), citing M. Kerandel, "Le tuberculose chez le Indigines dans les colonies français."

26. Stephen J. Maher, "Tuberculosis among the American Indians," *American Review of Tuberculosis* 19 (1929): 407–411, 411; Dr. D. A. Volume,

"Tuberculosis and the Indians," included in E. L. Stone, Director of Medical Services to R. G. Ferguson, 14 November 1932, R. G. Ferguson Papers, Saskatchewan Lung Association Archives, Saskatchewan Archives Board, VII, File 25 (hereafter Ferguson Papers and file number).

27. D. Drysdale Anderson, "Pulmonary Tuberculosis in a Native Population: The Development of Resistance," *Transactions of the Royal Society of Tropical Medicine and Hygiene* 21, no. 6 (1928): 463–472.

28. Peter Allan, *Report of Tuberculosis Survey of the Union of South Africa* (Cape Town: Cape Times Limited, Government Printers, 1924), 34.

29. Washington Matthews, "Consumption among the Indians," *Transactions of the American Climatological Association* 1886: 241.

30. S. Lyle Cummins, "Primitive Tribes and Tuberculosis," *Transactions of the Royal Society for Tropical Medicine and Hygiene* 5 (1912): 245–255, 248.

31. For the pre-Cummins use of the term see no author, "Tuberculosis among Indians," *Medical Record* 64 (5 December 1903): 900.

32. For an excellent discussion of virgin soil epidemics, both as a medically possible phenomenon and as a historian's fetish, see David S. Jones, "Virgin Soils Revisited," *William and Mary Quarterly* 60, no. 4 (2003), http://www.historycooperative.org/journals/wm/60.4/jones.html. See also Paul Kelton's consideration of virgin soil's limited utility when explaining the effects of what he calls the Great Southeastern Smallpox Epidemic in *Epidemics and Enslavement: Biological Catastrophe in the Native Southeast, 1492–1715* (Lincoln: University of Nebraska Press, 2007).

33. Cummins, "Primitive Tribes and Tuberculosis," 253.

34. Vint's work cited in E. Cochrane, "Tuberculosis in the Tropics: A Survey of Tuberculosis in the Tropics, Part I," *Tropical Diseases Bulletin* 34, no. 10 (1937): 743–772, 751.

35. Cummins, "Primitive Tribes and Tuberculosis," 249. Emphasis in original.

36. Mark Harrison and Michael Worboys, "A Disease of Civilization: Tuberculosis in Britain, Africa, and India, 1900–39," in Lara Marks and Michael Worboys, eds., *Migrants, Minorities and Health: Historical and Contemporary Studies* (New York: Routledge, 1997), 93–124, 104.

37. W. A. Chapple, discussion of Cummins, "Primitive Tribes and Tuberculosis," *Transactions of the Royal Society for Tropical Medicine and Hygiene* 5 (1912): 261–273, 261, 262.

38. Allan K. Krause, "Pathogenesis of Tuberculosis," *American Review of Tuberculosis* 18, no. 3 (1928): 224–225. Krause believed that if living conditions were more thoroughly investigated the cause of TB's rapid spread

among "primitive" peoples would be explained. See also Weston A. Price, "Some Causes for Changes in Susceptibility of Eskimos and Indians to Acute and Chronic Infections upon Contact with Modern Civilization," *Journal of Dental Research* 14 (1934): 230. Drawing on dental research, Price argued that malnutrition increased susceptibility. For worries over the troubling dominance of virgin soil see also R. J. Collins and G. L. Leslie, "The Treatment of Tuberculosis Lymphadenitis among American Indians," *American Review of Tuberculosis* 14 (1926): 647. For another dissenting view see Dr. E. L. Stone, "Tuberculosis among the Indians of the Norway House Agency," *Journal of Public Health* 16 (1925): 79. Stone noted that "these Indians have a remarkable resistance to tuberculosis." While he argued that Indians were more susceptible to TB, he also argued that Indians resisted active disease as greatly as anyone unless they lived under conditions conducive to its progress.

39. George Bushnell, *A Study in the Epidemiology of Tuberculosis* (New York: William Wood, 1920); C. D. De Langen, "Tuberculosis in the Dutch East Indies and in the Tropics," *Transactions of the Fourth Congress, Far Eastern Association of Tropical Medicine* (Batavia, 1921), esp. 230; for American Indians see McMillen, " 'The Red Man and the White Plague,' " esp. 620–625; Herbert Basedow, "Diseases of the Australian Aborigines," *Journal of Tropical Medicine and Hygiene* 35, no. 12 (1932): 211–212; E. Boltanski, "La tuberculose des Noirs," *La presse médicale* 43, no. 35 (1935): 709–710.

40. L. Cobbett, "The Resistance of Civilised Man to Tuberculosis: Is It Racial or Individual in Origin?" *Tubercle* (September 1925): 577–590, 588.

41. Randall Packard, *White Plague, Black Labor: Tuberculosis and the Political Economy of Health and Disease in South Africa* (Berkeley: University of California Press, 1989), 203; Wilcocks, "Notes on Tuberculosis in Dar-es-Salaam," 201; Wilcocks, "The Problem of Tuberculosis in East Africa," *East African Medical Journal* 9 (1932): 88–98, 93.

42. For the inchoate state of research see Aleš Hrdlička, "Contribution to the Study of Tuberculosis in the Indian," *Transactions of the Sixth International Congress on Tuberculosis*, vol. 3 (Philadelphia: William F. Fell, 1908), 481.

43. "Report of Supervisor Walter G. West, Fort Belknap Reservation, July 12, 1918," CCF 61806-18-700, reel 4; J. R. Collard to CIA, 19 November 1924, CCF 85437-24 Shoshone, reel 19; on misdiagnosing Hopi children at the Phoenix Indian School as having TB see Albert M. Wigglesworth, Senior Physician to CIA, 23 April 1925, CCF 1907-39 15668-25-700, Hopi, reel 6, both in IHD, part 1. On the unreliability of BIA data on tuberculosis see

Clifford E. Trafzer, "Coughing Blood: Tuberculosis Deaths and Data on the Yakima Reservation, 1911–1964," *Canadian Bulletin of Medical History* 15 (1998): 254.

44. C. C. Hickman to CIA, 7 July 1931, CCF 36518–31 Yankton, reel 26, IHD, part 1.

45. M. V. Ziegler, Medical Report on Yankton Agency, 13 June 1931, CCF 36518–31, reel 26, IHD, part 1.

46. Edgar Bates to F. E. Perkins, 10 October 1933, CCF 56071-33-700 Warm Springs, reel 23, IHD, part 1.

47. Earl Woodridge to CIA, 29 July 1931, CCF 64832-30-700 Rocky Boy, reel 16, IHD, part 1.

48. J. H. Crouch, "A Study of Tuberculosis among the Indians in Montana," *Public Health Reports* 47 (16 September 1932): 1907–1914.

49. L. R. Jones, "Report of a Tuberculosis Survey among the Indians of the Southwest," 1 November 1935, CCF 1907–39 58532-34-705, General Service (hereafter GS), box 58, Record Group 75 (hereafter RG 75), National Archives, Washington, D.C. (hereafter NA).

50. E. L Ross and A. L. Paine, "A Tuberculosis Survey of Manitoba Indians," *Canadian Medical Association Journal* 41, no. 2 (1939): 180–184, 180.

51. On blood and private property see Melissa L. Meyer, "American Indian Blood Quantum Requirements: Blood Is Thicker Than Family," in Blake Allmendinger and Valerie J. Matsumoto, eds., *Over the Edge: Remapping the American West* (Berkeley: University of California Press, 1999), 239; on insurance companies see Frederick L.Hoffman, *The Indian as a Life Insurance Risk* (New York: Prudential Press, 1928). For the myriad ways in which blood quantum has affected one tribe see Circe Sturm, *Blood Politics: Race, Culture, and Identity in the Cherokee Nation of Oklahoma* (Berkeley: University of California Press, 2002).

52. D. A. Sanford, "What Is Killing Our Indians?" *Indian's Friend* (September 1901): 10. Sanford wrote that the main cause of the high rate of TB is that it had been "inherited from past generations. It is in their blood"; Roy E. Thomas, "The Influence of Mixed Blood upon the Susceptibility to Infection in the American Indian," *Southern California Practitioner* 25 (1910): 576–577; for the connection between degree of Indian blood and TB, as well as Indians' lifestyle causing the disease, see Martha A. Waldron, "The Indian Health Question," *Lend a Hand* 5, no. 11 (1890): 766–774.

53. On the fear of "full bloods" not supporting the IRA, among other reforms, see Thomas Biolsi, *Organizing the Lakota: The Political Economy of the New*

Deal on the Pine Ridge and Rosebud Reservations (Tucson: University of Arizona Press, 1992), 80–83; for the related issue of progressive versus traditional Indians, which was often synonymous with blood quantum, see David Rich Lewis, "Reservation Leadership and the Progressive-Traditional Dichotomy: William Wash and the Northern Utes, 1865–1928," *Ethnohistory* 38, no. 2 (1991): 124–148; for a brief discussion in the context of the New Deal of the importance of blood quantum in determining who was and was not eligible to be considered an Indian by the government based on blood quantum see Elmer R. Rusco, *A Fateful Time: The Background and Legislative History of the Indian Reorganization Act* (Reno: University of Nevada Press, 2000), 267–269.

54. H. Hamlin, "A Health Survey of the Seminole Indians," *Yale Journal of Biology and Medicine* 6 (1933): 155.

55. H. J. Warner, "The Incidence of Tuberculosis Infection among School-Children on Five Montana Indian Reservations," *American Review of Tuberculosis* 26 (1932): 511.

56. Esmond R. Long, "A Brief Comparison of Tuberculosis in the White, Indian, and Negro Races," *American Review of Tuberculosis* 35 (1936): 2; see also Crouch, "A Study of Tuberculosis among the Indians in Montana"; R. G. Ferguson, "The Indian Tuberculosis Problem and Some Preventive Measures," *Transactions of the Twenty-Ninth Annual Meeting of the National Tuberculosis Association* (New York: NTA, 1933), 101. Interestingly, in an unpublished study on the Pine Ridge reservation done in 1939, Charles Davis found that while TB infection increased among "full-bloods," pathology did not; that is, degree of blood had nothing to do with whether one's infection became active. Charles Davis, Report on TB, 13 June 1939, CCF 55599-37-705 Pine Ridge, RG 75, reel 2, IHD, part 2.

57. Townsend to L. R. Jones, 22 January 1937, CCF 9962-35-705, part 1, box 59; for the research that revealed this see L. R. Jones, "Tabulated Report of Intracutaneous Tuberculin Tests Done at Turtle Mountain Agency," no date, but tests were done in August and October 1936, CCF 1907–39, 13223-36-705, Turtle Mountain, reel 3, part 2, IHD.

58. Forrest Clements, "Racial Differences in Mortality and Morbidity," *Human Biology* 3 (1931): first quote on 418, second on 406.

59. The 1932 study is Warner, "The Incidence of Tuberculosis Infection among School-Children on Five Montana Indian Reservations"; the 1945 study, from which the quote is drawn, is J. R. McGibony and A. W. Dahlstrom, "Tuberculosis among Montana Indians," *American Review of Tuberculosis*

52, no. 2 (1945): 109. It is worth noting that during discussions in the first decades of the twentieth century concerning tribal membership on the Colville reservation, Indians considered blood to be more a mark of Indian cultural traits than a quantifiable amount of actual blood. See Alexandra Harmon, "Tribal Enrollment Councils: Lessons on Law and Indian Identity," *Western Historical Quarterly* 33, no. 2 (2001), http://www.historycooperative.org/journals/whq/32.2/harmon.html, para. 52 (last accessed 13 July 2006).

60. For an example of how difficult accurate blood quantum data was to procure, and the resulting confusion see Frederick Hoffman, "Are the Indians Dying Out?" *American Journal of Public Health* 20 (June 1930): 609–614.

61. Charles H. A. Walton, "Racial Incidence of Tuberculosis in Manitoba," *American Review of Tuberculosis* 32, no. 1 (1935): 183–195, quote on 187. For the ways in which blood quantum operated within medical discourse, especially in regard to the notion that those with less Indian blood were healthier, see Mary Ellen Kelm, "Diagnosing the Discursive Indian: Medicine, Gender, and the 'Dying Race,'" *Ethnohistory* 52, no. 2 (2005): 392–396; on the importance of blood quantum in constructing Indian identities see Thomas Biolsi, "The Birth of the Reservation," in Frederick E. Hoxie, Peter C. Mancall, and James H. Merrell, eds., *American Nations: Encounters in Indian Country, 1850 to the Present* (New York: Routledge, 2001), 110–140, esp. 125–28; for how blood quantum is related to the question "Who is an Indian?" see Meyer, "American Indian Blood Quantum Requirements," 231–249. See also Pauline Tuner Strong and Barrik Van Winkle, "'Indian Blood': Reflections on Reckoning and Refiguring of Native American Identity," *Cultural Anthropology* 11, no. 4 (1996): 547–576. There are interesting parallels with studies done in the 1930s to determine whether or not sickle cell anemia was truly a black disease when cases began to turn up in whites. See Melbourne Tapper, "Interrogating Bodies: Medico-Racial Knowledge, Politics, and the Study of a Disease," *Comparative Studies in Society and History* 37, no. 1 (1995): 83–88; for work in the 1930s that called into question the utility of blood for determining racial type see also David McBride, *From TB to AIDS: Epidemics among Urban Blacks since 1900* (Albany: State University of New York Press, 1991), 50; for a brief history of changes in thinking regarding blood and its relationship to, among other things, disease see Michael G. Kenny, "A Question of Blood, Race, and Politics," *Journal of the History of Medicine and Allied Sciences* 61, no. 4 (2006): 473–478.

62. For an excellent demonstration of how complicated and ever shifting ideas about blood quantum were see Harmon, "Tribal Enrollment Councils."

63. Aronson had some experience with Indians and TB. He did a TB study in Michigan that included 176 Indians. Joseph D. Aronson, "Incidence of Tuberculous Infection in Some Rural Communities in Michigan," *American Journal of Hygiene* 21, no. 3 (1935): 543–561.

64. Aronson to Townsend, 5 May 1937; Townsend to Aronson, 22 May 1937; for Aronson wondering about the proof of blood quantum see his remarks in "Conference—B.C.G. Program," 13 October 1936, p. 3, all in CCF 9962-35-705, part 1, box 59, RG 75, NA.

65. For the Arapaho and Indian identity see Loretta Fowler, *Arapahoe Politics, 1851–1978: Symbols in Crises of Authority* (Lincoln: University of Nebraska Press, 1982), 164–166. Other work on blood quantum bears out the claim that it is more a social, and not a biological, construction. See William T. Hagan, "Full Blood, Mixed Blood, Generic, and Ersatz: The Problem of Indian Identity," *Arizona and the West* 27, no. 4 (1985): 309–326; David L. Beaulieu, "Curly Hair and Big Feet: Physical Anthropology and the Implementation of Land Allotment on the White Chippewa Reservation," *American Indian Quarterly* 8, no. 4 (1984): 281–314; Melissa L. Meyer, "Signatures and Thumbprints: Ethnicity among the White Earth Anishinaabeg, 1889–1920," *Social Science History* 14, no. 3 (1990): 305–345.

66. E. L. Stone, "Tuberculosis among the Indians of the Norway House Agency" (typescript), no date but included in Duncan C. Scott to Dr. R. E. Wodehouse, 25 March 1924, VII, 45, Ferguson Papers.

67. Albert M. Wigglesworth, Senior Physician to CIA, 23 April 1925, CCF 1907–39 15668-25-700, Hopi, reel 6, IHD, part 1. For Cummins's and Bushnell's influence regarding virgin soil see the various editions of Maurice Fishberg, *Pulmonary Tuberculosis* (Philadelphia: Lea and Febiger, 1922), 67–69.

68. For the quote see R. G. Ferguson, "Some Light Thrown on Infection, Resistance, and Segregation by a Study of Tuberculosis Among Indians," *Transactions of the American Clinical and Climatological Association* 50 (1934): 21; for another example of the same claim see R. G. Ferguson, "A Study of the Epidemiology of Tuberculosis in a Primitive People," *Edinburgh Medical Journal* 36 (1929): 199–206, 203; see also Ferguson, "Tuberculosis Research among the Qu'Appelle Indian Health Unit, 1933," VII, 45, 1933–39, Ferguson Papers; for a critique of Ferguson's methods, which calls into question the "virginity" of the population he studied, see Lux, "Perfect Subjects," 282–284; for a discussion of Ferguson and Cummins and their sympathetic views see Lux, *Medicine That Walks:*

Disease, Medicine, and Canadian Plains Native People, 1880–1940 (Toronto: University of Toronto Press, 2001), 205; also on Ferguson's TB/BCG work, but not calling into question his virgin soil theory, is Georgina D. Feldberg, *Disease and Class: Tuberculosis and the Shaping of Modern North American Society* (New Brunswick: Rutgers University Press, 1996), 162–165. Finally, on Ferguson and the acceptance of the connection between race and TB in Canada see James Daschuk, *Clearing the Plains: Disease, Politics of Starvation, and the Loss of Aboriginal Life* (Regina: University of Regina Press, 2014), esp. 177.

69. William Charles White to Linsly R. William, National Tuberculosis Association, CCF 9962-35-705, part 2b, GS, RG 75, NA.

70. R. G. Ferguson, M.D., "Progress Report of the Tuberculosis Research among the Indians, Carried on at Fort Qu'Appelle," VII, 25, 1932–35, Ferguson Papers. On the lack of good records and the difficulties of diagnosis in Manitoba see Charles H.A. Walton, "A Study of the Racial Incidence of Tuberculosis in the Province of Manitoba," *American Review of Tuberculosis* 32, no. 1 (1935): 183–195.

71. For the epidemic's effect on children see R. G. Ferguson, "Progress Report of the Tuberculosis Research among the Indians, Carried on at Fort Qu'Appelle," 27 May 1927, VII/5, Ferguson Papers.

72. R. G. Ferguson, "Suggested Plan of Qu'Appelle Indian Health Unit," n.d., VII/5, Ferguson Papers.

73. Wathena Myers Johnson and J. Arthur Myers, "Tuberculosis in Infants and Primitive Races," *American Review of Tuberculosis* 28 (1933): 381–409, 381, 383. For an early example of research that argued that Indian children, based on tuberculin testing, were equally resistant to TB as non-Indian children see Homer Davis, "Mantoux Observations in 629 Children," *Nebraska State Medical Journal* 17 (March 1932): 100.

74. C. J. Wilson, "Tuberculosis in the Natives of Kenya," *Kenya and East African Medical Journal* 1927 (4): 314; Dr. W. D. Inness, Memorandum by the Director of Medical and Sanitary Services Treatment of TB Gold Coast, 8 August 1928, CO 96-682-2, National Archives of the United Kingdom (hereafter NAUK).

75. A. J. R. O'Biren, Notes by the Medical Secretary of the Colonial Advisory Medical and Sanitary Committee, 14 September 1932, CO 691-125-2, NAUK.

CHAPTER 2. THE FALL OF RACE

1. Portions of the material on American Indians have been published in Christian W. McMillen, " 'The Red Man and the White Plague': Rethinking Race, Tuberculosis, and American Indians," *Bulletin of the History of Medicine* 82, no. 3 (2008): 608–645.

2. T. Wi Repa to Secretary, Maori Purposes Fund Board, no date, but this is a survey of living conditions of the "Maori Race for the period 1932 to 1933," MA 51, box 8, no. 61, National Archives of New Zealand.

3. J. G. Townsend to L. R. Jones, 9 November 1934, SW TB Survey, Central Classified Files (hereafter CCF) 58532-34-705, General Service (hereafter GS), Record Group 75 (hereafter RG 75), National Archives, Washington, D.C. (hereafter NA).

4. L. R. Jones, 23 July 1935, statistical data submitted to BIA; see also Jones, "Recommendations for Continuation and Expansion of the Tuberculosis Control Program in the Indian Service," 28 October 1935, both in CCF 58532-35-705 GS; Aronson to J. G. Townsend, CCF 9962-35-705 GS, all in RG 75, NA.

5. "Tuberculosis Research among the Indians of the Qu'Appelle Indian Health Unit, 1932," R. G. Ferguson Papers, Saskatchewan Lung Association Archives, Saskatchewan Archives Board, VII, File 5, 1922–33 (hereafter Ferguson Papers and file number).

6. Charles Wilcocks, report of activities carried out during 1931, in file "Tuberculosis Investigations under the C.D.F. [Colonial Development Fund]," 15 February 1932, CO 691-125-2, National Archives of the United Kingdom (hereafter NAUK). On the abundance of research on all manner of tropical diseases, of which, compared to the sleeping sickness, TB received only a paltry amount from Colonial Development Act grants, see Helen Tilley, *Africa as a Living Laboratory: Empire, Development, and Scientific Knowledge, 1870–1950* (Chicago: University of Chicago Press, 2011), 174–175.

7. Medical Department, Tanganyika Territory, "Tuberculosis in Tanganyika Territory," 1932, BY/13/238, Kenya National Archives (hereafter KNA).

8. H. Harold Scott, "Tuberculosis in the Tropics," *British Journal of Tuberculosis* (1929): 179–189.

9. Colony and Protectorate of Kenya, Annual Medical Report, 1945, p. 10.

10. C. J. Wilson, "Tuberculosis in the Natives of Kenya," *Kenya and East African Medical Journal 4* (1927): 296, 312. Wilson gathered much of his data from district medical officers all over Kenya; for their individual assessments of TB see BY/13/238, KNA.

11. Colony and Protectorate of Kenya, Annual Medical Report, 1937, p. 16.

12. Memorandum to Deputy of Sanitary Service, 7 November 1928, TB, Gold Coast, CO 323-1045-10, NAUK.

13. Aronson to Long, 19 May 1939, Esmond Long to James Townsend, 20 May 1939, CCF GS 33108–39, box 1457, RG 75, NA.

14. Tanganyika Territory, "Annual Medical Report for the Year Ending 31st December 1928" (Dar es Salaam: Government Printer, 1929), 14. See also H. N. Davies, "The Work of a Tuberculosis Unit in East Africa," *Tubercle* 20, no. 2 (1938): 76–88.

15. Tanganyika Territory, "Annual Medical Report for the Year Ending 31st December 1928," 14.

16. "Draft Scheme for a Tuberculosis Survey in an African Native Community," 1 October 1930, FD 1–3033, NAUK.

17. Cummins sent the "Draft Scheme" to at least one person involved in devising the plans for TB research in Africa. This does not of course mean he drafted the scheme, but the letter suggests he was at least involved in writing it. See A. Salisbury MacNalty to Landsborough Thomson, 30 September 1930, FD 1-1-33, NAUK.

18. "Draft Scheme for a Tuberculosis Survey in an African Native Community," 1 October 1930, FD 1–3033, NAUK.

19. Ibid.

20. Helen Tilley has done a considerable job exploring the multifaceted nature of scientific research in Africa between the wars. See generally her *Africa as a Living Laboratory*.

21. Much has been written about the overly technical assault on disease in the 1950s and 60s. For an excellent example see Randall Packard, *The Making of a Tropical Disease: A Short History of Malaria* (Baltimore: Johns Hopkins University Press, 2007), 111–149.

22. Wilcocks, report of activities carried out during 1931, in file "Tuberculosis Investigations under the C.D.F."

23. "Draft Scheme for a Tuberculosis Survey in an African Native Community," 1 October 1930, FD 1–3033, NAUK.

24. Wilcocks, report of activities carried out during 1931, in file "Tuberculosis Investigations under the C.D.F."

25. Ibid.

26. Charles Wilcocks, "Tuberculosis in Tanganyika Territory: Final Report on Investigations Carried out between 1930 and 1936 under the Auspices of the Colonial Development Fund" (Dar es Salaam: Government Printing Office, 1938), 44.

27. R. J. Matthews, "The State of Tuberculosis in the Protectorate of Zanzibar," *Tubercle* 16, suppl. 1 (1935): 48–87, 49.

28. For the argument regarding the transition to industrialization as the principal factor in TB's increase see Mark Harrison and Michael Worboys, "A Disease of Civilization: Tuberculosis in Britain, Africa, and India, 1900–39," in Lara Marks and Michael Worboys, eds., *Migrants, Minorities and Health: Historical and Contemporary Studies* (New York: Routledge, 1997), 93–124; S. Lyle Cummins, "Tuberculosis and the Empire," *British Journal of Tuberculosis* 31, no. 3 (1937): 140–143, 141; Charles Wilcocks, "Presidential Address on Tuberculosis and Industry in Africa," *Royal Sanitary Institute* 73, no. 5 (1953): 48–82, 81. Research into late nineteenth- and early twentieth-century hospital records in Uganda shows that it was not virgin soil as early as the turn of the twentieth century. See Thomas Daniel, "The Early History of Tuberculosis in Central East Africa: Insights from the Clinical Records of the First Twenty-Five Years of Mengo Hospital and Review of Relevant Literature," *International Journal of Tuberculosis and Lung Disease* 2, no. 10 (1998): 784–790.

29. B. A. Dormer, J. Friedlander, and F. J. Wiles, "A South African Team Looks at Tuberculosis," *Transvaal Mine Medical Officers Association* 23, no. 257 (November 1943): 71–114, 75–76, 82, 88.

30. A. W. Williams, "Tuberculosis in East Africa," Report to the DMS, Uganda, November 1945, A. W. Williams Papers, MSS Afr.s.1872, Oxford Development Records Project, Rhodes House Library, University of Oxford.

31. James Townsend to Joseph Aronson, 31 January 1941, CCG 9962-35-705, GS, RG 75, NA.

32. Aronson to Townsend, 6 August 1936, CCF 9962-35-705, part 1, GS, box 59, RG 75, NA.

33. Aronson to Townsend, 6 August 1936, CCF 9962-35-705, part 1, GS; "rural slum areas" in Joseph D. Aronson, Robert M. Saylor, Erma I. Parr, Summary of Tuberculosis Control Studies as of January 1st, 1940, CCF 9962-35-705, part 2, GS, box 59, RG 75, NA. "Bionomic" factors in J. G. Townsend, Joseph D. Aronson, Robert Saylor, and Irma Parr, "Tuberculosis Control among the North American Indians," *American Review of Tuberculosis* 45, no. 1 (1942): 46. Aronson had earlier considered racial susceptibility in relation to African Americans, but he came to no firm conclusion. See Aronson, "Incidence of Tuberculosis Infection in Some Communities of the South," *American Journal of Hygiene* 14, no. 2 (1931):

390. Aronson, while largely denying race as a factor, could not let it go entirely. In 1953, he speculated that the difference between the Arapaho and Shoshone rates of TB—both tribes lived on the Wind River reservation under what he considered similar conditions—might be due to race or degree of exposure. Samuel C. Stein and Joseph D. Aronson, "The Occurrence of Pulmonary Lesions in BCG-Vaccinated and Unvaccinated Persons," *American Review of Tuberculosis* 68, no. 5 (1953): 700.

34. S. Lyle Cummins, *Empire and Colonial Tuberculosis: A General Survey* (London: National Association for the Prevention of Tuberculosis, 1945), 35–36.

35. Frank Retief, "Random Notes and Observations on Tuberculosis," 12 August 1947, Pad 2, "Diseases and Epidemic Tuberculosis," Witwatersrand Native Labour Association archives, TEBA collection, University of Johannesburg.

36. S. Lyle Cummins, "Introduction to Studies of Tuberculosis among African Natives, Report to the Medical Research Council," *Tubercle* 16, suppl. 1 (January 1935): 12–13. Harrison and Worboys argue that Cummins expressed this view based on his experience in South Africa; this is partially true. But it's important to note, because it shows Cummins's views were more encompassing than Harrison and Worboys suggest, that he expresses the above sentiment while discussing East Africa; Lucien Hoebeke, "Tuberculose nègre et colonies africaines, chapitre III: La T. Parmi les populations de Congo Belge. Caractères de la T. Nègre," *Bruxelles-Médical* 14 (1934): 1603–1617, 1617.

37. Wathena Myers Johnson and J. Arthur Myers, "Tuberculosis in Infants and Primitive Races," *American Review of Tuberculosis* 28 (1933): 381–409.

38. R. G. Ferguson, "A Study of the Epidemiology of Tuberculosis in a Primitive People," *Edinburgh Medical Journal* 36 (1929): 203; Michael Worboys has argued that the association between race and TB grew stronger in Great Britain in the 1920s. See Worboys, "Tuberculosis and Race in Britain and Its Empire, 1900–1950," in Waltraud Ernst and Bernard Harris, eds., *Race, Science and Medicine, 1700–1960* (New York: Routledge, 1999), 144–166, esp. 155.

39. See R. G. Ferguson, "Progress Report of the Tuberculosis Research among the Indians, Carried on at Fort Qu'Appelle," 27 May 1927; quote from R. G. Ferguson, "Tuberculosis Research among the Indians of the Qu'Appelle Indian Health Unit," 1930, p. 7; both in VII/25, Ferguson Papers.

40. "Notes on Post-Mortem Examinations Performed by Dr. C. Wilcocks," Medical Officer, Moshi, Annual Medical Report, Tanganyika Territory,

1929, 204; see also Wilcocks, "Report for January to June 1931," 1 August 1931, CO 691-119-12, NAUK.

41. C. W. Hobley, Provincial Commissioner, Ukamba Province, to John Arthur, 6 June 1910; Arthur to Hobley, 7 September 1910, MOH/1/5690 KNA; see also Wilson, "Tuberculosis in the Natives of Kenya," 313-314.

42. Charles Wilcocks, "Tuberculosis in the Natives of Tropical and Subtropical Regions," *Transactions of the Royal Society of Tropical Medicine and Hygiene* 32, no. 6 (1939): 669-684, quote on 681.

43. First two quotes in H. F. Schrader to J. G. Townsend, CCF 60794-35 Blackfeet; "discarded" in H. F. Schrader, "Notes on a Study of Death Certificates, Blackfeet Reservation of Indians, with Special Attention to Tuberculosis," CCF 61267-35-700, no date, both in reel 1, IHD, part 1.

44. Louis I. Dublin, "The Mortality from Tuberculosis among the Race Stocks in the Southwest," *American Review of Tuberculosis* 45 (1942): 61-74, 70.

45. J. A. Carswell, "Poverty and Tuberculosis with Particular Reference to the Economic and Social Significance of High Death Rates among Alaskans," National Tuberculosis Association, *Transactions of the Thirty-Fourth Annual Meeting, June 21-23, 1938*, Los Angeles.

46. David A. Stewart, "The Red Man and the White Plague," *Canadian Medical Association Journal* 35 (December 1936): 675.

47. For evolutionary thinking and race in South Africa see Saul Dubow, *Scientific Racism in Modern South Africa* (Cambridge: Cambridge University Press, 1995); B. A. Dormer, "Tuberculosis in South Africa," *British Journal of Tuberculosis and Diseases of the Chest* 50, no. 1 (1956): 52-60, 54; Randall Packard, *White Plague, Black Labor: Tuberculosis and the Political Economy of Health and Disease in South Africa* (Berkeley: University of California Press, 1989), 208-209.

48. "Memorandum on Tuberculosis on the Gold Coast by Dr. Duff," 24 December 1928, CO 323-1045-10, NAUK.

49. R. G. Ferguson, "Progress Report of the Tuberculosis Research among the Indians, Carried on at Fort Qu'Appelle," 1934, VII, File 25, Ferguson Papers.

50. James Townsend to Rudolf Hertz, Dakota Indian Parish, CCF 9962-305-705, GS, RG 75, NA. It must be noted that Townsend did think American black pathology did differ; American blacks were prone to a severe, fulminating type of TB. The work Townsend relied on was John H. Korns, "Comparative Tuberculosis Findings among Indians and White Persons in Cattaraugus County, New York," *American Review of Tuberculosis* 34 (1936):

550–560, and Esmond R. Long and H. W. Hetherington, "A Tuberculosis Survey of the Papago Indian Area of Southern Arizona," Supplement to the *American Review of Tuberculosis* 33 (1936): 407–433.

51. Esmond R. Long, "Constitution and Related Factors in Resistance to Tuberculosis," *Archives of Pathology* 32, no. 1 (1941): 148. On chronic TB and the ability to heal in Nigeria see also J. E. Henshaw, "Observations on the Chronicity of Pulmonary Tuberculosis in Africans," *West African Medical Journal* 8 (1959): 229–236. Decades later, in 1968, chronic lesions were also seen as a measure of resistance to active disease. The discovery that 31 percent of Kenyans presenting with pulmonary TB for the first time had chronic lesions led the authors of one survey to claim that a "change has occurred in Kenya in the characteristics of newly-diagnosed tuberculosis lesions of the lungs." But there is no evidence that the authors had any sense that this had already been discovered thirty years before. East African and British Medical Research Council Co-Operative Investigation, "Tuberculosis in Kenya: A National Sampling Survey of Drug Resistance and Other Factors," *Tubercle* 49 (1968): 136–169, 159.

52. For the number of x-rays see Samuel Stein to Fred Foard, 18 August 1947, CCF 1940–57, 9698-45-705, GS; for the 17,500 figure see Fred T. Foard to various superintendents, 29 July 1949, CCF 1940–57 3832-45-705, part 1-B, GS, both in box 1129, Record Group (RG) 75, NA.

53. J. Arthur Myers and Virginia L. Dustin, "Albert Reifel and Tuberculosis among the American Indians," *Hygeia* (April 1947): 322.

54. Dr. Basil Anthony Dormer, conference remarks in *Chest and Heart Disease in the Commonwealth, 1958*, the Full Transactions of the NAPT Commonwealth Chest Conference, 1–4 July 1958 (London: National Association for the Prevention of Tuberculosis, 1958), 27.

55. Charles Wilcocks, "A Tropical Doctor in Africa and London: An Autobiography," 1977, Mss Afr.s. 1606, Rhodes House, University of Oxford.

56. Haynes to C. D. Rosenwald, Public Health Department, Mombasa, 25 August 1959, BY/13/239, KNA.

57. F. M. Burnet, "The Natural History of Tuberculosis," *Medical Journal of Australia* 1 (35th year), no. 3 (14 January 1948): 57–63, 57.

58. F. Marian Macken, "Initial Comments on Tuberculosis Case-Finding Survey among Australian Aboriginals," *Tubercle* 33 (1952): 376–381, 378.

59. J. C. Buchanan, "Tuberculosis as a Problem in Preventive and Social Medicine in Overseas Territories," *Tubercle* 36, no. 9 (1955): 272–276, 275.

60. J. Tenret, "Considérations sur la tuberculose pulmonaire des Noirs du Ruanda-Urundi, établies par la prospection antituberculeuse de Cemubac," *Acta Tuberculosea Belgica* 3 (June 1954): 293–301, 296. He also briefly discusses TB among American Indians and says that their living conditions are far worse than conditions in colonial countries.

61. A. C. Bruce Singleton, "Tuberculosis Control Measures in Civilised Communities and Their Application to Underdeveloped Areas in Africa," *Central African Journal of Medicine* 3, no. 1 (1957): 13–17, 14.

62. H. DeLien and J. Nixon Hadley, "How to Recognize an Indian Health Problem," *Human Organization* (Fall 1952): 30.

63. Johannes Holm, "Tuberculosis: A Problem of Different Races," text of a speech before the Fourth Commonwealth Health and Tuberculosis Conference, 3 October 1955, WHO/TBC/Int./28. This is not to say that worldwide speculating on the connections between race and TB had vanished. For the persistence of the view that some races were more susceptible see Alton S. Pope, "Tuberculosis in the Tropics," in *Industry and Tropical Health: Proceedings of the First Industrial Tropical Health Conference, Sponsored by the Harvard School of Public Health, December 8–10, 1950* (Cambridge, Mass.: Harvard School of Public Health for the Industrial Council for Tropical Health, 1950), 239–240.

64. Alfred L. Kroeber, "A Half Century of Anthropology," in *The Nature of Culture* (Chicago: University of Chicago Press, 1952), 139; for an earlier iteration of anthropology's rejection of race see "Resolution of the American Anthropological Association" (originally published in *Science* in 1938) in Ruth Benedict, *Race: Science and Politics* (New York: Modern Age Books, 1940), 260–261; for a discussion of changes in anthropology and biology see generally Elazar Barkan, *Retreat of Scientific Racism: Changing Concepts of Race in Britain and the United States between the World Wars* (Cambridge: Cambridge University Press, 1992).

65. David S. Jones, "Virgin Soils Revisited," *William and Mary Quarterly* 60, no. 4 (2003), http://www.historycooperative.org/journals/wm/60.4/jones.html (last accessed 29 June 2006); Alfred W. Crosby, "Virgin Soil Epidemics as a Factor in the Aboriginal Depopulation in America," *William and Mary Quarterly* 33, no. 2 (1976): 289–299.

66. This point is important for two reasons: first, to use as proof of virgin soil theory Indian people who were by no measure "virgin" is inappropriate; second, the bulk of work done on the susceptibility of indigenous people to European pathogens is generally restricted to the contact and immediate

postcontact periods, which includes epidemics of recently contacted peoples in the twentieth century. See, for example, Francis L. Black, "An Explanation of High Death Rates among New World Peoples When in Contact with Old World Diseases," *Perspectives in Biology and Medicine* 37, no. 2 (1994): 292–303; A. Magdalena Hurtado et al., "Longitudinal Study of Tuberculosis Outcomes among Immunologically Naïve Ache Natives of Paraguay," *American Journal of Physical Anthropology* 121 (2003): 134–150.

67. For an earlier critique of the use of Ferguson see George A. Clark et al., "The Evolution of Mycobacterial Disease in Human Populations," *Current Anthropology* 28, no. 1 (1987): 46–47. As early as 1941 Esmond Long called into question Ferguson's studies, noting that Ferguson did not take into account environmental conditions. See Long, "Constitution and Related Factors," 149; see also Lall G. Montgomery, "Tuberculosis among Pupils of a Canadian School for Indians," *American Review of Tuberculosis* 28, no. 4 (1933): 502–515, in which he noted that the Indian children he studied, when removed from infectious conditions, did not develop active TB; this, he noted, was in contradiction to the impression Ferguson gave that all Indians equally lack resistance and that environment is unimportant.

68. Alexandra O. Sousa et al., "An Epidemic of Tuberculosis with a High Rate of Tuberculin Anergy among a Population Previously Exposed to Tuberculosis, the Yanomami Indians of the Brazilian Amazon," *Proceedings of the National Academy of Sciences* 94 (1997): 13229.

69. Richard Bellamy, "Genetic Susceptibility to Tuberculosis in Human Populations," *Thorax* 53 (1998): 588. It should be noted that Bellamy cites, almost repeats verbatim, Arno G. Motulsky's citing of Ferguson. Motulsky, "Metabolic Polymorphisms and the Role of Infectious Diseases in Human Evolution," *Human Biology* 32, no. 1 (1960): 35. Motulsky noted in a table that Indians upon first exposure were the most susceptible to TB; the Irish "race" was seventh.

70. The work of William W. Stead is again important. See "The Origin and Erratic Global Spread of Tuberculosis: How the Past Explains the Present and Is the Key to the Future," *Clinics in Chest Medicine* 18, no. 1 (1997): 70; see also Stead et al., "Racial Differences in Susceptibility to Infection by Mycobacterium Tuberculosis," *New England Journal of Medicine* 322, no. 7 (1990): 422–427; Stead, "Genetics and Resistance to Tuberculosis: Could Resistance Be Enhanced by Genetic Engineering?" *Annals of Internal Medicine* 116 (1992): 937–941. For other citations to Ferguson's work as evidence for virgin soil epidemics, which is then embedded in a larger argument

about the possible racial basis for TB infection as well as TB's effect on natural selection, see Marc Lipsitch and Alexandra O. Sousa, "Historical
Intensity of Natural Selection for Resistance to Tuberculosis," *Genetics* 161
(2002): 1599–1607. There are valuable critiques of the acceptance of racial
susceptibility that come from the biomedical community. For a sensible critique of race-based theories see, for example, Masahiro Kushigemachi,
"Racial Differences in Susceptibility to Tuberculosis: Risk of Disease after
Infection," *Journal of Chronic Diseases* 37, no. 11 (1984): 853–862. See also
Barry Bloom's editorial in the *New England Journal of Medicine* in which he
says: "Establishing genetic susceptibilities to infectious diseases in humans
poses formidable scientific obstacles because of variations in the prevalence
of infection among populations and the confounding effects of social and
economic factors." Bloom, "The Evolving Relationship between Humans
and Mycobacterium Tuberculosis," *NEJM* 338, no. 10 (1998): 667–678. For a
study that considers a range of factors which might contribute to susceptibility, including genetics, see A. Magdalena Hurtado, Inés Hurtado, and Kim
Hill, "Public Health and Adaptive Immunity among Natives of South
America," in Francisco M. Salzano and A. Magdalena Hurtado, eds., *Lost
Paradises and the Ethics of Research and Publication* (New York: Oxford
University Press, 2004), 164–190; for the variations in severity of TB among
First Nations in the late nineteenth century see J. W. Daschuk, P. Hackett,
and S. MacNeil, "Treaties and Tuberculosis: First Nations People in Late
19th-Century Western Canada, a Political and Economic Transformation,"
Canadian Bulletin of Medical History 23, no. 2 (2006): 307–330.
71. Jay S. Kaufman and Richard S. Cooper, "Commentary: Considerations for
Use of Racial/Ethnic Classification in Etiologic Research," *American
Journal of Epidemiology* 154, no. 4 (2001): 291.
72. For an example of this type of research that argues for the validity and continued use of race because of clear genetic differences based on race see Neil
Risch et al., "Categorization of Humans in Biodmedical Research: Genes,
Race, and Disease," *Genome Biology* 3, no. 7 (2002): 1–12; for a strong refu-
tation of research based on race see Richard S. Schwartz, "Racial Profiling in
Medical Research," *New England Journal of Medicine* 344, no. 18 (2001):
1392–1393; for a critical view of the persistence of "race talk" in modern biomedicine, especially in light of recent discoveries in genetics, see Lundy
Braun, "Race, Ethnicity, and Health: Can Genetics Explain Disparities?"
Perspectives in Biology and Medicine 45, no. 2 (2002): 159–174; for the view
that race/ethnicity is still a category with great purchase among geneticists

see Simon M. Outram and George H. T. Ellison, "Anthropological Insights into the Use of Race/Ethnicity to Explore Genetic Contributions Disparities in Health," *Journal of Biosocial Science* 38, no. 1 (2006): 83–102; for an excellent analysis of the flawed thinking involved in genetic/evolutionary approaches to disease susceptibility see Gilles Bibeau and Duncan Pedersen, "A Return to Scientific Racism in Medical Social Sciences: The Case of Sexuality and the AIDS Epidemic in Africa," in Margaret Lock and Mark Nichter, eds., *New Horizons in Medical Anthropology: Essays in Honour of Charles Leslie* (New York: Routledge, 2002), 141–171; Lundy Braun, Anne Fausto-Sterling, Duana Fullwiley, Evelynn M. Hammonds, Alondra Nelson, William Quivers, Susan M. Reverby, and Alexandra E. Shields, "Racial Categories in Medical Practice: How Useful Are They?" *PLoS Medicine* 4, no. 9 (2007): 1423–1428. For reasons of space, citing all the research and commentary on contemporary studies of race and medicine is not possible.

73. Bellamy et al., "Genetic Susceptibility to Tuberculosis in Africans: A Genome-Wide Scan," *Proceedings of the National Academy of Sciences* 97, no. 4 (2000): 8005–8009; Celia M. T. Greenwood et al., "Linkage of Tuberculosis to Chromosome 2q35 Loci, Including NRAMP1, in a Large Aboriginal Canadian Family," *American Journal of Human Genetics* 67 (2000): 405–416; Yung-Hsiang Hsu et al., "Association of NRAMP1 Gene Polymorphism with Susceptibility to Tuberculosis in Taiwanese Aboriginals," *Journal of the Formosan Medical Association* 105, no. 5 (2006): 363–369; Jodene Fitness et al., "Large-Scale Candidate Gene Study of Tuberculosis Susceptibility in the Karonga District of Northern Malawi," *American Journal of Tropical Medicine and Hygiene* 71, no. 3 (2004): 341–349. For the trouble geneticists run into when trying to tie ethnicity to genetics see Scott MacEachern, "Genes, Tribes, and History," *Current Anthropology* 41, no. 3 (2000): 357–371.

74. Marlo Möller, Erika de Wit, and Eileen G. Hoal, "Past, Present and Future Directions in Human Genetic Susceptibility to Tuberculosis," *FEMS Immunology and Medical Microbiology* 58, no. 1 (2010): 3–26, 4.

75. Caitlin Pepperell et al., "Dispersal of *mycobacterium tuberculosis* via the Canadian Fur Trade," *Proceedings of the National Academy of Science* 108, no. 16 (2011): 6526–6531.

76. For this point see Mike Bamshad, M.D., "Genetic Influences on Health: Does Race Matter?" *Journal of the American Medical Association* 294, no. 8 (2005): 937–946.

77. There are several studies that investigate this question. They are summarized in Daniel Elias et al., "Are Intestinal Helminths Risk Factors for Developing Active Tuberculosis?" *Tropical Medicine and International Health* 11, no. 4 (2006): 551–558; see also Zvi Bentwich et al., "Can Eradication of Helminthic Infections Change the Face of AIDS and Tuberculosis?" *Immunology Today* 21, no. 11 (1999): 485–487.

CHAPTER 3. THE CHALLENGE OF TB

1. WHO Press Release, "Vaccination against Tuberculosis, WHO Experts to Meet in Copenhagen," 27 November 1953, Press Release WHO/70, MOH 3/742, Kenya National Archives (hereafter KNA).

2. WHO Expert Committee on Tuberculosis, Seventh Report, World Health Organization Technical Report Series, Report No. 195 (Geneva: World Health Organization, 1960), 4.

3. Herbert Moller, BCG Advisor, Eastern Mediterranean Office, UNICEF, "Suggestions for WHO Activity in the Field of BCG in 1953 with Special Reference to the Eastern Mediterranean Region," 3 February 1952, Programme Division, Eastern Mediterranean, CF/RA/BX/PD/1952/T019, UNICEF Archives.

4. E. A. Trim, Director of Medical Services, *Annual Medical Report*, Kenya (Nairobi: Government Printing Office, 1952), first quote 1952, pp. 7–8; second quote 1952, p. 16; East African High Commission, East African Medical Survey, Annual Report, 1951, p. 50; Paul Hutton et al., "Acute Pulmonary Tuberculosis in East Africans: A Controlled Trial of Isoniazid in Combination with Streptomycin and PAS," *Tubercle* 37, no. 3 (1956): 151–165, 151.

5. "Public Health-Increase in Tuberculosis and Leprosy in British East Africa," Edward M. Groth, American Consul General, Nairobi, 26 May 1950, 845P.55/5–2650, Central Files, box 1576, RG 59, Records of the U.S. Department of State, National Archives, Washington, D.C. (hereafter NA).

6. For the goals of TB research in East Africa see P. D'Arcy Hart, "Possible Short List of Trials for Consideration in East Africa," 1 July 1959, FD 1–8773, National Archives of the United Kingdom (hereafter NAUK).

7. Dr. Hugh Stott, M.D., "African Tuberculosis," East African Medical Survey, Annual Report, 1951, East Africa High Commission, Nairobi. See also Comments by Dr. Frederick Heaf, 28 March 1950, Extract from C.A.M.C. Minutes of 453rd Meeting, CO 859-210-5, NAUK.

8. "Plan for a BCG Programme in a Hypothetical Country as Requested in HQ's Letter AS.CDS.TB. DC.TB. 16 of April '53," Asia-BCG, Programme Division, Subject Files, Asia Region, 1947–55, CF/RA/BX/PD.1962/T004, UNICEF Archives.

9. R. Neubauer, "Report on Visit to West and Central African Territories," October–December 1953, p. 147, DC-TB-AFRO, WHO Archives, Geneva.

10. WHO Press Release, "Executive Board: Tuberculosis an Increasingly Important Problem in Africa," 27 January 1954, WHO Library, Geneva.

11. Randall M. Packard, *The Making of a Tropical Disease: A Short History of Malaria* (Baltimore: Johns Hopkins University Press, 2007), 224.

12. World Health Organization, "Plan for WHO Tuberculosis Control Projects," 19 January 1953, Tub. Cent/53/1, WHO Archives.

13. Secretary of Health to Secretary of the Treasury, 1 August 1956, BY/13/188, KNA.

14. J. Pepys to Harold Himsworth, 2 October 1957, TB Chemotherapy Trials, East Africa, FD 1–8770, NAUK.

15. J. Pepys to P. O. Williams, "East African Tuberculosis Investigation. Outline of proposed trial." No date, but filed with papers dated between December 1956 and January 1957, FD 1/8770, NAUK.

16. Johannes Holm, "Report on a Visit to India, February–April, 1951," Programme Division—Asia-General, CF/RA/BX/PD/1947/T021; for the importance of India as a demonstration project see also B. Fraser to Myron Schmittlinger, 18 July 1950, BCG-General, 1949–1950, A648, LF-WYH–05, both in UNICEF Archives. For the view that research with controlled trials was desired, but that "attempts of this kind are often opposed as 'experimenting' on human beings," see I-Chin Yuan and Carroll E. Palmer, "The WHO Tuberculosis Research Office: A Review of the First Four Years," *Public Health Reports* 68, no. 7 (July 1953): 679.

17. Fox's comments were recorded at the following meeting: "Medical Research Council: Future Studies in East Africa, minutes of a meeting held at 20, Park Crescent, W.1., on Monday, the 16th September, 1963, at 2p.m.," TRU.63/C.130 (24.9.63), FD 12/553/1, NAUK.

18. J. Paviot, "Report on a Visit to Kenya, 5–11 February, 1967," Kenya–4, AFR/TB/89, WHO Archives.

19. B. K. Sikand, S. S. Goyal, and G. P. Mathur, "A Clinical Trial of p-Acetylaminobenzaldehyde Thiosemicarbazone in the Treatment of Pulmonary Tuberculosis," *Indian Journal of Tuberculosis Research* 11, no. 1 (1964): 38–50.

20. William Stott, "Drug Acceptability and Chemoprophylaxis in Under-Developed Countries," 3 April 1959, BY/ 7/189, KNA. This is a draft version of published article of the same name that appeared in the *Bulletin of the International Union Against Tuberculosis* 29 (1959).

21. No author, 24 June 1957, British Somaliland Protectorate, Tuberculosis Control, Programming Notes, CF/RA/BX/PD/1962/T054, UNICEF Archives.

22. Pierce Kent, "Thiacetazone Investigation," 20 January 1963, BY/13/243, KNA.

23. Thus I would suggest that it was not the case, as Sunil Armith argued, that "by disseminating universal norms (what sociologists have called the assumptions of 'world society') the WHO could govern what it meant to speak of 'health policy' (and, of course, what fell beyond the realm of 'health policy') to such an extent that modern public health meant something similar in states with widely different political cultures." Sunil S. Amrith, *Decolonizing International Health: India and Southeast Asia, 1930–65* (London: Palgrave Macmillan, 2006), 12.

24. Ibid., 150.

25. P. P. Turner, "Presidential Address: The Physician and the Public Health," *East African Medical Journal* 41 (1964): 541–550, esp. 547–548.

26. "Hand to mouth" in Comments of Pierce Kent at "Committee for Research on Tuberculosis in the Tropics," TRU.63/C.144, 1 November 1963; "barely viable" in "Future Administration of the East African Tuberculosis Chemotherapy Trials," no date but filed with other papers from October and November 1963, both in FD 12/553/1, NAUK.

27. In a handwritten note on a transcript of a conversation between Hart of the MRC and Mahler, Harold Himsworth noted that: "Hart added in confidence, that contributing governments to WHO had restricted their allocations for tuberculosis work on the grounds that WHO had had too much for too long for this—hence their inability to offer anything for a bacteriologist in Nairobi." Harold Himsworth, 8 February 1962, FD 12/552, NAUK. This tantalizing thread cannot be followed very far, as WHO does not allow researchers to access materials on donations and on possible restrictions on a given subject. On the budgetary problems of WHO in the early years see Amy L. S. Staples, *The Birth of Development: How the World Bank, Food and Agriculture Organization, and World Health Organization Changed the World, 1945–1965* (Kent, Ohio: Kent State University Press, 2006), 150–153.

28. "'Outline of the WHO-Assisted Research Programme in Tuberculosis,' by Halfdan Mahler," Committee for Research on Tuberculosis in the Tropics, TRU.64/C.25, 28 February 1964, NAUK FD 12/554, NAUK.

29. Chambourac, Dir. of WHO to Fendall, DMS-Kenya, 1 July 1963, BY/7/192; Fraenkel, BBC to DMS, Kenya, 4 October 1963, BY/7/193, KNA.

30. "Extract from Dr. Lush's report on his visit to East Africa," FD 12–557, NAUK.

31. Waksman's solitary win did not reflect the efforts of the many to find antibiotics that cured TB, it only acknowledged his role in the development of streptomycin. See Frank Ryan, *The Forgotten Plague: How the Battle against Tuberculosis was Won—and Lost* (Boston: Little, Brown, 1992), 365–376.

32. Ibid., 342–364.

33. T. Aidan Cockburn, "Eradication of Infectious Disease," *Science* 133, no. 3458 (7 April 1961): 1050–1058, 1058. For an insightful exploration of this era's rise and demise see Frank M. Snowden, "Emerging and Reemerging Diseases: A Historical Perspective," *Immunological Reviews* 225 (2008): 9–26.

34. He may or may not have said this, but it's been attributed to him many times. Brad Spellberg, "Dr. William H. Stewart: Mistaken or Maligned?" *Clinical Infectious Diseases* 47, no. 2 (2008): 294.

35. Packard, *The Making of a Tropical Disease*, esp. 111–176.

36. Walsh McDermott, "The Role of Biomedical Research in International Development," The National Institutes of Health International Lecture (Bethesda, 1963), 2; for a trenchant critique of the way this worked in one country see Timothy Mitchell, "Can the Mosquito Speak?" in *Rule of Experts: Egypt, Techno-Politics, and Modernity* (Berkeley: University of California Press, 2002). See also Nancy Leys Stepan, *Eradication: Ridding the World of Diseases Forever?* (Ithaca: Cornell University Press, 2011).

37. Walsh McDermott, "Modern Medicine and the Demographic-Disease Pattern of Overly Traditional Societies: A Technological Misfit," *Journal of Medical Education* 41 (September 1966): 137.

38. Walsh McDermott, "Tuberculosis at Home and Abroad," *Bulletin of the National Tuberculosis and Respiratory Disease Association* 54, no. 10 (1968): 7–11, 11. Emphasis in original.

39. Van Zile Hyde, memo from 12 December 1954 in Office of International Health, Correspondence 1949–1969, Information-Meetings, 1949–1959, box 5, RG 90, National Archives, College Park, Md. On fighting communism

under the guise of public health see also Harry Cleaver, "Malaria Control and the Political Economy of Public Health," *International Journal of Health Services* 7, no. 4 (1977): 557–579.

40. Fred L. Soper, "Problems to Be Solved if the Eradication of Tuberculosis Is to Be Realized," *American Journal of Public Health* 52, no. 5 (May 1962): 735. The paper was published in 1962; the speech was delivered in 1961.

41. Carroll E. Palmer, "Tuberculosis: A Decade in Retrospect and Prospect," *Journal-Lancet* 78 (June 1958): 257–260; James E. Perkins, "Global Tuberculosis Eradication," International Symposium of the Deborah Sanatorium and Hospital, Philadelphia, Pennsylvania, November 20–22, 1958, in *American Review of Respiratory Diseases* 80, no. 4 (October 1959): 138–139. See also Niels Brimnes, "BCG Vaccination and WHO's Global Strategy for Tuberculosis Control, 1948–83," *Social Science and Medicine* 67, no. 5 (2008): 863–873. Brimnes argues that the WHO's approach was "high modernist" and fixated on technology. "BCG vaccination was high modernism on the cheap" (866).

42. See especially Packard, *The Making of a Tropical Disease*, 136–149.

43. On the multiple meanings of modernization see Frederick Cooper, "Modernity," in *Colonialism in Question: Theory, Knowledge, History* (Berkeley: University of California Press, 2005); on modernization see, for example, the essays in David C. Engerman, Nils Gilman, Mark H. Haefele, and Michael E. Latham, *Staging Growth: Modernization, Development, and the Global Cold War* (Amherst: University of Massachusetts Press, 2003); Nicole Sackley, "Passage to Modernity: American Social Scientists, India, and the Pursuit of Development, 1945–1961" (Ph.D. dissertation, Princeton University, 2004); Nick Cullather, "Miracles of Modernization: The Green Revolution and the Apotheosis of Technology," *Diplomatic History* 28, no. 2 (2004): 227–254; Cullather, " 'The Target Is the People': Representations of the Village in Modernization and National Security Doctrine," *Cultural Politics* 2, no. 1 (2006): 29–48; Michael E. Latham, *Modernization as Ideology: American Social Science and "Nation Building" in the Kennedy Era* (Chapel Hill: University of North Carolina Press, 2000); see also the essays in Frederick Cooper and Randall Packard, eds., *International Development and the Social Sciences: Essays on the History and Politics of Knowledge* (Berkeley: University of California Press, 1997). For these applied to medical interventions see Randall Packard, " 'No Other Logical Choice': Global Malaria Eradication and the Politics of International Health in the Post-war Era," *Parassitologia* 40 (1998): 217–229, 220; Amrith, *Decolonizing International Health*, 99–120.

44. James C. Scott, *Seeing Like a State: How Certain Schemes to Improve the Human Condition Have Failed* (New Haven: Yale University Press, 1998); Michael Adas, *Dominance by Design: Technological Imperatives and America's Civilizing Mission* (Cambridge, Mass.: Harvard University Press, 2006).

45. "Speech by Dr Johs. Holm as Official Representative of WHO at the Annual General Meeting of the British Tuberculosis Association and the Tuberculosis Society of Scotland in Glasgow, Scotland, 26–29 June 1957," WHO/TBC/Int./40, 13 August 1957, WHO Archives.

46. P. D'Arcy Hart, "Recent Trends in Tuberculosis Research," Spring 1958, FD 1/8772, NAUK.

47. Hart to P. O. Williams, 10 June 1959, FD 1–8773, NAUK.

48. Remarks of Dr. G. Sicault, "How Can the Voluntary Bodies Best Assist in the Global Attack on Tuberculosis: A Panel Discussion Held in Paris on September 20th and 21st 1962," *Bulletin of the International Union Against Tuberculosis* 33, no. 2 (1963): 2–135, 11.

49. Medical Department Circular No. 13/1961, "Control of Tuberculosis," BY/7/174, KNA.

50. G. Canetti, "The Eradication of Tuberculosis: Theoretical Problems and Practical Solutions." *Tubercle* 43 (1962): 301–321, 315, 318, 321.

51. In a generally excellent essay Frank Snowden unfairly calls the era the "age of hubris." Frank M. Snowden, "Emerging and Reemerging Diseases: A Historical Perspective," *Immunological Reviews* 225 (2008): 9–26, esp. 9–12.

CHAPTER 4. PREVENTING TB

1. L. R. Jones, "Tuberculosis Control Through the Indian Service, Read Before the Southwest Indian Education Conference, Ft. Wingate, New Mexico, 31 August 1934," Central Classified Files (hereafter CCF) 58532-34-705 General Service (hereafter GS), Record Group 75, Records of the Bureau of Indian Affairs (hereafter RG 75), National Archives, Washington, D.C. (hereafter NA).

2. Commentary on how little was known concerning Indian health, and its relationship to lack of adequate care, was common; see Joseph A. Murphy (medical director, Bureau of Indian Affairs), "Health Problems of the Indians," *Annals of the American Academy of Political and Social Science* 37, no. 2 (1911): 347. The two major reports on disease among Indians noted the lack of reliable data. See first from 1913: Contagious and Infectious Diseases among the Indians, 62nd Cong., 3rd Sess., S. Doc. 1038, 1913, 72.

Tuberculosis among the North American Indians: Report of a Committee of the National Tuberculosis Association (Sen. Comm. Print, 67th Cong., 4th Sess., 1923) contained reports, in response to a questionnaire, from thirty-nine affiliates of the national organization, state boards of health, and public health agencies; almost none had any statistics on the incidence of TB. The responses of 178 agency physicians and superintendents to the questionnaire were not included. The Meriam Report rightly called this report, despite its length and seeming thoroughness, "somewhat cursory" (Meriam Report, 205). For the Meriam Report's discussion of the problem see pp. 260, 266–270, 273–274. The commissioner of Indian Affairs noted in 1934 that the "statistics on the tuberculosis rate have never been reliable." Annual Report of the Commissioner of Indian Affairs, 1934, 92.

3. J. W. Levy, physician in charge at Yakima Sanitarium, to C. R. Whitlock, Superintendent, CCF 10730–31 Yakima, reel 25, Indian Health and Disease, part 1, Reports on Medical and Nursing Activities (Lexis-Nexis, 2005) (hereafter IHD, part 1). On this point see also Clifford E. Trafzer, *Death Stalks the Yakima: Epidemiological Transitions and Mortality on the Yakama Indian Reservation, 1888–1964* (East Lansing: Michigan State University Press, 1997), 129.

4. J. Arthur Myers and Virginia L. Dustin, "Albert Reifel and Tuberculosis among the American Indians," *Hygeia* (April 1947): 319.

5. J. G. Townsend, Joseph D. Aronson, Robert Saylor, and Irma Parr, "Tuberculosis Control among the North American Indians," *American Review of Tuberculosis* 45, no. 1 (1942): 41, 46.

6. Bertram S. Kraus (with the collaboration of Bonnie M. Jones), *Indian Health in Arizona* (Second Annual Report of the Bureau of Ethnic Research, Department of Anthropology, University of Arizona, 1954), 135–136. For a contemporary example of the importance of epidemiological research in being able to understand and treat disease see Jon Cohen, "Haiti: Making Headway under Hellacious Circumstances," *Science* 313, no. 5786 (28 July 2006): 470–473, on the GHESKIO (Haitian Group for the Study of Kaposi's Sarcoma and Opportunistic Infections) clinic's pioneering AIDS work; see also Nulda Beyers et al., "The Use of Geographical Information System (GIS) to Evaluate the Distribution of Tuberculosis in a High-Incidence Community," *South African Medical Journal* 86, no. 1 (1996): 40; for this point regarding TB and Alaska Natives historically see Nicholas E. Flanders, "Tuberculosis in Western Alaska, 1900–1950," *Polar Record* 23, no. 145 (1987): 383–396.

7. David S. Jones, *Rationalizing Epidemics: Meanings and Uses of American Indian Mortality since 1600* (Cambridge, Mass.: Harvard University Press, 2004), 155–556.

8. Robert A. Trennert, "The Federal Government and Indian Health in the Southwest: Tuberculosis and the Phoenix East Farm Sanatorium, 1909–1955," *Pacific Historical Review* 65, no. 1 (1996): 61–84; for TB hospitals see also Leonard G. Wilson, "The Rise and Fall of Tuberculosis in Minnesota: The Role of Infection," *Bulletin of the History of Medicine* 66 (1992): 43–44. On the growing awareness of TB and the efforts employed by the BIA to combat it see Joseph A. Murphy, M.D., *Manual on Tuberculosis: Its Cause, Prevention and Treatment* (Washington, D.C.: Government Printing Office, 1910). For an overview see Diane T. Putney, "The Tuberculosis Crusade Expands," in "Fighting the Scourge; American Indian Morbidity and Federal Policy, 1897–1928" (Ph.D. dissertation, Marquette University, 1980); for the view that little was done by the BIA to combat TB in the first few decades of the twentieth century see also Todd Benson, "BCG and the Demand for Federal Indian Health Care," in "Race, Health, and Power: The Federal Government and American Indian Health, 1909–1955" (Ph.D. dissertation, Stanford University, 1994), esp. 186–192.

9. Lewis Meriam et al., *The Problem of Indian Administration* (Baltimore: Johns Hopkins University Press, 1928), 207, 10.

10. "Neglectful murder" in Jones, *Rationalizing Epidemics*, 158; Fred T. Foard, "The Federal Government and American Indians' Health," *Journal of the American Medical Association* 142, no. 5 (1950): 328.

11. J. C. Hancock, "Diseases among the Indians," *Southwestern Medicine* 17 (April 1933): 127.

12. For the role of nurses in combating TB see Clifford E. Trafzer, "Medicine Circles Defeating Tuberculosis in Southern California," *Canadian Bulletin of the History Medicine* 23, no. 2 (2006): 489–492.

13. Elinor Gregg to Joseph D. Aronson, 26 October 1936, Central Classified Files (hereafter CCF) 9962-35-705, part 1, GS, box 59, RG 75, NA.

14. Aronson and Long to CIA, 11 November 1935, CCF 9962-35-705 GS, box 59, RG 75, NA. The interest in studying and preventing TB was part of a newfound interest on the part of the BIA in basic medical research, most of which was actually carried out under contract with research physicians affiliated with universities. See *Annual Report of the Secretary of the Interior* (Washington: GPO, 1937), 237–238.

15. For an example of such research, which led to a more accurate picture of TB among the Kiowas, see L. R. Jones, "List of Names of Tuberculous Patients and Report of Their Disposition; Number of Their Contacts and Their Disposition. Kiowa Agency; Miss Abbruzzese' District," 27 November 1939, CCF 1907–39 16096-38-705, Kiowa, reel 1; on locating spreaders and getting an accurate picture of TB as a route to treatment see also Esmond Long to Townsend, 11 July 1938, CCF 55599-37-705, Pine Ridge, reel 2, both in part 2, IHD; on increased sophistication in the epidemiology of Indian TB generally see Esmond R. Long and H. W. Hetherington, "A Tuberculosis Survey of the Papago Indian Area of Southern Arizona," Supplement to the *American Review of Tuberculosis* 33 (March 1936): 407.

16. For the effectiveness and accuracy of x-rays in helping to find cases see Esmond Long to J. G. Townsend, 2 August 1938; for mapping see Esther M. Sandstrom and Violet L. Sobers, Memo on Tuberculosis Spot Map, 12 April 1940; for home visits and mileage see "Tuberculosis Case Finding Survey, 1938," all in CCF 19333-38-705, Navajo, reel 2, IHD, part 2.

17. For tattooing Navajos see Memo from Medical Director, Navajo Area, to Navajo Area Physicians, 17 July 1935; W. W. Peter to Joseph Aronson and Esmond Long, 31 July 1935, both in Surveys/Tuberculosis Control—BCG, Correspondence Relating to Health Surveys, Phoenix Area Office (PAO), RG 75, NA, Laguna Niguel. Linus Pauling famously suggested that carriers of the gene for sickle cell anemia be tattooed across the forehead. See Keith Wailoo, *Dying in the City of Blues: Sickle Cell Anemia and the Politics of Race and Health in America* (Chapel Hill: University of North Carolina Press, 2001), 186.

18. Townsend to Aronson, 7 November 1936, CCF 9962-35-705 GS, RG 75, NA.

19. For BCG's coverage see Alice Zwerling, Marcel A. Behr, Aman Verma, Timothy F. Brewer, Dick Menzies, and Madhukar Pai, "The BCG World Atlas: A Database of Global BCG Vaccination Policies and Practices," *PLoS Medicine* 8, no. 3 (2011): 1–8; George W. Comstock, "Field Trials of Tuberculosis: Vaccines: How Could We Have Done Them Better?" *Controlled Clinical Trials* 15 (1994): 247–276; Graham A. Colditz et al., "Efficacy of BCG Vaccine in the Prevention of Tuberculosis: Meta-analysis of the Published Literature," *Journal of the American Medical Association* 271, no. 9 (1994): 698–702.

20. Ian Sutherland, "State of the Art in Immunoprophylaxis in Tuberculosis," in *Status of Immunization in Tuberculosis: Report of a Conference on Progress to*

Date, Future Trends, and Research Needs (Bethesda: National Institutes of Health, 1971), 113–128, 124.

21. P. Menut, "The Lübeck Catastrophe and Its Consequences for Anti-Tuberculosis BCG-Vaccination," in A. M. Moulin and A. Cambrioso, eds., *Singular Selves: Historical Issues and Contemporary Debates in Immunology* (Paris: Elsevier, 2001), 202–210.

22. Available at http://www.who.int/vaccine_research/diseases/tb/vaccine_development/bcg/en/.

23. G. Kayne, "BCG in Western Europe," *American Review of Tuberculosis* 33 (1936): 10–42, 10.

24. H. G. ten Dam, "Research on BCG Vaccination," *Advances in Tuberculosis Research* 21 (1984): 79–106, 79.

25. On the controversies surrounding BCG see Linda Bryder, " 'We Shall Not Find Salvation in Inoculation': BCG Vaccination in Scandinavia, Britain and the USA, 1921–1960," *Social Science and Medicine* 49, no. 9 (1999): 1157–1167; Georgina Feldberg, *Disease and Class: Tuberculosis and the Shaping of North American Society* (New Brunswick: Rutgers University Press, 1995), especially chapters 4–6.

26. Charles Nagel to CIA, 3 September 1933, CCF 403051933–700 Ft. Belknap; M. C. Guthrie to Kendall Emerson, 16 November 1933, CCF 9962-35-705 GS, RG 75, NA.

27. L. R. Jones, "A Few Salient Points Concerning Its [BCG] Application to the Children of a People Whose Environment Is so Unusual as Is Found in the Navajo Area," 20 Febraury 1935, CCG 58532-34-705 GS, RG 75, NA.

28. Jones to Townsend, 11 February 1935, CCF 58532-35-705, RG 75, NA.

29. L. R. Jones, "Recommendations for Continuation and Expansion of the Tuberculosis Control Program in the Indian Service," 28 October 1935, CCF 585-32-35-705 GS, RG 75, NA.

30. Heterick to Townsend, 22 October 1935, CCF 996235–705 GS, part I, RG 75, NA.

31. L. R. Jones, "Recommendations for Continuation and Expansion of the Tuberculosis Control Campaign in the Indian Service," 28 October 1935, CCG 58532-34-705 GS, RG 75, NA.

32. See Todd Benson, "BCG and the Demand for Federal Indian Health Care," 205–225.

33. W. W. Peter to CIA, 19 February 1935, CCF 9962-35-705 GS, part I, RG 75, NA.

34. Esmond Long, "Report of the Committee on B.C.G. in the Navajo Area," 15 May 1935, CCF 9962-35-705, RG 75, NA.

35. La Farge to Haven Emerson, director of the National Tuberculosis Association, 14 December 1935, reel 3, Papers of the American Association on Indian Affairs (hereafter AAIA Papers).

36. Sniffen to La Farge, 23 December 1935, reel 3, AAIA Papers. On the failed trachoma experimental treatment see Todd Benson, "Blinded with Science: American Indians, the Office of Indian Affairs, and the Federal Campaign against Trachoma, 1924–1927," *American Indian Culture and Research Journal* 23, no. 3 (1999): 119–142.

37. Townsend to La Farge, 3 January 1936, reel 3, AAIA Papers.

38. W. W. Peter to CIA, 19 February 1935; see also Esmond Long's comments in the "Report of the Committee on BCG in the Navajo Area," 15 May 1936, both in CCF 9962-35-705 GS, RG 75, NA.

39. Long to White, 18 October 1935, CCG 9962-35-705 GS, RG 75, NA.

40. Memo to CIA from Aronson, 8 November 1935, CCF 9962-35-705 GS, RG 75, NA.

41. Townsend to W. W. Peter, 1 August 1935; W. W. Peter to Lloyd Arnold, 28 January 1936, both in CCF 9962-705-35, part 1, GS, box 59, RG 75, NA. For a thorough examination of the TB program among the Navajos, including their being left out of the BCG trial, see Sandra Varney MacMahon, "Tuberculosis among the Navajos in the 1930s: Disease and Politics," in "Tuberculosis, the Navajos, and Western Healthcare Providers, 1920–1960" (Ph.D. dissertation, University of New Mexico, 2003).

42. For choosing Pima and Shoshone, as well as getting tribal council support, see Memo to CIA from Aronson, "Recommendations for the Study of the Control of Tuberculosis among Indians," 8 November 1935; for Aronson's and Long's interest in the qualities noted above see Memo to CIA from Long and Aronson, "Outline of a Tuberculosis Control Program," 19 November 1935; on getting tribal council support at Pima see Gertrude Sturges to CIA, 16 December 1935; see also Aronson to Townsend, 8 January 1936; for comparative value as they considered moving into Alaska see Townsend to Long, 12 August 1936, all in CCF 9962-705-35, part 1, GS, box 59, RG 75, NA.

43. On the difficulties of setting up a trial in Europe and the controversy over BCG there see Clifford Rosenberg, "The International Politics of Vaccine Testing in Interwar Algiers," *American Historical Review* 117, no. 3 (2012): 671–697.

44. Herbert A. Burns, "Tuberculosis in the Indian," *American Review of Tuberculosis* 26 (1932): 498.

45. For this concern see especially Long to L. W. White, Asst. to the Dir. of Health, 18 October 1935, CCF 9962-705-35, part 1, GS, box 59, RG 75, NA.

46. J. G. Townsend, "Report on the Tuberculosis Program in the United States Indian Service," August 1943, CCF 1907–39 4405-34-705, GS, box 58. The TB research program could be put to political ends, too. Three years later, when the American Medical Association was investigating the poor state of Indian health and the BIA was under increasing fire for its neglect of disease—and feared losing control of medical matters to the PHS—the bureau hoped to use the TB research as an example of at least one thing it had done right. See Memo from John Provinse to Ralph Snavely, 3 October 1947, CCF 1940–57 3832-45-705, GS, box 1129, both in RG 75, NA.

47. For Emerson, see minutes of a meeting on BCG, 11 May 1936, CCF 9962-705-35, part 1, GS, RG 75, NA.

48. 17 March 1939, Aronson to H. Muench, Rockefeller Foundation, CCG 9963-35-705 GS, RG 75, NA; on Shah's experience in the United States see S. R. A Shah, "Modern Measures in the Mass Control of Tuberculosis in the United States of America," *Indian Medical Gazette* 75 (October 1940): 617–624.

49. Aronson to Townsend, 2 December 1939, CCG 9962-35-705, GS, RG 75, NA.

50. Aronson to Carroll Palmer, 23 September 1946, CCF 1940–57 9698-45-705, GS, RG 75, NA.

51. For Long's reporting on Indian BCG work see remarks of Esmond Long in *Tuberculosis in the Commonwealth, 1947: Complete Transactions of the Commonwealth and Empire Health and Tuberculosis Conference* (London: National Association for the Prevention of Tuberculosis, 1947), 148–153. See also Joseph D. Aronson and Charlotte Ferguson Aronson, "Appraisal of Protective Value of BCG Vaccine," *Journal of the American Medical Association* 149, no. 4 (1952): 335.

52. Aronson to Townsend 5 August 1936; Townsend to Aronson, 12 August 1936; Townsend to Long, 12 August 1936; Long to Townsend, 19 August 1936; Townsend to Aronson, 24 August 1936; Memo to Dr. Townsend from John Collier, 28 August 1936, CCF 9962-705-35, part 1, GS, box 59, RG 75, NA.

53. Esmong Long to Townsend, 18 March 1937, CCF 9962-305-705, part 1, GS, NARA. I am not providing box numbers because many files were reboxed during and since my research. File numbers do not change, and so these documents can be found via file number.

54. For the numbers see BCG meeting minutes, 11 May 1938, CCF 9962-35-705, GS, RG 75, NA.

55. For expanding the program see discussion in BCG meeting, 11 May 1938, CCG 9962-35-705, GS, RG 75, NA.

56. Miriam Brailey to Townsend, 17 May 1938, CCF 9962-35-705, GS, RG 75, NA.

57. J. D. Aronson and C. E. Palmer, "Experience with BCG Vaccine in the Control of Tuberculosis among North American Indians," *Public Health Reports* 61 (1946): 802–820, 819.

58. Joseph D. Aronson, "Protective Vaccination against Tuberculosis with Special Reference to BCG Vaccination" *American Review of Tuberculosis* 58, no. 3 (1948): 255–281, 264.

59. On the decline of TB between 1955 and 1982 see H. L. Rieder, "Tuberculosis among American Indians of the Contiguous United States," *Public Health Reports* 104, no. 6 (1989): 653–657; see also Albert Reifel, "Tuberculosis among Indians of the United States," *Diseases of the Chest* 16, no. 2 (1949): 234–247, table 1 on 235. Feldberg discusses this issue; see *Disease and Class*, 171.

60. Aronson, "Protective Vaccination," 267–268.

61. On some of these methodological points see Carroll Palmer and Lawrence Shaw, "Present Status of BCG Studies," *American Review of Tuberculosis* 68, no. 3 (1953): 462–466.

62. See tables in Aronson to Townsend, 6 January 1940, CCG 9962-35-705, GS, RG 75, NA.

63. Joseph D. Aronson and Helen C. Taylor, "The Trend of Tuberculous Infection among Some Indian Tribes and the Influence of BCG Vaccination on the Tuberculin Test," *American Review of Tuberculosis* 72, no. 1 (1955): 35–52, 49.

64. J. G. Townsend, J. D. Aronson, R. Saylor, and I. Parr, "Tuberculosis Control among the North American Indians," *American Review of Tuberculosis* 45 (1942): 41–52, 47.

65. Aronson and Taylor, "The Trend of Tuberculous Infection among Some Indian Tribes," 47.

66. J. R. McGibony and A. W. Dahlstrom, "Tuberculosis among Montana Indians," *American Review of Tuberculosis* 52 (1945): 104–120.

67. J. D. Aronson, C. F. Aronson, and H. C. Taylor, "A Twenty-Year Appraisal of BCG Vaccination in the Control of Tuberculosis," *Archives of Internal Medicine* 101, no. 5 (1958): 881–893, 892.

68. Aronson, Aronson, and Taylor, "A Twenty-Year Appraisal," 892.

CHAPTER 5. BCG GOES GLOBAL

1. Joseph Aronson to Director of Health, Office of Indian Affairs, 19 April 1946, Central Classified Files (hereafter CCF), 3832-45-705, Record Group 75 (hereafter RG 75), National Archives, Washington, D.C. (hereafter NA).

2. So, too, did R.G. Ferguson's BCG studies, though they seem to have been less influential than Aronson's based on the frequency with which Aronson was cited and the infrequency of citations to Ferguson. R. G. Ferguson and A. B. Simes, "BCG Vaccination of Indian Infants in Saskatchewan," *Tubercle* 30, no. 1 (1949): 5–11.

3. Hugh Stott, "B.C.G. Vaccination in Kenya," no date but filed with papers in 1950, CO 927-181-5; Wilcocks, "A Note on the Possible Use of BCG Vaccine in the Colonies," CO 859-210-6, National Archives of the United Kingdom (hereafter NAUK). See also Haynes and Stott, "Preliminary Investigation into the Use of BCG in Kenya," *Tubercle* 32, no. 6 (1951): 127–136, 129.

4. Santon Gilmour, "Tuberculosis in Uganda: A Short Survey," 1950, CO 822-140-1, NAUK.

5. Dr. F. Retief, "Tuberculosis Conference—King George 5th Hospital—Durban, Monday, 10th November to Friday 14th November, 1952," Pad 2: "Diseases and Epidemics, Tuberculosis," Witwatersrand Native Labour Association Archives, TEBA collection, University of Johannesburg, South Africa.

6. There are several reviews of the early history of BCG and the debates over its efficacy. The most recent, and the best at discussing the work done in French, is Clifford Rosenberg, "The International Politics of Vaccine Testing in Interwar Algiers," *American Historical Review* 117, no. 3 (2012): 671–697.

7. J. B. McDougall, *Tuberculosis: A Global Study in Social Pathology* (Baltimore: Williams and Wilkins, 1949), 390. Linda Bryder, "'We Shall Not Find Salvation in Inoculation': BCG Vaccination in Scandinavia, Britain and the USA, 1921–1960," *Social Science and Medicine* 49 (1999): 1158–1159.

8. William Johnston, *The Modern Epidemic: A History of Tuberculosis in Japan,* Harvard East Asian Monographs 162 (Cambridge, Mass.: Harvard University Press, 1995), 258–259; on Jamaica see John Farley, *To Cast Out Disease: A History of the International Health Division of the Rockefeller Foundation (1913–1951)* (New York: Oxford University Press, 2004), 185–89; Proceedings of the First Inter-American Congress of Public Health, 26 September–1 October 1952, Havana, Cuba; on China see Dr. Marcel Junod,

Chief UNICEF China Mission, Nanking, "B.C.G. Campaign in China," 14 May 1948, CF/RA/BX/N9/PD/F/RG/1983/T040, UNICEF Archives; on Peru see "Preliminary Report by Prof. C. Gyllensward on Visit to Peru Regarding BCG Work," 30 April 1949, CF/RA/BX/PD/1947/T024, UNICEF Archives; on Vietnam see Laurence Monnais, "Preventive Medicine and 'Mission Civilisatrice': Uses of the BCG Vaccine in French Colonial Vietnam between the Two World Wars," *International Journal of Asia Pacific Studies* 2, no. 1 (2006): 40–66.

9. J. Cerf et al., "Premiers résultats de la vaccination BCG indiscriminée à Léopoldville," *Annales de la Société Belge de Médecine Tropicale* 40, no. 3 (1960): 457–468; on Tanganyika see MacMichaal, Governor of Tanganyika to Philip Cunliffe-Lister, Sec. of State for the Colonies, 21 December 1934, CO 691-143-4, NAUK; on South Africa see Peter Allan, Medical Superintendent, Kelsport Sanatorium to Sec. for Public Health, Cape Town, 2 February 1926, Witwatersrand Native Labour Association archives, TEBA collection, University of Johannesburg.

10. Charles Wilcocks, "A Note on the Possible Use of the BCG Vaccine in the Colonies," 1 May 1950, CO 858-210-6, NAUK.

11. R. Neubauer, "Report on Visit to West and Central African Territories," October–December 1953, DC-TB-AFRO, WHO Archives, Geneva, pp. 1, 33–34. He noted a "small tuberculin testing and BCG vaccination campaign" in Congo-Brazzaville.

12. E. Sergent et al., "Prémunition antituberuleuse par le BCG: Campagne con-trôlée poursuivie à Alger depuis 1935," *Archives de L'Institut Pasteur d'Algérie* 38, no. 2 (1960): 131–137; Rosenberg, "The International Politics of Vaccine Testing in Interwar Algiers."

13. The quotes are from International Tuberculosis Campaign, "The What, How and Why of the International Tuberculosis Campaign," 1 December 1948, first quote on 12, second on 13, Far East, BCG, CF/RA/BX/ PD/1947/T012, UNICEF Archives; for the figure of seventeen million see "International Tuberculosis Campaign: Fours Years of Work on Five Continents," *United Nations Bulletin* 11, no. 5 (1951): 232–234.

14. Niels Brimnes, "Vikings against Tuberculosis: The International Tuberculosis Campaign in India, 1948–1951," *Bulletin of the History of Medicine* 81, no. 2 (2007): 407–430, 409; see also George Comstock, "The International Tuberculosis Campaign: A Pioneering Venture in Mass Vaccination and Research," *Clinical Infectious Diseases* 19, no. 3 (1994): 528–540.

15. G. S. Wilson, "The Value of B.C.G. Vaccination in Control of Tuberculosis," *British Medical Journal* 2, no. 4534 (1947): 855–859, 855.

16. G. Kayne, "BCG in Western Europe," *American Review of Tuberculosis* 33 (1936): 10–42, 11.

17. See Bryder, "We Shall Not Find Salvation," and Feldberg, *Disease and Class*, 176–207; R. J. Anderson and C. E. Palmer, "BCG," *Journal of the American Medical Association* 143 (1950): 1048.

18. My argument owes a debt to Niels Brimnes's superb work on the history of BCG. See his essential "BCG Vaccination and WHO's Global Strategy for Tuberculosis Control 1948–1983," *Social Science and Medicine* 67, no. 5 (2008): 863–873.

19. Frasier to Pate, 7 August 1950, UNICEF Archives.

20. Carroll Palmer to Maurice Pate, UNICEF, 15 January 1952, BCG General, 1952–53, A649, LF-NYH–05, UNICEF Archives.

21. Hugh Stott, "BCG Vaccination Trial in Kenya," 1950 (no precise date), CO 927-181-5, NAUK.

22. Brock Chisholm to C. Man, Dir. Regional Office for Southeast Asia, 11 February 1952, BCG General, 1952–53, A649, LF-NYH–05, UNICEF Archives.

23. Halfdan Mahler, 3rd Quarterly Report, India-BCG Project, 20 October 1953, Programme Division, Asia Region, CF/RA/BX/PD/1962/T0008. UNICEF Archives.

CHAPTER 6. QUESTIONING BCG

1. Portions of this chapter have been published in Christian W. McMillen and Niels Brimnes, "Medical Modernization and Medical Nationalism: Resistance to Mass Tuberculosis Vaccination in Postcolonial India, 1948–1955," *Comparative Studies in Society and History* 52, no. 1 (2010): 180–209.

2. Johannes Holm, "Report on a Visit to India, February–April, 1951," Programme Division—Asia-General, CF/RA/BX/PD/1947/T021; on the importance of India for the success of other programs see also B. Fraser to Myron Schmittlinger, 18 July 1950, BCG-General, 1949–1950, A648, LF-WYH–05, UNICEF Archives. For the view that research with controlled trials was desired, but that "attempts of this kind are often opposed as 'experimenting' on human beings," see I-Chin Yuan and Carroll E. Palmer, "The WHO Tuberculosis Research Office: A Review of the First Four Years," *Public Health Reports* 68, no. 7 (July 1953): 679.

3. There was organized, local resistance at the sites of vaccination in Iraq: see J. K. Henriksen, "The UNICEF/WHO/Iraq BCG campaign in Iraq (Iraq 10): Evaluation and Assessment Report, April 1952–August 1954, in Iraq-BCG-1954-55, Program Division, Eastern Mediterranean, Subject Files, 1952–56, CF/RA/BX/PD/1962/T024; in Vietnam there was an organized newspaper campaign: see Dr. M. Gauthier, "Final Report on the BCG Campaign in Vietnam, 30 June 1956, Vietnam-BCG, Program Division, Subject Files, Asia Region, CF/RA/BX/PD/1962/T080; for Mexico see L. Eloesser, "Notes Mexico-January 20 to February 15, 1951 (Confidential)," Mexico-BCG, Program Division, Latin America Region, CF/RA/BX/PD/1962/T145, UNICEF Archives.

4. David Arnold, "Cholera and Colonialism in British India," *Past and Present* 113 (1986): 118–151, 147, 149.

5. David Arnold, *Colonizing the Body: State Medicine and Epidemic Disease in Nineteenth-Century India* (Berkeley: University of California Press 1993), 139–144; Sanjoy Bhattacharya, Mark Harrison, and Michael Worboys, *Fractured States: Smallpox, Public Health and Vaccination Policy in British India 1800–1947* (New Delhi: Orient Longman, 2005), 52–69, 203–225.

6. Veena Das and Abhikit Dasgupta, "Scientific and Political Representations: Cholera Vaccine in India," *Economic and Political Weekly* (19–26 February 2000): 633–644; Sarah K. Wallace, "Global Health in Conflict: Understanding Opposition to Vitamin A Supplementation in India," *American Journal of Public Health* 102, no. 7 (2012): 1286–1297. See also Sanjoy Bhattacharya, *Expunging Variola: The Control and Eradication of Smallpox in India, 1947–1977* (New Delhi: Orient Longman, 2006), 230–247, especially 237–238; P. Greenough, "Intimidation, Coercion and Resistance in the Final Stages of the South Asian Smallpox Eradication Campaign, 1973–1975," *Social Science and Medicine* 41, no. 5 (1995): 633–645, particularly 638.

7. These figures were routinely referred to around 1950. See, for instance, *Report of the Health Survey and Development Committee* (Calcutta: Government of India Press, 1946), vol. I, 97.

8. Mark Harrison and Michael Worboys, "A Disease of Civilisation: Tuberculosis in Britain, Africa and India, 1900–39," in Lara Marks and Michael Worboys, eds., *Migrants, Minorities and Health: Historical and Contemporary Studies* (London: Routledge, 1997), 113–114. Brimnes, "Vikings," 414–415.

9. Undated Press Note (but the note is accompanied by a covering letter dated 28 May 1948). Tamil Nadu State Archive (hereafter TNSA), Health Department, no. 809, 1950.

10. *Second Annual Report of the International Tuberculosis Campaign* (Copenhagen: ITC, n.d.) 47–48. J. Frimodt Moller, "Second Report on the Tuberculosis Survey at Madanapalle," *Proceedings of the Seventh Tuberculosis Workers Conference Held in Bombay November 1949* (n.p.: n.d.), 80.

11. Not much is known about Raman. Apparently he was a long-standing servant of the Madras government and had a close relationship to Congress leadership. He claimed to have been influential in directing Gandhi's attention to sanitation in the 1920s. The magazine *People's Health* seems very much to have been his own enterprise. See A. V. Raman to C. Rajagopalachari, 2 October 1948, and C. Rajagopalachari to A. V. Raman, 15 September 1949. Installment V, Correspondence with: *People's Health*, editor of, Rajaji Papers, Jawarlahal Nehru Memorial Library, New Delhi (hereafter RP).

12. I shall refer to the government of India in New Delhi as the Union government in order to distinguish it from the government of the Madras Province, which in 1950 became the State of Madras.

13. *People's Health*, vol. III, no. 2, 53. The expert was not from ITC. It is more likely that reference is made to a WHO consultant present when BCG was first used in India in August 1948.

14. *People's Health*, vol. III, no. 5, 195.

15. See for instance the *Hindu*, 14 February 1949. Articles that referred to Raman's critique of BCG from the *Indian Express, Nagpur Times*, and *Sunday Times* were all reproduced in *People's Health*, vol. III, 5, 206–208.

16. *Indian Express*, 5 February 1949, in *People's Health*, vol. III, no. 5, 198. See also the *Hindu*, 5 February 1949. It should be noted that newspaper articles were reproduced in *People's Health* with reference to the day they were written, not the day of publication. Here, it is generally assumed that they appeared in the newspaper the day after they were written.

17. *Hindu*, 14 February 1949, in *People's Health*, vol. III, no. 5, 204.

18. Ibid. Emphasis in original.

19. *Hindu*, 14 February 1949, in *People's Health*, vol. III, no. 5, 205.

20. *Hindu*, 16 February 1949, in *People's Health*, vol. III, no. 5, 212. See also *Madras Mail*, 16 February 1949.

21. See, for instance, Elizabeth TenBroek, "The BCG Campaign in India," *People's Health*, vol. III, no. 11, 499–510.

22. *People's Health*, vol. IV, no. 2, 56. Palmer quote: American "Public Health Abstract," 7 October 1949. The phrase "uninformed criticism" was used by

the Union Minister of Health Rajkumari Amrit Kaur to describe the opposition to BCG.

23. Editorial, *People's Health*, vol. I, no. 1, 4.

24. *People's Health*, vol. IV, no. 11, 459.

25. Speeches in *People's Health*, vol. III, no. 5, 213–226. See also *Hindu*, 17 February 1949.

26. *People's Health*, vol. III, no. 5, 222. That BCG could not stand alone in the effort to control TB had always been the official position of the WHO. See, for instance, "Expert Committee on Tuberculosis: Report of the Fourth Session," WHO Technical Report Series, 7 (1950), 19.

27. Editorial, *People's Health*, vol. III, no. 5, 188–189.

28. Amrith, *Decolonizing International Health* (London: Palgrave Macmillan, 2006), 57–63. John Farley, *Bilharzia: A History of Imperial Tropical Medicine* (Cambridge: Cambridge University Press, 1991), 179.

29. *Report of the Health Survey and Development Committee*, vol. II, 1–2.

30. Ibid., vol. II, 3. For the advice to plan boldly, see vol. I, 2.

31. Ibid., vol. II, 3–4.

32. Ibid., vol. II, 159.

33. Ibid., vol. II, 7.

34. *People's Health*, vol. III, no. 5, 203–204.

35. Warwick Anderson has argued that vaccination—although often seen as epitomizing the interventionist aspirations of the colonial state—was in fact a very limited intervention compared to other hygienic measures. Warwick Anderson, "Immunization and Hygiene in the Colonial Philippines," *Journal of the History of Medicine and Allied Sciences* 62, no. 1 (2007): 1–20.

36. *People's Health*, vol. IV, no. 2, 46. The expression "black magic" first appeared in an unpublished letter to Henry S. L. Polak, 14 October 1909, see *Collected Works of Mahatma Gandhi* (hereafter CWMG), vol. IX, 479. Gandhi later used the expression several times in more public statements. See CWMG, vol. XIX, 357, and vol. LXV, 361.

37. For a reading of Gandhi that highlights his opposition to Western medicine see David Arnold, *Colonizing the Body*, 285–288. For treatments that mention Gandhi's acceptance of elements of science—although with an emphasis on nutrition rather than sanitation—see Joseph S. Alter, *Gandhi's Body: Sex, Diet and the Politics of Nationalism* (Philadelphia: University of Pennsylvania Press, 2000), 3–27, and Amrith, *Decolonizing International Health*, 32–36.

38. "Speech at Opening of Tibbi College," Delhi, *Bombay Chronicle*, 15 February 1921, in CWMG, vol. XIX, 358. See also Shamsad Khan, "Systems

of Medicine and Nationalist Discourse in India: Towards 'New Horizons' in Medical Anthropology and History," *Social Science and Medicine* 62 (2006): 2786–2797.

39. "General Knowledge about Health—XXIV," *Indian Opinion*, 14 June 1913, in CWMG, vol. XII, 111. Letter to Manilal and Sushila Gandhi, 30 June 1929, in CWMG, vol. XLI, 146. While Gandhi was referring specifically to vaccination against smallpox, the term "vaccination" in the public debate referred to the injection of various immunizing agents into the body. Also, BCG was based on bacteria from bovine tuberculosis and thus—like the smallpox vaccine—was a product derived from the cow.

40. See, for instance, "Speech at Opening of Tibbi College, Delhi," *Bombay Chronicle*, 15 February 1921, in CWMG, vol. XIX, 357.

41. "Smallpox and Cholera," *Navajivan*, 30 June 1929, in CWMG, vol. XLI, 141.

42. Svend K. Svendsen, "Indberetning om The International Tuberculosis Campaign i Indien og Ceylon," 13 March 1949, *Svenska Röda Korsets Arkiv. Internationella Avdeling. Tuberkulos bekämmandet 1947–51. Overstyreslsens Tuberkuloskommittee B*, vol. 2. Riksarkivet, Stockholm. Translation courtesy of Niels Brimnes.

43. Quoted in *Hindustan Times*, 22 April 1949.

44. Handwritten note and memorandum of 4 June 1949. Health Department, no. 2617, 1949, TNSA.

45. T. S. S. Rajan was a Congress veteran, minister for public health in Madras from 1949 and clearly more skeptical toward BCG than his colleague A. B. Shetty, who was health minister in the same government. On Rajan, see http://www.thehindu.com/2003/10/28/stories/2003102800001900.htm.

46. Rajan to Benjamin, typed-up draft letter, 15 October 1949. Health Department, no. 1313, 1950, TNSA.

47. Note written by Additional Secretary, Public Health Department, 5 October 1949. Health Department, no. 1313, 1950, TNSA.

48. C. Mani to Dr. James McDougal, 1? October 1949, Tuberculosis: Collaboration with Regional Offices, South East Asia Region, File 458/13/2, WHO Archives, Geneva.

49. Letter no. 1461, Ministry of Health, Government of Madras to Government of India, 26 April 1950. Health Department, no. 1461, 1950, TNSA.

50. "Draft Plan of Operations—for Continuation and Expansion of BCG Vaccination Programme in India during 1952 and 1953." Health Department, no. 1216, 1953, TNSA.

51. ITC ceased to operate in India on 30 June 1951, but WHO and UNICEF continued the enterprise on roughly the same lines.

52. Mahler, "Final Report on India BCG," 36, India-BCG, FEP 30, 1955, Program Division, Asia Region, CF/RA/BX/PD/1962/T008, UNICEF Archives.

53. Mahler, Quarterly Field Report, 1st Quarter, 1954, India BCG Project, 23 April 1954; Inger Mundt-Petersen, WHO BCG Nurse, "Final Report: BCG Work in India, 5 May 1954–31 December 1955," both in India-BCG, FEP 30, 1955, Program Division, Asia Region, CF/RA/BX/PD/1962/T071, UNICEF Archives. UNICEF headquarters was aware of the potential dangers of anti-BCG sentiment. See U.N. Economic and Social Council, "India: Recommendation of the Executive Director for Continuation and Expansion of the BCG Anti-Tuberculosis Vaccination Campaign," E/ICEF/L.597, 13 July 1954. On "Birth Control Germ" being a popular epithet as well as the belief that BCG was being used to sterilize young Indians see Kul Bhushan, "My Experience of Mass BCG Campaign," *Bulletin Devoted to the Prevention of Tuberculosis* 9 (1964): 12–14, 17–18.

54. Mahler, India BCG 2nd Quarterly Field Report, 11 August 1954, India-BCG, FEP 30, 1954, Program Division, Asia Region, CF/RA/BX/PD/1962/T008, UNICEF Archives.

55. See Mahler, India BCG Project, 3rd Quarterly Report, 1953, 20 October 1953.

56. In a private letter, Raman described himself as "one, who has ruined one's own health in an attempt to serve People's Health." A. V. Raman to C. Rajagopalachari, 15 March 1951. Installment V, Correspondence with: People's Health, editor of, RP.

57. Poul Larsen, "Report on the Annual BCG Conference in India Held at Coimbatore on 13th November 1954, and the Inauguration of the Mass BCG Campaign in the State of Madras," CF/RA/BX/PD/1962/T008, UNICEF Archives.

58. Mahler, India BCG 4th Quarterly Field Report, 20 January 1955, India-BCG, FEP 30, 1954, Program Division, Asia Region, CF/RA/BX/PD/1962/T008, UNICEF Archives.

59. On public health campaigns as responses to crises and thus not part of most Indians' experience see Bhattacharya, *Expunging Variola*, 63.

60. "Minister Deplores Mass Hysteria against B.C.G.," *Indian Express*, 20 August 1955.

61. A. M. Rosenthal, "Indian Battles TB Vaccine Critic; Struggle May Affect Health Drive," *New York Times*, 3 September 1955, A3.

62. Poul Larsen to Brian Jones, 13 September 1955, India-BCG, FEP 30, 1955, Program Division, Asia Region, CF/RA/BX/PD/1962/T008, UNICEF Archives.

63. Amrith, *Decolonizing International Health*, 141–142; for greater India figures see Poul Larsen to T. G. Davies, 17 September 1955, India-BCG, FEP 30, 1955, Program Division, Asia Region, CF/RA/BX/PD/1962/T008, UNICEF Archives. For the precipitous decline in numbers caused by the anti-BCG forces see also U.N. Economic and Social Council, "Recommendation to the Executive Director for an Allocation-India-BCG Anti-Tuberculosis Campaign," E/ICEF/L.939, 29 August 1956.

64. I. N. Saxena to C. Rajagopalachari, 30 July 1955, Installment V, Subject File 135, RP.

65. "Rapport for the Third Quarter of 1955 for the Work in the BCG Campaign of India by Inger Mundt-Petersen, BCG-Nurse," India-BCG, Program Division, Asia Region, CF/RA/BX/PD/1962/T008, UNICEF Archives.

66. [Illegible], Secretary of the Reddy Young Men's Association, to Rajaji, 1 August 1955, RP.

67. "Rapport for the Third Quarter of 1955 by Inger Mundt-Petersen, BCG-Nurse."

68. Benifrasad Bansal to Rajaji, 9 August 1955, RP.

69. See M. Beddow-Bayly to Rajaji, 5 December 1956, Installment V, Subject File 138, RP; M. Beddow-Bayly, "B.C.G. Vaccination Deflated," November 1956; Beddow-Bayly, "B.C.G. Vaccination: Why You Should Wait before Having Your Child Tested and Vaccinated," *Anti-Vivisection News*, April 1954. For news of Rajaji's movement in England see also "Sixtieth Annual Report of the National Anti-Vaccination League, Report for the Year 1955," 13; see also D. C. Desai to Rajaji, 6 September 1955, Installment V, Subject File 135, RP. Though Desai was government inspector of railways in Bangalore he was also a member of the Anti-Vaccination League of London. Similar links with antivaccinationist bodies in Britain were forged in the first half of the twentieth century, when Indians opposed vaccinations against smallpox. See Bhattacharya, Harrison, and Worboys, *Fractured States*, 214–217.

70. "Keeper of My Conscience," in Ramachandra Guha, "The Wisest Man in India: Aspects of C. Rajagopalachari," in Guha, *The Last Liberal and Other Essays* (New Delhi: Permanent Black, 2004), 34.

71. Rajmohan Gandhi, *The Rajaji Story, 1937–1972*, vol. 2 (Bombay: Bharatiya Vidya Bhavan, 1984), 258. The friendship between Raman and Rajagopalachari might also help to explain why Raman's opposition died down around the time Rajagopalachari assumed control of the Madras government.

72. Rajagopalachari to R. Amrit Kaur, 23 May 1952. Health Department, no. 1216, 1953, TNSA.

73. Rajmohan Gandhi, *The Rajaji Story;* A. R. H. Copley, *The Political Career of C. Rajagopalachari, 1937–54: A Moralist in Politics* (Madras: Macmillan Company of India, 1978).

74. P. Parkash [sp.?], M.A. to the B. Advocate to Rajaji, 9 August 1955, Installment V, Subject File 135, RP.

75. P. Mohamed Ali, 20 July 1955, Quarterly Field Report, 2nd Quarter 1955, India BCG Project, India-BCG, FEP 30, 1955, Program Division, Asia Region, CF/RA/BX/PD/1962/T008, UNICEF Archives. For Rajaji's embrace of English and other aspects of his modernity see Antony Copley, "The Indo-British Encounter: Perspectives of an Indian Conservative," *20th Century Studies* 10 (December 1973): 63, 60–75.

76. N. K. Iyengar, "B.C.G.," 23 June 1955, *Statesman*.

77. N. K. Iyengar to Rajaji, 2 July 1955, Installment V, Subject File 135, RP.

78. [Illegible] to Reverend Rajaji, 5 September 1955, Installment V, Subject File 135, RP.

79. S. Soundararajan to Rajaji, 3 August 1955, Installment V, Subject File 135, RP.

80. T. V. Subramanian to Rajaji, 30 July 1955, Installment V, Subject File 135, RP.

81. S. R. Srinivasa Raghavan to Rajaji, 6 September 1955, Installment V, Subject File 135, RP.

82. Rajagopalachari to R. Amrit Kaur, 23 May 1952. Health Department, no. 1216, 1953, TNSA.

83. Rajkumari Amrit Kaur to Rajaji, 5 June 1952, Installments VI–XI, Subject File 28, RP.

84. *Hindu*, 8 May and 23 November 1955.

85. *Hindu*, 8 May 1955. Raman, who leaned much more on Gandhian positions, did express some skepticism toward vaccination against smallpox. See *People's Health*, vol. III, no. 5, 191.

86. As reported in the *Hindu*, 17 May and 1 July 1955.

87. C. Rajagopalachari, *B.C.G. Vaccination—Why I Oppose It* (Madras: Jupiter Press, 1955), 6.

88. K. S. Ranganathan, "The Principles of B.C.G. Vaccination," Indian Medical Forum, February 1950, 57–60; Ranganathan, "First Results of Mass Vaccination with B.C.G.," *Indian Medical Gazette*, February 1952, 62–69.

89. *Hindu*, 16 June 1955.

90. Ibid., 3 July 1955.

91. Ibid., 22 July 1955.

92. Ibid., 28 July 1955.

93. Ibid., 3 August 1955.

94. *Truth about B.C.G.: Why Government Have Launched a Mass Campaign* (Director of Information and Publicity, Government of Madras, 1955).

95. Ibid., 7.

96. Ibid., 8. Frimodt-Moller's statement from 3 August was printed in extenso as an appendix to the pamphlet, see 25–26.

97. C. Rajagopalachari, *B.C.G. Vaccination—Why I Oppose It*, 9.

98. *Truth about B.C.G.*, 9–10, where the following is cited: Carroll E. Palmer, "B.C.G. Vaccination and Tuberculin Allergy," *Lancet* 259, no. 6715 (10 May 1952): 935–940, see esp. 940.

99. Carroll E. Palmer, "Dr. Palmer on BCG," *Bulletin: Dedicated to the Prevention of Tuberculosis* (Issued by the Tuberculosis Section, Directorate General of Health Services, Ministry of Health, Government of India, New Delhi, December 1956), 7; see also *Truth about B.C.G.*, 8–9; for Rajaji's original use of Palmer see *B.C.G. Vaccination—Why I Oppose It*, 25.

100. Resolution included in Dr. Ved Prakash Khanna to Rajaji, 10 August 1955, Installment VI, Subject File 136; for an early example see Vinayakarao Bapat, "B.C.G. Vaccination and Prevention of Tuberculosis According to Ayurveda," pamphlet reprinted from *Medical Digest*, no date, Installments VI–XI, Subject File 25, RP.

101. Ralph C. Croizer, "Medicine, Modernization, and Cultural Crisis in China and India," *Comparative Studies in Society and History* 12, no. 3 (1970): 275–291.

102. A. B. Parisad to Rajaji, 12 August 1955, Installment V, Subject File 136, RP.

103. Dr. T. R. Savan to Rajaji, 31 July 1955, Installment V, Subject File 135, RP.

104. Second quote: Rajaji to Rajkumari Amrit Kaur, 10 June 1955, Installments VI–XI, Subject File 28, RP.

105. "Efficacy of B.C.G.," 20 August 1955, *Hindu;* "Minister Deplores Mass Hysteria against B.C.G.," 20 August 1955, *Indian Express*.

106. See the following documents: Memo from A. B. Shetty, Madras Minister of Health, to Rajaji, "Tuberculosis-Report of Ill-Health of Two Children of Sri Virayya Servai . . . after B.C.G. Vaccination," 12 September 1955; "Copy

of D.O.H. No.H.3/19673/55 dated 24-8-1955 from the Municipal Health Officer, Madurai; Memo from A. B. Shetty to Rajaji, "Tuberculosis—B.C.G. Vaccination—Alleged After Effects," 10 September 1955; "Copy of D.O.No. H3/39573/55 dated 15-8-1955 from Dr. P. M. Rajaratnam, Municipal Health Officer, Madurai," all in Installments VI–XI, Subject File 27, RP.

107. Prit Singh to Rajaji, 20 May 1955, Installments VI–XI, Subject File 26, RP; excerpt of same letter in *B.C.G. Vaccination—Why I Oppose It*, 39.

108. "Report of Suri Rizwan Ullah Siddiqi, referred to the Director of Medical and Health Services, vide his letter No. 1014–16/C. dated 27th August, 1955"; Faizan Ullah Siddiqi to Rajaji, 15 and 20 August 1955, all in Installments VI–XI, Subject File 27, RP. See also "U.P. Inquiry into B.C.G. Vaccination," 4 September 1955, *Sunday Statesman*.

109. C. Rajagopalachari, *B.C.G. Vaccination–Why I Oppose It*, 2.

110. Raghavan to Rajaji, 6 September 1955, Installment V, Subject File 135, RP. See also D.C. Mazumdar, "Problem of Tuberculosis in India with Special Reference to B.C.G. Vaccination," *Journal of the Indian Medical Association* 20, no. 6 (March 1951): 220–223.

111. Rajkumari Amrit Kaur to Rajaji, 2 June 1955, Installments VI–XI, Subject File 28, RP.

CHAPTER 7. FAITH, FAILURE, AND THE BCG VACCINE

1. The global history of vaccination is marked by a multitude of responses to vaccines as old as vaccination itself—antivaccination sentiment directed, often, at a strong state; fear of a vaccine's safety; the popularity of injections; and quotidian acceptance of vaccination. This last element, as Paul Greenough notes, is perhaps the most mysterious of all—why "should most publics around the world willingly accept sometimes painful injections of unknown substances intended to do invisible things to their bodies in ways that are usually unexplained?" See Paul Greenough, "Social Science and Immunization: New Possibilities and Projects," *Items: Social Science Research Council* 52, no. 1 (1998): 1–9, 5. Regarding more contemporary vaccination programs, most people either "actively demand" or "passively accept" vaccines. Acute forms of large-scale resistance are exceptional; resistance is more often passive—simply not showing up for vaccination, for instance. See Mark Nichter, "Vaccinations in the Third World: A Consideration of Community Demand," 617–623, and Paul Greenough, "Global Immunization and Culture: Compliance and Resistance in Large-

Scale Public Health Campaigns," 605–607, both in *Social Science and Medicine* 41, no. 5 (1995).

2. For an example of this elsewhere see Marcos Cueto, "Appropriation and Resistance: Local Responses to Malaria Eradication in Mexico, 1955–1970," *Journal of Latin American Studies* 37, no. 3 (2005): 533.

3. P. Mohamed Ali, India B.C.G. Project, Third Quarterly Report, 30 October 1955, India BCG, Program Division, Asia Region, CF/RA/BX/PD/1962/T008. P. Mohamed Ali, India B.C.G. Project. Fourth Quarterly Report, 20 January 1956. CF/RA/BX/PD/1962/T033. See also Sunil S. Amrith, *Decolonizing International Health: India and Southeast Asia, 1930–65* (London: Palgrave Macmillan, 2006).

4. Dr. Chabaud to H.E. Blatta Zaoude Belaineh, Ethiopian Minister of Health, 27 March 1952, Ethiopia-BCG, 1952–1953, Program Division, Eastern Mediterranean Region, box CF/RA/BX/PD/1962/T022, UNICEF Archives.

5. Carroll Palmer, Lawrence W. Shaw, and George W. Comstock, "Community Trials of BCG Vaccination," *American Review of Tuberculosis* 77, no. 6 (1958): 877–907, 879. See also chapter 6, note 3.

6. Hans C. H. Beringer, Assignment Report—Tuberculosis Control, 31 May 1967, AFR/TB/92, WHO Archives.

7. Initially it was thought that the program was costing considerably more than other programs, such as the one in neighboring Eritrea. Upon further exploration UNICEF found that this was not the case and the program had been shut down under false pretenses. Resident Representative, Addis Ababa to Chief, EMAO, UNICEF, Beirut, 4 October 1957, BCG Ethiopia, Programme Division, Eastern Mediterranean region, CF/RA/BX/PD/1962/T022, UNICEF Archives.

8. Wallace Fox, "Research on Tuberculosis in the Tropics," 1962, FD 7/1186, National Archives of the United Kingdom (hereafter NAUK).

9. Mahler's thoughts are from minutes of a meeting of the "Committee for Research on Tuberculosis in the Tropics," 28 February 1964, FD-12–554, NAUK.

10. "Notes on Research in the Field of Tuberculosis Immunization in Man," WHO/TBC/Int./49, 29 October 1962. WHO Library, Geneva. Emphasis added.

11. Niels Brimnes, "BCG Vaccination and the WHO's Global Strategy for Tuberculosis Control, 1948–1983," *Social Science and Medicine* 67 (2008): 863–873, 869.

12. A. H. Taba to Sam Keeny, 26 May 1961, Pakistan-BCG Reports, 1958–61, box CF/RA/PD/1962/T113, UNICEF Archives.

13. "Report of the WHO/CCTA Tuberculosis Seminar, Nairobi, Kenya, 16–22 November 1960," Basutoland, TB AFP-139 Correspondence, WHO Archives.

14. Official policy in "B.C.G. Vaccination," Medical Department Circular No. 11/1965, 14 June 1965, FD 12/555, NAUK; "must have priority" in W.H.O. Tuberculosis Centre (Chemotherapy and BCG), "Tuberculosis Control in Kenya—A Children's Problem," July 1964, BY/7/174, Kenya National Archives (hereafter KNA).

15. First Quarterly Report of the Kenya/WHO Tuberculosis Control Project (Kenya-4), 5 April 1966, Kenya 4, WHO Archives.

16. See, for example, J. B. McDougall, Head of Tuberculosis Section, WHO to Dear Sir, no date but probably 1949, Tuberculosis—BCG Immunization Campaign in India, 458-6-1, WHO Archives.

17. Dr. P. Mohamed Ali, "A Note on the Future of BCG Vaccination in India," no date but filed with a covering letter of 1 May 1959, India, BCG Correspondence, Programme Division, Asia Region, CF/RA/BX/PD/1962/T070, UNICEF Archives. Ali had made this point previously. See P. Mohamed Ali, "The Place of BCG Vaccination in the Control of Tuberculosis in India," *Indian Journal of Tuberculosis* 4, no. 1 (1956): 31–37.

18. Georges Canetti, "The Eradication of Tuberculosis: Theoretical Problems and Practical Solutions," *Tubercle* 43 (1962): 301–321, 314.

19. Carroll Palmer, Lawrence W. Shaw, and George W. Comstock, "Community Trials of BCG Vaccination," *American Review of Tuberculosis* 77, no. 6 (1958): 877–907, 896.

20. Ibid., 899. For a discussion of this point see also Georgina Feldberg, *Disease and Class: Tuberculosis and the Shaping of Modern North American Society* (New Brunswick: Rutgers University Press, 1995), 190–191, 197–198.

21. W.H.O. Tuberculosis Centre (Chemotherapy and BCG), "Tuberculosis Control in Kenya—A Children's Problem," July 1964, BY/7/174, KNA.

22. By the mid-1970s the view that BCG had very limited, if any, value in places where infection rates were low had become well accepted. See A. Rouillon and H. Waaler, "BCG Vaccination and Epidemiological Situation: A Decision Making Approach to the Use of BCG," *Advances in Tuberculosis Research* 19 (1976): 64–126, 69.

23. Editorial, "Fifty Years of BCG," *Tubercle* 52, no. 4 (1971): 303–305; "B.C.G. and Vole Bacillus Vaccines in the Prevention of Tuberculosis in Adolescence and Early Adult Life," *British Medical Journal* 1, no. 5336 (1963): 973–978.

24. George Comstock, "Long-Term Results of BCG Vaccination in the Southern United States," *Public Health Reports* 93, no. 2 (1966): 171–183, 172.

25. S. Willis and M. Vandiviere, "The Heterogeneity of BCG," *American Review of Respiratory Disease* 84 (1961): 288–290.

26. George W. Comstock, Verna T. Livesay, and Shirley F. Woolpert, "Evaluation of BCG Vaccination among Puerto Rican Children," *American Journal of Public Health* 64, no. 3 (1974): 283–291, 291.

27. P. D. Hart, "Efficacy and Applicability of Mass B.C.G. Vaccination in Tuberculosis Control," *British Medical Journal* 1, no. 5540 (1967): 587–592. Much was subsequently written on this. See, for example, H. G. ten Dam, K. Toman, K. L. Hitze, and J. Guld, "Present Knowledge of Immunization against Tuberculosis," *Bulletin of the World Health Organization* 54, no. 3 (1976): 255–269, esp. 259.

28. Brimnes, "BCG Vaccination and the WHO's Global Strategy for Tuberculosis Control, 1948–1983," 869.

29. Ibid., 870.

30. H. G. ten Dam, "Research on BCG Vaccination," *Advances in Tuberculosis Research* 21 (1984): 79–106, 90.

31. It seems that hope colored, too, a meta-analysis of BCG's efficacy. Published in the *Journal of the American Medical Association* in 1994 (and revisited in *Clinical Infectious Diseases* in 2000), the study came to the conclusion that BCG had a protective effect of 50 percent. Indeed, if half of those treated with BCG were living disease free because of the vaccine then its value was clear. Yet the percentage of cases prevented was the average calculated from all trials—which as we know ranged from zero to 80 percent. The authors noted, too, that questions remained, such as BCG's "overall efficacy"— whatever that might mean. Finally, it was clear that BCG worked better the farther one got from the equator. But rather than allow for the possibility of a social explanation for this finding—there might, after all, be one to explain high infection rates in tropical countries—several of the authors went on to explore biological reasons. See G. A. Colditz, T. F. Brewer, C. S. Berkey, M. E. Wilson, E. Burdick, H. V. Fineberg, and F. Mosteller, "Efficacy of BCG Vaccine in the Prevention of Tuberculosis: Meta-Analysis of the Published Literature," *Journal of the American Medical Association* 271, no. 9 (1994): 698–702; Timothy F. Brewer, "Preventing Tuberculosis with Bacillus Calmette-Guérin Vaccine: A Meta-Analysis of the Literature," *Clinical Infectious Diseases* 31, suppl. 3 (2000): S64–S67; M. E. Wilson, H. V.

Fineberg, and G. A. Colditz, "Geographic Latitude and the Efficacy of Bacillus Calmette-Guérin Vaccine," *Clinical Infectious Diseases* 20, no. 4 (1995): 982–991.

32. Global Tuberculosis Programme and Global Programme on Vaccines, "Statement on BCG Revaccination for the Prevention of Tuberculosis," *Weekly Epidemiological Record* 32, no. 11 (1995): 229–231.

33. Brimnes, "BCG Vaccine and the WHO's Strategy," 870.

34. Mangtani Punam, Ibrahim Abubakar, Cono Ariti, Rebecca Beynon, Laura Pimpin, Paul E. M. Fine, Laura C. Rodrigues, et al., "Protection by BCG Vaccine against Tuberculosis: A Systematic Review of Randomized Controlled Trials," *Clinical Infectious Diseases* 58, no. 4 (2014): 470–480.

35. Paul E. M. Fine, "The BCG Story: Lessons from the Past and Implications for the Future," *Reviews of Infectious Diseases* 11, suppl. 2 (1989): S353–S359, S358.

CHAPTER 8. CURING TB

1. Director of Medical Services to All Medical Officers, 17 July 1950, MOH/3/306, Kenya National Archives (hereafter KNA).

2. A. W. Williams, "Tuberculosis Problem in East Africa (with Special Reference to Uganda)," in folder "Tuberculosis in East Africa, Report to the DMS, Uganda, November 1945," Oxford Development Records Project, MSS Afr.s 1872, Rhodes House Library, University of Oxford.

3. John Lonsdale and D. A. Low quoted in Joseph Morgan Hodge, *The Triumph of the Expert: Agrarian Doctrines of Development and the Legacies of British Colonialism* (Athens: Ohio University Press, 2007), 209. See generally Hodge's chapter 7 for a superb treatment of this period in East Africa generally.

4. George Oduor Ndege, *Health, State, and Society in Kenya* (Rochester, N.Y.: University of Rochester Press, 2001), 128–134.

5. Robert M. Maxon, "Social and Cultural Changes," in B. A. Ogot and W. R. Ochieng', eds., *Decolonization and Independence in Kenya, 1940–93* (London: James Currey, 1995), 110–147, esp. 132–135.

6. Kenneth S. Ombongi, "The Historical Interface between the State and Medical Science in Africa: Kenya's Case," in P. Wenzel Geissler and Catherine Molyneux, eds., *Evidence, Ethos and Experiment: The Anthropology and History of Medical Research in Africa* (New York: Berghahn Books, 2011).

7. Ross Upshur, Jerome Singh, and Nathan Ford, "Apocalypse or Redemption: Responding to Extensively Drug-Resistant Tuberculosis," *Bulletin of the World Health Association* 87 (2009): 481–483.

8. For fairly recent treatments of Mau-Mau see David Anderson, *Histories of the Hanged: The Dirty War in Kenya and the End of Empire* (New York: W. W. Norton, 2005); Caroline Elkins, *Imperial Reckoning: The Untold Story of Britain's Gulag in Kenya* (New York: Henry Holt, 2005); for a broader view of Kenyan history that included Mau-Mau see Bruce Berman and John Lonsdale, *Unhappy Valley: Conflict in Kenya and Africa, Book Two: Violence and Ethnicity* (London: James Currey, 1992).

9. On this point concerning researchers operating above the fray of politics, and being encouraged to do so by the Colonial Office, see Sabine Clarke, "A Technocratic Imperial State? The Colonial Office and Scientific Research, 1940–1960," *Twentieth Century British History* 18, no. 4 (2007): 453–480, esp. 457; see also Clarke, "The Research Council System and the Politics of Medical and Agricultural Research for the British Colonial Empire, 1940–52," *Medical History* 57, no. 3 (2013): 338–358.

10. P. Wenzel Geissler, "Parasite Lost: Remembering Modern Times with Kenyan Government Medical Scientists," in Geissler and Molyneux, eds., *Evidence, Ethos and Experiment*, 297–332, 304.

11. Walsh McDermott, "Tuberculosis at Home and Abroad," *Bulletin of the National Tuberculosis and Respiratory Disease Association* 54, no. 10 (1968): 7–11, 11. Emphasis in original.

12. While not the first article to report on the problem, this is a good summary of it up to 1948: John Crofton and Dennis A. Mitchison, "Streptomycin Resistance in Pulmonary Tuberculosis," *British Medical Journal* 2, no. 4588 (1948): 1009–1015; see also Medical Research Council, "Prevention of Streptomycin Resistance by Combined Chemotherapy: A Medical Research Council Investigation," *British Medical Journal* 1, no. 4769 (1952): 1157–1162.

13. D. R. Blomfeld to DMS, Nairobi, 11 November 1952; Haynes to Dr. Wright, 17 November 1952; Medical Department Circular No: 56/52, "Isoniazid," 5 December 1952, all in MOH/3/306, KNA; "The Treatment of Pulmonary Tuberculosis with Isoniazid: An Interim Report to the Medical Research Council by Their Tuberculosis Chemotherapy Trials Committee," *British Medical Journal* 2, no. 4787 (4 October 1952): 735–746; see also M. Buck and R. J. Schnitzer, "The Development of Drug Resistance of M. Tuberculosis to Isonicotinic Acid Hydrazide," *American Review of Tuberculosis* 65, no. 6

(1952): 759–760; E. J. Grace, V. Bryson, W. Szbalski, and M. Demerec, "Potential Danger of Isoniazid Resistance through Failure to Use Multiple Chemotherapy in Treatment of Tuberculosis," *Journal of the American Medical Association* 149, no. 13 (1952): 1241.

14. A. J. Walker, "Scheme for the Control of Tuberculosis," 28 July 1955, OP/EST/1/632, KNA.

15. World Health Organization, "Ambulatory Chemotherapy in Tuberculosis Control," WHO/TBC/Int./26, 17 June 1955, esp. 6–8, WHO Archives.

16. "DRAFT, RE: Allocation of Beds at Port Reitz Chest Hospital, Mombasa, for the Treatment of Cases Admitted from the Various District Hospitals, Coast," no date but filed with materials from fall 1953, MOH/3/306; see also J. C. R. Buchanan to Farnsworth Anderson, 15 March 1954, MOH/3/742, both in KNA. For the ad hoc nature of treatment see also W. S. Haynes to Principal Medical Officer, Coast Province, 4 September 1958, BY/13/239, KNA.

17. For these figures see "East African Tuberculosis Investigation," 22 September 1959, BY/13/242, KNA; for more on Ghana see W. J. Bell and P.P. Brown, "Bacterial Resistance to Steptomycin, PAS and Isoniazid in Untreated Patients with Symptomatic Pulmonary Tuberculosis in Ashanti," *Tubercle* 41 (1960): 247–252; for East Africa see J. Pepys, D. A. Mitchison, and B. J. Kinsley, "The Prevalence of Bacterial Resistance to Isoniazid and to PAS in Patients with Acute Pulmonary Tuberculosis Presenting for Treatment in East Africa," *Tubercle* 41 (1960): 32–36.

18. Peter Cavanagh, "The Sensitivity to Streptomycin, PAS and Isoniazid of Strains of Myco. Tuberculosis Isolated from Patients in Khartoum and Wad Medani," *Tubercle* 46, no. 3 (1965): 250–255.

19. Wallace Fox to W. M. Arnott, 4 March 1960, FD 23-1087, NAUK. On the prevalence see Hong Kong Government Tuberculosis Service/British Medical Research Council Co-Operative Investigation, "Drug-Resistance in Patients with Pulmonary Tuberculosis Presenting at Chest Clinics in Hong Kong," *Tubercle* 45 (1964): 77–95.

20. J. Frimodt-Moller, "The Tuberculosis Situation in India Today," *Tubercle* 43 (1962): 88–94, 94.

21. W. S. Haynes to PMO [Principal Medical Officer], Coast Province, 4 September 1958, BY/13/239, KNA.

22. A. W. Williams to Harold Himsworth, 17 June 1959, FD 1-8773, NAUK.

23. Williams to A. J. Walker, DMS, Kenya, 22 September 1959, BY/13/242, KNA.

24. Pierce Kent, "Report: Kenya 1957/1958—Tuberculosis Treatment Results at the End of One Year (10% Sample Survey)," BY/13/240, KNA.

25. PMO, Central Province, to Permanent Secretary/Chief Medical Officer, 3 October 1960, BY/13/242, KNA.

26. J. Pepys, D. A. Mitchison, and B. J. Kinsley, "The Prevalence of Bacterial Resistance to Isoniazid and to PAS in Patients with Acute Pulmonary Tuberculosis Presenting for Treatment in East Africa," *Tubercle* 41 (1960): 32–36, 35.

27. P. D'Arcy Hart, Confidential Memo, "Possible short list of trials for consideration in East Africa," 21 June 1959, FD 1-8773, NAUK.

28. A. W. Williams, "East African Tuberculosis Therapy Trials—A Review," *East African Medical Review* 37, no. 12 (1960): 744–764. For a thorough review of all the published literature on the trials see Wallace Fox, G. A. Ellard, and D. A. Mitchison, "Studies on the Treatment of Tuberculosis Undertaken by the British Medical Research Council Tuberculosis Units, 1946–1986, with Relevant Subsequent Publications," *International Journal of Tuberculosis and Lung Disease* 3, no. 10, suppl. 2 (1999): S231–S279; for a summary of the thiacetazone with isoniazid trials see Joan Heffernan, "A Summary of the Results of East African–British Medical Research Council Studies of Thiacetazone-containing Regimens," *Tubercle* 49, suppl. (1968): 23–26.

29. A. J. Walker, "Cost to the local health authorities for the care of tuberculosis," 26 June 1958; on the high costs see Memo "Cost to local health authorities for the care of tuberculosis," File No. SAN.709/IX, no date, giving projections for number of TB cases by end of 1958, both in BY/13/239, KNA.

30. For the number of cases see Annual Medical Report, Colony and Protectorate of Kenya, 1956, 24; for the number on treatment see ibid., 1957, 18.

31. W. Fox, P. W. Hutton, I. Sutherland, and A. W. Williams, "A Comparison of Acute Extensive Pulmonary Tuberculosis and Its Response to Chemotherapy in Britain and Uganda," *Tubercle* 37, no. 6 (1956): 435–450, 435.

32. Medical Research Council, "Cooperative Trial of Tuberculosis in East Africa," 20 August 1956, FD 1-8770, NAUK.

33. P. Hutton, Y. K. Lutalo, A. W. Willaims, I. M. Tonkin, and W. Fox, "Acute Pulmonary Tuberculosis in East Africans: A Controlled Trial of Isoniazid in Combination with Streptomycin or PAS," *Tubercle* 37, no. 3 (1956): 151–165;

P. D'Arcy Hart to Harold Himsworth, "Anti-tuberculosis Chemotherapy Trials in East Africa, Conference on Tuberculosis in East Africa, January, 1957," 10 December 1956, FD 1-8770, NAUK. See also A. I. L Turnbull, "The Effect of Chemotherapy on Pulmonary Tuberculosis in the Central African," *Central African Journal of Medicine* 15 (1955): 228–234.

34. "Confidential Memo: Possible Short List of Trials for Consideration in East Africa," 21 June 1959, FD 1-8773, NAUK.

35. Hutton et al., "Acute Pulmonary Tuberculosis in East Africans," 151.

36. For a good overview of postwar British medical research see Hellen Valier and Carsten Timmermann, "Clinical Trials and the Reorganization of Medical Research in Post–Second World War Britain," *Medical History* 52, no. 4 (2008): 493–510.

37. A. W. Williams to P. D'Arcy Hart, 10 December 1956, FD 1-8770, NAUK; for Williams's earlier work on East Africa, the records for which are frustratingly slim, see A. W. Williams Papers, Oxford Development Records Project, MSS Afr.s 1872, Rhodes House Library, University of Oxford.

38. Arthur Williams, "Note on the Medical Research Council/East Africa Tuberculosis Investigation, 1953–1959," in Colonial Medical Research Committee, CMR (59) 41, FD 1/8773, NAUK.

39. "Report of the WHO/CCTA Tuberculosis Seminar," Nairobi, Kenya, 16–22 November 1960, Basutoland-TB AFP-139, Correspondence, 1961, WHO Archives.

40. J. S. Owen, N. M. O'Beirn, and J. R. Lauckner, "Some Problems in the Treatment of Ambulatory Treatment of Pulmonary Tuberculosis in Nigeria," *West African Medical Journal* 7, no. 2 (June 1958): 97–105, 103; for the views that antibiotics inappropriately administered could do more harm than good see also S. B. Sachs, "The Domiciliary Treatment of Pulmonary Tuberculosis: A Socio-Economic and Clinical Review," *South African Medical Journal* 30, no. 31 (1956): 735–739, 738.

41. J. Pepys to P. O. Williams, 10 December 1956, FD 1/8770, NAUK.

42. This had been an actively investigated question in Kenya since the early 1950s. See W. S. Haynes, "The Treatment of Pulmonary Tuberculosis in Kenya Africans with Thiacetazone," *East African Medical Journal* 29, no. 9 (1952): 339–355; for the development of this class of drugs see Z. Ahmad, N. H. Makaya, and J. Grosset, "History of Drug Discovery: Early Evaluation Studies and Lessons Learnt from Them," in P. R. Donald and P. D. van Helden, eds., *Anti-Tuberculosis Chemotherapy*, vol. 40 of *Progress in Respiratory Research* (2012): 2–9.

43. MRC, "East African Tuberculosis Investigation, Outline of Proposed Trial," no date but filed with papers from December 1956 to January 1957; "Confidential Draft Protocol, Trial of Isoniazid Alone and in Combination with Thiosemicarbazone in Pulmonary Tuberculosis in East Africa," 11 December 1956, both in FD 1-8770, NAUK.

44. Quote in P. D'Arcy Hart to Harold Himsworth, "Anti-tuberculosis Chemotherapy Trials in East Africa, Conference on Tuberculosis in East Africa, January, 1957," 10 December 1956; see also Pepys to P. O. Williams, 10 December 1956; Tuberculosis Research Unit, Confidential, "Trial of Isoniazid Alone & in Combination with Thiosemicarbazone in Pulmonary Tuberculosis in East Africa," 11 December 1956, all in FD 1-8770, NAUK. For the WHO's views on the pros and cons of isoniazid alone and the need to answer the questions see World Health Organization Technical Report Series, no. 141, "Chemotherapy and Chemoprophylaxis in Tuberculosis Control" (Geneva: World Health Organization, 1957), 11–12.

45. P. D'Arcy Hart, "Recent Trends in Tuberculosis Research," 1958, FD 1/8772, NAUK.

46. Niels Brimnes, "The Community Approach," unpublished manuscript in author's possession, 21.

47. John Goodall, "Tuberculosis in Nyasaland: A Record of Two Years' Experience," *Tubercle* 36, no. 2 (1955): 43–49, 48.

48. For example: P. P. Turner, Coast Province Provincial Physician, to N. R. E. Fendall, DMS, 23 March 1961, BY/13/240, KNA; for most East African doctors opposing isoniazid alone see James Deeny, "Report Made on a Visit to British Somaliland Protectorate, 8 September 1957 to October 9, 1957," Somaliland-2, WHO Archives; on the WHO recommending isoniazid alone see World Health Organization, "Ambulatory Chemotherapy in Tuberculosis Control," WHO/TBC/Int./26, 17 June 1955, p. 13, WHO Archives.

49. First two quotes in DMS to J. R. Buchanan, MRC, 6 April 1956; "astonished" in DMS to Pierce Kent, 18 April 1956, both in MOH/3/813, KNA. On Holm and the WHO advocating the use of isoniazid alone see Holm, "The Ideas and Plans of the World Health Organization in Connexion with Chemotherapy in Tuberculosis Control in Under-Developed Countries," WHO/TBC/Int./40, 13 August 1957, p. 7, WHO Archives.

50. Hugh Stott, "The Organisation of a Tuberculosis Chemotherapy Pilot Project in Kenya Colony. To Be Undertaken Jointly by the Government of Kenya, the World Health Organisation and the United Nations Children's

Fund," 26 June 1956, BY/13/188, KNA; H. Stott, "The Case for the Use of Isoniazid Alone in the Treatment of Pulmonary Tuberculosis in East Africa," *East African Medical Journal* 34, no. 7 (1957): 325–338; Walsh McDermott, "Antimicrobial Therapy of Pulmonary Tuberculosis," *Bulletin of the World Health Organization* 23 (1960): 427–461, esp. 457; on McDermott's influence over the WHO regarding monotherapy see John Crofton's remarks in *Short-Course Chemotherapy for Tuberculosis: The Transcript of a Witness Seminar Held by the Wellcome Trust Centre for the History of Medicine at UCL, London, on 3 February 2004*, edited by D. A. Christie and E. M. Tansey (London: Wellcome Trust Centre for the History of Medicine at UCL, 2005), 38.

51. James Deeny, "Report Made on a Visit to British Somaliland Protectorate, 8 September 1957 to October 9, 1957," Somaliland-2, WHO Archives.

52. K. Deuschle, L. Ormond, D. Elmendorf, C. Muschenheim, and W. McDermott, "The Course of Pulmonary Tuberculosis During Long-term Single-drug (Isoniazid) Therapy," *American Review of Tuberculosis* 70, no. 2 (1954): 228–265, 251–252. See especially the note on p. 230 that "all patients were hospital inpatients who were kept on bed rest with some individual modifications such as the allowance of bathroom privileges."

53. Pierce Kent, "Tuberculosis—Bacillary Drug Resistance," for attention of Dr. Fendall, 6 March 1961, BY/13/240, KNA.

54. David S. Jones, "Technologies of Compliance: Surveillance of Self-Administration of Tuberculosis Treatment, 1956–1966," *History and Technology* 17, no. 4 (2001): 279–318; Jones, "The Health Care Experiments at Many Farms: The Navajo, Tuberculosis, and the Limits of Modern Medicine, 1952–1962," *Bulletin of the History of Medicine* 76, no. 4 (2002): 749–790.

55. A Cooperative Investigation in East African Hospitals and Laboratories with the Collaboration of the British Medical Research Council, "Comparative Trial of Isoniazid Alone in Low and High Dosage and Isoniazid Plus PAS in the Treatment of Acute Pulmonary Tuberculosis in East Africans," *Tubercle* 41 (1960): 83–102. The MRC found that also in India isoniazid should not be used alone, as it was less effective than a PAS/isoniazid combination. See "A Concurrent Comparison of Isoniazid Plus PAS with Three Regimens of Isoniazid Alone in the Domiciliary Treatment of Pulmonary Tuberculosis in South India," *Bulletin of the World Health Organization* 23 (1960): 535–585.

56. East African/British M.R.C. Tuberculosis Therapy Studies, "Proposed Research Programme 1964–65," 27 January 1965, FD 12/554, NAUK.

57. "Report by Dr. H. M. Foreman, Brief Survey of Tuberculosis in Kenya," 1958, BY/7/174, KNA.

58. Kent to DMS, 12 July 1965, BY/13/243, KNA.

59. J. Pepys to Harold Himsworth, 2 October 1957;? [written on MRC letterhead] to Lewthwaite, 16 October 1957, both in FD 1-8770, NAUK.

60. P. D'Arcy Hart to A. W. Williams, 3 April 1959, FD 1-8773, NAUK.

61. "Confidential: British M.R.C./East African Tuberculosis Investigations," 30 November 1959, FD 1-8773, NAUK; on the desire to begin unrestricted use of the new combination see A. W. Williams to E. P. Rigby, "E.A. Tuberculosis Therapy Trials," 3 February 1960, BY/13/242, KNA.

62. Tuberculosis Chemotherapy Centre, "A Concurrent Comparison of Home and Sanatorium Treatment of Pulmonary Tuberculosis in South India," *Bulletin of the World Health Organization* 21, no. 1 (1959): 51–144. On the MRC's work see Helen Valier, "At Home in the Colonies: The WHO-MRC Trials at the Madras Chemotherapy Centre in the 1950s and 1960s," in Flurin Condrau and Michael Worboys, eds., *Tuberculosis Then and Now: Perspectives on the History of an Infectious Disease* (Montreal: McGill-Queen's University Press, 2010), 213–234; Niels Brimnes, "Magic Bullets: Chemotherapy," unpublished manuscript in author's possession, esp. 6–7; Sunil Amrith, "In Search of a 'Magic Bullet' for Tuberculosis: South India and Beyond, 1955–1965," *Social History of Medicine* 17, no. 1 (2004): 113–130.

63. PMO, Central Province, to Permanent Secretary/Chief Medical Officer, 3 October 1960; see also the same concerns of the Principal Physician in Nyanza Province, R. M. Foster to Provincial Medical Officer, 17 August 1960, both in BY/13/242, KNA.

64. PMO, Central Province, to Permanent Secretary/Chief Medical Office, 13 February 1960, BY/13/242, KNA.

65. On the "well-oiled machinery" see J. Pepys to Harold Himsworth, 19 May 1960, FD 1/8773, NAUK; A. W. Williams, "East African Thiacetazone Trials," 26 October 1960; on hospitals opting out of the trial see Kent to Permanent Secretary/Chief Medical Officer, 4 January 1961, both in BY/13/242, KNA.

66. "Isoniazid with Thiacetazone in the Treatment of Pulmonary Tuberculosis in East Africa—Second Investigation: Co-operative Studies in East African Hospitals and Laboratories with the Collaboration of the East African and British Medical Research Councils," *Tubercle* 44, no. 3 (1963): 301–333.

67. C. G. Gordon, "A Method of Controlled Home Treatment of Pulmonary Tuberculosis in Tanganyika," *Tubercle* 42 (1961): 148–158, 150.

CHAPTER 9. THE LOST PROMISE OF ANTIBIOTICS

1. WHO Expert Committee on Tuberculosis, Eighth Report, World Health Organization Technical Report Series, no. 290 (Geneva: WHO, 1964), 14.

2. WHO Press Release, "Vaccination against Tuberculosis, WHO Experts to Meet in Copenhagen," 27 November 1953, Press Release WHO/70, MOH 3/742, Kenya National Archives (hereafter KNA).

3. Niels Brimnes, "Magic Bullets: Chemotherapy," 30. Unpublished manuscript in author's possession.

4. J. R. Lauckner, "Domiciliary Chemotherapy for Pulmonary Tuberculosis in Developing Countries (Based on Experience in Nigeria)," *Bulletin of the International Union Against Tuberculosis* 35 (1964): 268–273, 271.

5. Wallace Fox, "Notes on the Tuberculosis Chemotherapy Centre, Madras," May 1958, FD 7/1020, National Archives of the United Kingdom (hereafter NAUK).

6. T. Egsmose, P. Kent, C. Munch-Jensen, and J. Thillemann, "Drug Acceptability in Domiciliary Tuberculosis Control Programmes," *Bulletin of the World Health Organization* 29 (1963): 627–636.

7. Remarks of Johannes Holm in "How Can the Voluntary Bodies Best Assist in the Global Attack on Tuberculosis? A Panel Discussion Held in Paris on September 20th and 21st 1962," *Bulletin of the International Union Against Tuberculosis* 33, no. 2 (1963): 2–135, 29.

8. W. J. Bell, "Memorandum on Tuberculosis Research," 1960, in Tuberculosis Research at Kumasi, West Africa, FD 7-1263, NAUK.

9. Brandon Lush, "East African Tuberculosis Trials," 20 February 1962, FD 12/552, NAUK.

10. East African Tuberculosis Investigations, Annual Report—1965, FD 12/555, NAUK; see also Pierce Kent to DMS, 21 July 1966, BY/7/195, KNA.

11. "Minutes of the First Meeting of the Kenya Advisory Committee on Tuberculosis Held on Wednesday, 8th February, 1967 in the Conference Room, Ministry of Health, Nairobi," BY/7/195, KNA; for the 50 percent figure see also P. W. Kent, "Tuberculosis Control—Counting the Cost," *Tubercle* 49, suppl. (1968): 6–9, 8.

12. P. W. Kent, W. Fox, A. B. Miller, A. J. Nunn, R. Tall, and D. A. Mitchison, "The Therapy of Pulmonary Tuberculosis in Kenya: A Comparison of the Results Achieved in Controlled Clinical Trials with Those Achieved by the Routine Treatment Services," *Tubercle* 51, no. 1 (1970): 24–38.

13. Wallace Fox, "Self-Administration of Medicaments: A Review of the Published Work and a Study of the Problems," Proceedings of the XVI International Tuberculosis Conference, 1961, *Excerpta Medica, International Congress Series* 44, no. 1 (1962): 307–331, 328.

14. Niels Brimnes, "The Community Approach," 20. Unpublished manuscript in author's possession.

15. Wallace Fox, "Organisational and Administrative Considerations in the Diagnosis and Treatment of Pulmonary Tuberculosis in the Developing Countries," *Tubercle* 49, no. 3 (1968): 332–346, 341; I. L. Briggs, "Drug Resistance in Patients with Pulmonary Tuberculosis: Presenting for Treatment at the Infectious Diseases Hospital, Salisbury," *Central African Journal of Medicine* 9 (1963): 87–90, 89.

16. P. P. Turner, "Home Treatment of Tuberculosis in the Nyeri District of Kenya," *Tubercle* 43 (1962): 76–82.

17. C. G. Gordon, "A Method of Controlled Home Treatment of Pulmonary Tuberculosis in Tanganyika," *Tubercle* 42 (1961): 148–158, 158.

18. Pierce Kent, "Domiciliary Tuberculosis," 23 March 1961, BY/13/240, KNA.

19. C. G. Gordon, "The Tuberculosis Situation in an Area of Tanganyika, Following a Five-Year Period of Prevention and Treatment," *Tubercle* 43 (1962): 43–54.

20. Gordon, "A Method of Controlled Home Treatment of Pulmonary Tuberculosis in Tanganyika," 150.

21. Ibid., 151.

22. Ibid.

23. Ibid., 158.

24. Randall Packard, *White Plague, Black Labor: Tuberculosis and the Political Economy of Health and Disease in South Africa* (Berkeley: University of California Press, 1989); Sunil S. Amrith, *Decolonizing International Health: India and Southeast Asia, 1930–65* (London: Palgrave Macmillan, 2006), see esp. chapter 6.

25. Anderson quoted in Brimnes, "The Community Approach," 30.

26. Pierce Kent, "Tuberculosis—Domiciliary Treatment," Medical Department Circular No.3/1957, 4 January 1957, BY/7/174, KNA.

27. Wallace Fox, "Research on Tuberculosis Overseas," Address to Tropical Medicine Research Board, no date, 1962, Medical Research Council, FD 7-1186, NAUK.

28. Ibid.

29. Wallace Fox, "Realistic Chemotherapeutic Policies for Tuberculosis in the Developing Countries," 2 July 1964, WHO/TB/Techn.Information/20, WHO Archives.

30. Ibid., 6.

31. Ibid., 8–9.

32. Ibid.

33. WHO, "Preliminary Report Regarding the Drug-Sensitivity Pattern of Tubercle Bacilli in Kenya," 29 November 1961, Kenya-4 Quarterly Reports, WHO Archives.

34. Pierce Kent to Permanent Secretary/Chief Medical Officer, 25 January 1961, BY/7/190, KNA.

35. Pierce Kent to Perm Sec., Ministry of Health, 13 February 1961, BY/13/240, KNA.

36. Expert Committee on Tuberculosis, Seventh Report, World Health Organization Technical Report Series, no. 195 (Geneva: World Health Organization, 1960), 11.

37. James O.W. Ang'Awa, "The Problem and Management of Drug-Resistant Cases of Pulmonary Tuberculosis in Kenya," *East African Medical Journal* 41, no. 9 (1964): 436–440, 438; "Preliminary Report Regarding the Drug-Sensitivity Pattern of Tubercle Bacilli in Kenya," WHO Tuberculosis Chemotherapy Research Centre, Nairobi—Kenya 4, 29 November 1961, Quarterly Reports, 1961–64, Kenya 4, WHO Archives.

38. "Informal Meeting of Advisers on Laboratory Methods for Drug Sensitivity/Resistance Determination of Mycobacteria, WHO Cooperative Studies on the Classification of Mycobacteria, Preliminary Results of Drug Sensitivity/Resistance Tests for INH, PAS, and Thiosemicarbazone (TB1), 4–7 December 1961," WHO/TB/Techn.Information/4, 21 November 1961, WHO Archives.

39. Remarks of Halfdan Mahler in "How Can the Voluntary Bodies Best Assist in the Global Attack on Tuberculosis? A Panel Discussion held in Paris on September 20th and 21st 1962," *Bulletin of the International Union Against Tuberculosis* 33, no. 2 (1963): 2–135, 59.

40. Mahler to various, 23 August 1963, 8th Session of the WHO Expert Committee on TB (Pre-session Planning), T 9/81/8 (a), WHO Archives.

41. N. L. Bordia to Mahler, 21 September 1963, 8th Session of the WHO Expert Committee on TB (Pre-session Planning), T 9/81/8 (a), WHO Archives.

42. On this point, the MRC was well aware. See Notes of Kent's Proposals, comments of Brandon Lush, 8 April 1964, FD 12/554, NAUK.

43. Expert Committee on Tuberculosis, "The Public Health Significance of Drug Resistance (Review of Data)," WHO/TB/Techn.Information/34, 6 August 1964, WHO Archives.

44. Ibid.

45. WHO Expert Committee on Tuberculosis, Ninth Report, *World Health Organization Technical Report Series*, no. 552 (Geneva: World Health Organization, 1974), 9, 20.

46. A. F. Tuboku-Metzger, "Pulmonary Tuberculosis in Sierra Leone," *Tubercle* 43 (1962): 454–455.

47. James O. W. Ang'Awa to Dr. Timms, "Case for a New Central Tuberculosis Laboratory," 19 May 1965, BY/13/241, KNA.

48. L. B. Reichman, "Tuberculosis Elimination—What's to Stop Us? Counterpoint," *International Journal of Tuberculosis and Lung Disease* 1, no. 1 (1997): 3–11, 11; on the history of the term "noncompliance" see Jeremy A. Greene, "Therapeutic Infidelities: 'Noncompliance' Enters the Medical Literature," *Social History of Medicine* 17, no. 3 (2004): 327–343.

49. B. H. Lerner, "From Careless Consumptives to Recalcitrant Patients: The Historical Construction of Noncompliance," *Social Science and Medicine* 45, no. 9 (1997): 1423–1431; for an excellent overview of the research see Salla A. Munro, Simon A. Lewin, Helen J. Smith, Mark E. Engel, Atle Fretheim, and Jimmy Volmink, "Patient Adherence to Tuberculosis Treatment: A Systematic Review of Qualitative Research" *PLoS Medicine* 4, no. 7 (2007): 1230–1245.

50. Paul Farmer and colleagues call compliance an "analytically flimsy concept." I agree. P. Farmer, S. Robin, S. L. Ramilus, and J. Y. Kim, "Tuberculosis, Poverty, and 'Compliance': Lessons from Rural Haiti," *Seminars in Respiratory Infections* 6, no. 4 (1991): 254–260, 259.

51. W. Fox, "The Problem of Self-Administration of Drugs: With Particular Reference to Pulmonary Tuberculosis," *Tubercle* 39, no. 5 (1958): 269–274, 273.

52. A. Toczek, H. Cox, P. du Cros, G. Cooke, and N. Ford, "Strategies for Reducing Treatment Default in Drug-resistant Tuberculosis: Systematic Review and Meta-analysis," *International Journal of Tuberculosis and Lung Disease* 17, no. 3 (2012): 299–307.

53. N. W. Horne, "Drug-resistant Tuberculosis: A Review of the World Situation," *Tubercle* 50, suppl. (1969): 2–12, 5–6.

54. "A Preliminary Report Regarding the Drug Sensitivity Pattern of Tubercle Bacilli in Kenya," 29 November 1961, Kenya 4, Jacket 5, WHO Archives;

Pierce Kent to Permanent Secretary, District Medical Officer, 15 February 1961, BY/13/240, KNA; on patients not reporting previous treatment see P. P. Turner, "A Detailed Survey of One Hundred Cases of Pulmonary Tuberculosis on Domiciliary Treatment in the Nyeri District of Kenya," *East African Medical Journal* 40 (1963): 58–63; see also A. Meyer, "Influence of Pretreatment Bacterial Resistance to Isoniazid, Thiacetazone, or PAS on the Response to Chemotherapy of African Patients with Pulmonary Tuberculosis," *Tubercle* 44 (1963): 393–416, 394. The problem was not limited to Kenya; patients in India did the same. See Brimnes, "Magic Bullets: Chemotherapy," 37.

55. See, for example, the affidavits from 1958 in DC/GRSSA/3/22/8, KNA.

56. See R. Macpherson, "Project for mobile medical unit in South Kiambu with particular reference to a survey of T.B incidence and the promotion of home treatment and follow up facilities," 25 April 1956, BY/4/249; Medical Officer in Charge, Kiambu District, "The Problem of Pulmonary Tuberculosis in the Kiambu District," 26 November 1954, MOH/3/742, both in KNA. For the effect of the Emergency on treatment see also R. D. Harland, "The Revolution of Tuberculous Treatment amongst the Meru Tribe of Kenya," no date but probably 1965, MSS Afr.s.1872, Oxford Development Records Project, Rhodes House Library, University of Oxford,

57. On illegal isoniazid in Nigeria see J. S. Owen, N. M. O'Beirn, and J. R. Lauckner, "Some Problems in the Ambulatory Treatment of Pulmonary Tuberculosis in Nigeria," *West African Medical Journal* 7, no. 2 (1958): 97–105, 100, 103; for Kenya see A. C. Waine, signed for Secretary of Local Government, Health, and Housing to Secretary for Community Development, Nairobi, 5 September 1955; T. G. Askwith, Sec. for Community Development, Nairobi to Secretary of Local Government, Health, and Housing, 3 October 1955, both in MOH/3/813, KNA; on the black market in Free Town, Senegal, see Tuboku-Metzger, "Pulmonary Tuberculosis in Sierra Leone"; for more on illicit drugs see Fox, "Organisational and Administrative Considerations in the Diagnosis and Treatment of Pulmonary Tuberculosis in the Developing Countries," 342; for the current problem see R. Bate, P. Jensen, K. Hess, L. Mooney, and J. Milligan, "Substandard and Falsified Anti-tuberculosis Drugs: A Preliminary Field Analysis" *International Journal of Tuberculosis and Lung Disease* 17, no. 3 (2013): 308–311.

58. On sharing drugs see Briggs, "Drug Resistance in Patients with Pulmonary Tuberculosis," 89.

59. "Tuberculosis in Kenya: A National Sampling Survey of Drug Resistance and Other Factors," *Tubercle* 49, no. 2 (1968): 136–169, 157.

60. Horne, "Drug-resistant Tuberculosis," 5–6.

61. "Tuberculosis in Kenya" (1968).

62. "Tuberculosis in Kenya: A Second National Sampling Survey of Drug Resistance and Other Factors, and a Comparison with the Prevalence Data From the First National Sampling Survey. An East African and British Medical Research Council Co-operative Investigation," *Tubercle* 59, no. 3 (1978): 155–177, table V.

63. On Southern Rhodesia see D. H. Shennan, "Resistance of Tubercle Bacilli to Isoniazid, PAS and Streptomycin, Related to History of Previous Treatment," *Tubercle* 45 (1964): 1–6; on Hong Kong see A. Pines and R. J. Richardson, "Drug Resistance in Patients with Pulmonary Tuberculosis Presenting at Chest Clinics in Hong Kong," *Tubercle* 45 (1964): 77–95.

64. "Tuberculosis in Kenya: A Second National Sampling" (1978), 175. In both of the surveys, when noting that they did not do work on the chronic failures almost the exact same language was used. From 1968: "A more comprehensive survey to obtain information on the pool of chronic infection would, however, be a formidable undertaking, both organizationally and in terms of workload in the laboratories" (157). From 1978: "A more comprehensive survey to obtain information on these aspects would be a formidable undertaking, both organisationally and in terms of the laboratory work-load" (175).

65. "Tuberculosis in Tanzania: A National Sampling Survey of Drug Resistance and Other Factors," *Tubercle* 56, no. 4 (1975): 269–294, 291. The same exact language used in the Kenya survey was used in the Tanzania survey.

66. "Tuberculosis in Kenya" (1968), 157. On thinking about surveying chronic infectious patients see "Dr. Kent's Visit, June 18th–26th 1964, Notes on a Meeting Held at the T.R.U., Hampstead," FD 12/554; see also Pierce Kent and Joan Herffernan, "M.R.C. East African Tuberculosis Investigations, Memorandum on further studies and their organisation," 27 May 1963, FD 12/553/1, both in NAUK.

67. "Tuberculosis in Kenya" (1968). "The prevalence of initial resistance in 86 patients who gave a history of having been in contact with a patient who had been under treatment for tuberculosis was 23% compared with 13% for 546 patients with no history of such contact, a statistically significant difference ($P < 0.05$). Similar differences were found in surveys in Great Britain (Fox and others, 1957) and in France (Canetti and others, 1964). These three surveys thus provide good evidence of infection of contacts by index patients

excreting resistant strains. The possibility, however, cannot be completely excluded that some patients under treatment may share medicament with contacts who are also suffering from the disease and that some of these contacts have, in fact, developed acquired drug resistance" (158).

68. Gordon, "A Method of Controlled Home Treatment of Pulmonary Tuberculosis in Tanganyika," 149.

69. Stig Anderson and D. Banerji, "A Sociological Inquiry into an Urban Tuberculosis Control Programme in India," *Bulletin of the World Health Organization* 29 (1963): 685–700, 697. On their work see Sunil Amrith, "In Search of a 'Magic Bullet' for Tuberculosis: South India and Beyond, 1955–1965," *Social History of Medicine* 17, no. 1 (2004): 113–130.

70. J. H. Darbyshire, "Kenya Tuberculosis Surveys in 1964 and 1974: Comparison of Methods of Treatment and Results Obtained," *Bulletin of the International Union Against Tuberculosis* 54, no. 2 (1979): 147–148.

71. See, for example, Quarterly Report, March–June, 1960, Kenya 4, BY/7/190, KNA; see also Egsmose et al., "Drug Acceptability in Domiciliary Tuberculosis Control Programmes," 630.

72. Kent to DMS, 6 May 1958, BY/13/239, KNA.

73. Kent to DMS, 20 May 1958, BY/13/239, KNA.

74. W.S. Haynes to Principal Medical Officer, Coast Province, 4 September 1958, BY/13/239, KNA.

75. W. J. Bell, "Memorandum on Tuberculosis Research," confidential memo, May/June, 1962, FD 7/1263, NAUK.

76. "Tuberculosis in the Kiambu District: A Preliminary Report by Dr. A. R. Shaw," 25 July 1968; 30 percent of patients on treatment in Narok were lost sight of in 1967: see Pierce Kent to Dr. Singh, "Tuberculosis in Narok District," 9 August 1967, both in BY/13/241, KNA.

77. Fernando Sadek, "Tuberculosis Work," 30 December 1970, BY/13/102, KNA.

78. Malcolm Clark, "Preliminary Report on an Investigation of Pulmonary Tuberculosis in an African Reserve," *East African Medical Journal* 28, no. 9 (1951): 355–379; Clark, "District Tuberculosis Work," 29 February 1952; Clark, "RE: Tuberculosis in Fort Hall District," 10 April 195, both in MOH/3/306, KNA; author's name illegible, Education Officer, Fort Hall, "A Rehabilitation Hospital for Pulmonary Tuberculosis at Muriranja's Hospital," 10 August 1954; MUR/3/15/24, KNA; see also D. R. Blomfeld, "Report on TB," 5 May 1955, MOH/3/742, KNA, in which he writes that Clark's work at Fort Hall should be "vigorously, pressed"; Fort Hall was

selected as one of the first areas to roll out TB1: E. P. Rigby, for Permanent Secretary/Chief Medical Officer, "Tuberculosis—The Use of TB1," 3 February 1960, BY/13/242, KNA.

79. K. Toman, Private and Strictly Confidential, Preliminary Assignment Report, 5 December 1965 to 16 January 1966, FD 12/555, NAUK. This is what came to be known as the "Toman Report." Copies of it are found in multiple archives.

80. J. Rogowski, Quarterly Field Report, Second Quarter 1971, Kenya 4, WHO Archives.

81. On the lack of key supplies, such as bacteriological kits and the departure of the project's microscopist see N. Cobbold, Technical Officer, Kenya 4, Notes of the Quarterly Report: 3rd Quarter 1968, 22 September 1968; on concerns over the program, including wondering who was in charge, see "Minutes of the Second Meeting of the Kenya Co-ordination Team on Tuberculosis Held Monday, 18th March, 1968 in the Conference Room, Ministry of Health, Nairobi," both in Kenya 4, WHO Archives.

82. Final Report, Tuberculosis Control in Kenya, Dr. J. J. Rogowski, AFR/TB/132, 19 January 1973, WHO Archives.

83. Kenya National Tuberculosis Programme, Evaluation of a Test-Run in the Murang'a District—July 1968–March 1971, AFRO Technical Papers, no. 9, WHO Library.

84. DRAFT Amendment to the Third Plan of Operation for the Tuberculosis Control Project in Kenya, no date but filed with third quarterly report for 1970, Kenya 4, BY/13/102, KNA.

85. W. Koinange Karuga to Permanent Sec., Ministry of Health, 19 April 1971, BY/13/102, KNA.

86. K. Abderrahim, A. Zirout, P. Chaulet, and D. Larbaoui. "L'organisation du traitement ambulataire de la tuberculose pulmonaire en Algérie," *La Tunisie médicale* 50, no. 1 (1972): 27–31, 28.

87. "Tuberculosis in Lesotho," *Epidemiological Bulletin* 1, no. 1 (1985): 6, Disease Control Unit, Maseru, Government of Lesotho. In REAP HTM1-STB-TBS, folder 124, Lesotho, WHO Archives.

88. K. Brudney and J. Dobkin, "Resurgent Tuberculosis in New York City: Human Immunodeficiency Virus, Homelessness, and the Decline of Tuberculosis Control Programs," *American Review of Respiratory Disease* 144, no. 4 (1991): 745–749.

89. M. A. Quigley, A. Mwinga, M. Hosp, I. Lisse, D. Fuchs, J. D. H. Porter, and P. Godfrey-Faussett, "Long-term Effect of Preventive Therapy for

Tuberculosis in a Cohort of HIV-infected Zambian Adults," *AIDS* 15, no. 2 (2001): 215–222, 220.

90. For the figures on loss and mortality see tables 1 and 2, respectively, in Martin W. G. Brinkhof, Mar Pujades-Rodriguez, and Matthias Egger, "Mortality of Patients Lost to Follow-up in Antiretroviral Treatment Programmes in Resource-Limited Settings: Systematic Review and Meta-Analysis," *PloS* 4, no. 6 (2009): e5790; on overall mortality being underreported see Stéphane Verguet, Stephen S. Lim, Christopher J. L. Murray, Emmanuela Gakidou, and Joshua A. Salomon, "Incorporating Loss to Follow-up in Estimates of Survival Among HIV-infected Individuals in Sub-Saharan Africa Enrolled in Antiretroviral Therapy Programs," *Journal of Infectious Diseases* 207, no. 1 (2013): 72–79, 73.

91. Wallace Fox, "Compliance of Patients and Physicians: Experience and Lessons from Tuberculosis-I," *British Medical Journal* 287, no. 6384 (1983): 33–35, 33.

92. David S. Jones, "Technologies of Compliance: Surveillance of Self-administration of Tuberculosis Treatment, 1956–1966," *History and Technology* 17, no. 4 (2001): 279–318.

93. Fox, "Compliance of Patients and Physicians," 34.

94. Anderson and Banerji, "A Sociological Inquiry into an Urban Tuberculosis Control Programme in India," 691, emphasis in original. One problem reported by two others was the large number of patients still on clinic registers who were in the "maintenance" phase of treatment and thus not required to come to the clinic but whom clinics called defaulters. This was purely an administrative problem. Their "noncooperation was more 'procedural' than real." S. P. Pamra and G. P. Mathur, "Drug Default in an Urban Community," *Indian Journal of Tuberculosis* 14 (1967): 200–203, 202.

95. Brimnes, "Magic Bullets: Chemotherapy," 34.

96. Koinange Karuga, Report of a Safari in Coast Province, 20 December 1971, BY/13/102, KNA.

97. D. R. Nagpaul, M. K. Vishwanath, and G. Dwarakanath, "A Socio-Epidemiological Study of Out-Patients Attending a City Tuberculosis Clinic in India to Judge the Place of Specialized Centres in a Tuberculosis Control Programme," *Bulletin of the World Health Organization* 43, no. 1 (1970): 17–34.

98. Salla A. Munro, Simon A. Lewin, Helen J. Smith, Mark E. Engel, Atle Fretheim, and Jimmy Volmink, "Patient Adherence to Tuberculosis Treatment: A Systematic Review of Qualitative Research," *PLoS Medicine* 4, no. 7 (2007): 1230–1245.

99. Paul Farmer, "Immodest Claims of Causality: Social Scientists and the 'New' Tuberculosis," in Paul Farmer, ed., *Infections and Inequalities: The Modern Plagues* (Berkeley: University of California Press, 1999), 228–261, 255.

100. K. Ndeti, "Sociocultural Aspects of Tuberculosis Defaultation: A Case Study," *Social Science and Medicine* 6, no. 3 (1972): 397–412.

101. Ibid., 402.

102. Ibid., 404–405.

103. Ibid., 407.

104. W. Koinange Karuga, "Report on a Visit to Machakos, on 16-4-71 to meet John Muia," BY/13/102, KNA.

105. The following is the third in a series and sums up the previous two: H. Nsanzumuhire, J. A. Aluoch, W. K. Karuga, E. A. Edwards, H. Stott, W. Fox, and I. Sutherland, "A Third Study of Case-finding Methods for Pulmonary Tuberculosis in Kenya, Including the Use of Community Leaders," *Tubercle* 62, no. 2 (1981): 79–94.

106. No author, "Short Course Treatment in Pulmonary Tuberculosis," *East African Medical Journal* 49, no. 7 (1972): 494–501.

107. A. Lottel, F. Hatton, S. Perdrizet, and A. Rouillon, "A Concurrent Comparison of Intermittent (Twice Weekly) Isoniazid Plus Streptomycin and Daily Isoniazid Plus PAS in the Domiciliary Treatment of Pulmonary Tuberculosis: Tuberculosis Chemotherapy Centre, Madras," *Bulletin of the World Health Organization* 31 (1964): 247–271.

108. On the development of drugs see Z. Ahmad, N. H. Makaya, and J. Grosset, "History of Drug Discovery: Early Evaluation Studies and Lessons Learnt from Them," *Progress in Respiratory Research* 40 (2012): 2–9; Wallace Fox, "The Scope of the Controlled Clinical Trial, Illustrated by Studies of Pulmonary Tuberculosis," *Bulletin of the World Health Organization* 45, no. 5 (1971): 559–572, esp. 570.

109. W. Fox and D. A. Mitchison, "Short-course Chemotherapy for Pulmonary Tuberculosis," *American Review of Respiratory Disease* 111, no. 3 (1975): 325–353.

110. Johannes Holm to Dr. M. G. Candau, Director General, WHO, 2 January 1967, ETH-MBD-001 [Ethiopia], WHO Archives.

111. "1967–68 East Africa TB Centre Report," FD 12/557, NAUK.

112. E. Roelsgaard, E. Iverson, and C. Bløcher, "Tuberculosis in Tropical Africa," *Bulletin of the World Health Organization* 30 (1964): 459–518, 495.

113. J. A. Aluoch to Director of Medical Services, 11 July 1978, BY/13/336, KNA.

114. "Report of a Committee Set Up by the Medical Research Council to Study Future Prospects," *Bulletin of the International Union Against Tuberculosis* 55, nos. 3–4 (1980): 86–92, 86.

115. W. G. Allan, "Tuberculosis in Hong Kong Ten Years Later," *Tubercle* 54, no. 3 (1973): 234–246, 242.

116. *Tuberculosis Control: Report of a UIAT/WHO Study Group*, World Health Organization Technical Report Series, no. 671 (Geneva: WHO, 1982), 21. WHO Library.

117. Dr. J. Dekker RTLC Kigoma, Tanzania National Tuberculosis/Leprost Programme, Kigoma Region, Annual Report, 1987, Archives of the International Union Against Tuberculosis and Lung Disease, Paris, France.

CHAPTER 10. THE MAKING OF THE HIV/TB PANDEMIC

Epigraphs: Gnana Sunderam, Reynard J. McDonald, Theodore Maniatis, James Oleske, Rajendra Kapila, and Lee Reichman, "Tuberculosis as a Manifestation of the Acquired Immunodeficiency Syndrome," *Journal of the American Medical Association* 256, no. 3 (1986): 362–366, 365; J. Prignot and J. Sonnet, "AIDS, Tuberculosis, and Mycobacterioses," *Bulletin of the International Union Against Tuberculosis and Lung Disease* 62, no. 4 (1987): 7–10; Richard Chaisson, "Tuberculosis and HIV Infection—New Opportunities for an Old Pathogen," *Western Journal of Medicine* 150, no. 6 (1989): 687–689, 689; J. L. Stanford, J. M. Grange, and A. Pozniak, "Is Africa Lost?" *Lancet* 338, no. 8766 (1991): 557–558; USAID, *HIV/AIDS: The Evolution of the Pandemic, the Evolution of the Response* (Washington, D.C.: USAID, 1993), 7; "HIV and Tuberculosis: Implications for TB Control Strategies and Agenda for Collaboration of AIDS and TB Programmes," WHO/TB/CARG(4)/94.4, Archives of the International Union Against Tuberculosis and Lung Disease (hereafter IUATLD Archives), Paris, France.

1. WHO, "WHO Three Is Meeting, Intensified Case Finding (ICF), Isoniazid Preventive Therapy (IPT), and TB Infection Control (IC) for People Living with HIV," Report of a Joint World Health Organization HIV/AIDS and TB Department Meeting, 2–4 April 2008, Geneva, Switzerland, p. 2.

2. Michael Sidibé, "HIV and TB: Untangling a Deadly Knot," *Huffington Post*, 25 March 2013, http://www.huffingtonpost.com/michel-sidib/hiv-tb_b_2927149.html.

3. Cheri Vincent, "To Win the Fight against AIDS, We Must First Defeat TB," USAID IMPACT Blog, http://blog.usaid.gov/2013/12/to-win-the-fight-against-aids-we-must-first-defeat-tb/.

4. Anthony D. Harries, Rony Zachariah, Elizabeth L. Corbett, Stephan D. Lawn, Ezio T. Santos-Filho, Rhehab Chimzizi, Mark Harrington, Dermot Maher, Brian G. Williams, and Kevin M. De Cock, "The HIV-Associated Tuberculosis Epidemic—When Will We Act?" *Lancet* 375, no. 9729 (2010): 1906–1919, 1906.

5. A. D. Harries, "Tuberculosis and Human Immunodeficiency Virus Infection in Developing Countries," *Lancet* 335, no. 8686 (1990): 387–390.

6. "Guidelines for National Tuberculosis Control Programmes in View of the HIV Epidemic," IUATLD Archives; Gary Slutkin, WHO/GPA, commented on the slow movement of the WHO and speculated that it might be due to disagreement over priorities or inadequate staffing in WHO's TB section. Gary Slutkin, memo on TUB-GPA collaboration, 11 August 1989, A20/180/16.29, WHO Archives.

7. Global Tuberculosis Programme, "Tuberculosis and HIV Research: Working Towards Solutions," Results of a WHO Workshop on the Formulation of a New TB/HIV Research Strategy, Geneva, 29–31 May 1995, WHO/TB/95.193, p. 2, WHO Library.

8. Stanford, Grange, and Pozniak, "Is Africa Lost?"

9. Kevin De Cock, "The New Tuberculosis," *Africa Health* 8 (1994): 8–10.

10. For the first mention of IPT see Arthur E. Pitchenik and Margaret A. Fischi, "Disseminated Tuberculosis and Acquired Immunodeficiency Syndrome," *Annals of Internal Medicine* 97, no. 1 (1983): 112; J. Sonnet et al., "High Prevalence of Tuberculosis in HIV Infected Black Patients from Central Africa," *Annales de la Société Belge de Médicin Tropicale* 67 (1987): 299–300; Lee B. Reichman, "HIV Infection—A New Face of Tuberculosis," *Bulletin of the International Union Against Tuberculosis and Lung Disease* 63, no. 3 (1988): 19–26, 23; H. van Deutekom, "Chemoprophylaxis and Chemotherapy of Tuberculosis in HIV Infected Patients," *Bulletin of the International Union Against Tuberculosis and Lung Disease* 65, nos. 2–3 (1990): 84–85. For an early look at a somewhat primitive, but suggestive, version of the Three *I*'s see Joint Working Group on HIV Infection and Tuberculosis of the World Health Organization (WHO), Global Programme on AIDS (WHO/GPA), Tuberculosis Unit (WHO/TUB), and the International Union Against Tuberculosis and Lung Disease (IUATLD), "Geneva, 18–19 January 1988, Meeting Report and

Recommendations," *Bulletin of the International Union Against Tuberculosis and Lung Disease* 63, no. 3 (1988): 16–18, 17.

11. Among others cited in the notes, a 1997 review by Mario Raviglione and others reads as if it were written in 2010. The year-to-year repetition in these kinds of reviews leaves one wondering what kind of progress has been, or can be, made when over the course of twenty years the recommendations remain the same. This is not to suggest that the recommendations themselves are insufficient or are not state-of-the-art. It is to point out that what often seems new is actually old. M. C. Raviglione, A. D. Harries, R. Msiska, D. Wilkinson, and P. Nunn, "Tuberculosis and HIV: Current Status in Africa," *AIDS* 11, suppl. B (1997): S115–S123.

12. Paul Nunn, Alasdair Reid, and Kevin M. De Cock, "Tuberculosis and HIV Infection: The Global Setting," *Journal of Infectious Diseases* 196, suppl. 1 (2007): S5–S14, S5.

13. E. L Corbett, B. Marston, G. J. Churchyard, and K. M. De Cock, "Tuberculosis in Sub-Saharan Africa: Opportunities, Challenges, and Change in the Era of Antiretroviral Treatment," *Lancet* 367, no. 9514 (2006): 926–937.

14. Simon J. Tsiouris et al., "Tuberculosis and HIV, Needed: A New Paradigm for the Control and Management of Linked Epidemics," *Journal of the International AIDS Society* 9 (2007): 62–66.

15. Elizabeth L. Corbett et al., "The Growing Burden of Tuberculosis: Global Trends and Interactions with the HIV Epidemic," *Archives of Internal Medicine* 163 (2003): 1009–1021.

16. Gerald Friedland et al., "Implementation Issues in Tuberculosis/HIV Program Collaboration and Integration: 3 Case Studies," *Journal of Infectious Diseases* 196, suppl. 1 (2007): S114–S123.

17. WHO, "Global Tuberculosis Control 2009: Epidemiology, Strategy, Financing." WHO/HTM/TB/2009.411 (Geneva: WHO, 2009).

18. The literature on the origins of HIV is immense. For the most accessible see Jacques Pepin, *The Origins of AIDS* (Cambridge: Cambridge University Press, 2011); David Quammen, "The Chimp and the River," in *Spillover: Animal Infections and the Next Human Pandemic* (New York: W. W. Norton, 2012).

19. A. Rouillon, "The Mutual Assistance Programme of the IUATLD: Development, Contribution and Significance," *Bulletin of the International Union Against Tuberculosis and Lung Disease* 66 (1991): 159–172, 168.

20. Memorandum from Arata Kochi, Chief TUB, WHO, to R. Widdus and G. Slutkin, GPA, WHO, 30 June 1989, A20/181/130, WHO Archives.

21. Bretton quoted in Kenneth B. Noble, "AIDS Linked to TB Outbreak in Africa," *New York Times*, 29 April 1990.

22. "Le Lutte antituberculeuse dans un pays en développement: La Côte d'Ivoire des origines à 1991, l'apparition du Sida-Tuberculose, pas les Dr Raymond Bretton et Geneviève Bretton le 10 Janvier 1991," A20/180/16AF.1, WHO Archives.

23. Zhi-Yi Hu, Trip Report: Study of HIV-1 and HIV-2 infection in patients attending TB centers in Abidjan, 2–5 October 1991, A20/181/131, Jacket 2, WHO Archives.

24. Jean Felix Ganaga, "Projet de Recherche Tuberculose-SIDA au Congo," A20/180/16AF.4, WHO Archives.

25. Peter Eriki, Presentation during TB/AIDS Managers' Meeting, Lake Victoria Hotel, Entebbe-Uganda, 27–30 April 1992, IUATLD Archives. Emphasis in original.

26. J. W. Pape, B. Liautaud, F. Thomas, J. R. Mathurin, M. M. St. Amand, M. Boncy, V. Pean, M. Pamphile, A. C. Laroche, and W. D. Johnson, "Characteristics of the Acquired Immunodeficiency Syndrome (AIDS) in Haiti," *New England Journal of Medicine* 309, no. 16 (1983): 945–950; A. E. Pitchenik, M. A. Fischl, G. M. Dickinson, D. M. Becker, A. M. Fournier, M. T. O'Connell, R. M. Colton, and T. J. Spira, "Opportunistic Infections and Kaposi's Sarcoma among Haitians: Evidence of a New Acquired Immunodeficiency State," *Annals of Internal Medicine* 98, no. 3 (1983): 277–284.

27. J. Mann, D. E. Snider, H. Francis, T. C. Quinn, R. L. Colebunders, P. Piot, J. W. Curran, N. Nzilambi, N. Bosenge, and M. Malonga, "Association between HTLV-III/LAV Infection and Tuberculosis in Zaire," *Journal of the American Medical Association* 256, no. 3 (1986): 346; Bob Colebunders to Jonathan Mann, 28 January 1988, A20.180.16.56, WHO Archives; see also J. C. Willame, "Tuberculose et Sero-Positive Anti-VIH à Kinshasa, Zaire," *Annales de la Société Belge de Médicin Tropicale* 68 (1988): 165–167; for an earlier recognition of the connection see A. E. Pitchenik, C. Cole, B. W. Russell, M. A. Fischl, T. J. Spira, and D. E. Snider, "Tuberculosis, Atypical Mycobacteriosis, and the Acquired Immunodeficiency Syndrome among Haitian and Non-Haitian Patients in South Florida," *Annals of Internal Medicine* 101, no. 5 (1984): 641–645.

28. Project SIDA, Department of Public Health, Kinshasa, Zaire, "Secondary Mycobacterium Tuberculosis in Household Contacts of HIV Seropositive Individuals with Pulmonary Tuberculosis," proposal submitted to UNDP/

WORLD BANK/WHO Special Programme for Research and Training in Tropical Diseases, June 1988, A20/181/124.9, WHO Archives.

29. Mads Melbye et al., "Evidence for Heterosexual Transmission and Clinical Manifestations of Human Immunodeficiency Syndrome and Related Conditions in Lusaka, Zambia," *Lancet* 328, no. 8516 (1986): 1113–1115.

30. Sunderam et al., "Tuberculosis as a Manifestation of the Acquired Immunodeficiency Syndrome (AIDS)."

31. Prignot and Sonnet, "AIDS, Tuberculosis, and Mycobacterioses," 710; see also G. Slutkin, J. Leowski, and J. Mann, "Effects of the AIDS Epidemic on the Tuberculosis Problem and Tuberculosis Programmes," *Bulletin of the International Union Against Tuberculosis and Lung Disease* 63, no. 2 (1988): 20–24. They wrote that when TB and HIV meet the "result may be an increased number of cases of tuberculosis in some regions of the world" (20).

32. Paul Farmer, *AIDS and Accusation: Haiti and the Geography of Blame* (Berkeley: University of California Press, 1992), 107–108, 117.

33. R. L. Colebunders, "HIV Infection in Patients with Tuberculosis in Kinshasa, Zaire," *American Review of Respiratory Disease* 139, no. 5 (1989): 1082–1085, 1085.

34. Review of Tuberculosis Control Programme, South Africa, 1995/96, Part 4: Preparation for a Situational Analysis of the TB Programme, HIV AND TB, in South Africa, TB Control Programme—Part of a Collection of Guidelines, Plans, Reports, Data of 46 African Countries, 1960–2000, REAP HTM1-STB-TBS, WHO Archives.

35. "Report of Informal Consultation on Chemoprophylaxis to Prevent Tuberculosis among Persons Infected with Human Immunodeficiency Virus," Geneva, 6–8 February 1990, A20-180-16.7, WHO Archives.

36. L. Mbengerenwa et al., "Association between Human Immunodeficiency Virus (HIV) and Tuberculosis in Zimbabwe," no date but included with Paul Neill to Fabio Luelmo, GPA, 14 March 1989, A20/181160/3, WHO Archives.

37. "Technical Report of the Activities of the Institute of Phthisiology and Pneumology, Rio De Janeiro Federal University, February 1988 to May 1991, Topic: Study of the Association between Tuberculosis and HIV Infection in Rio de Janeiro," A20.180.16BRA.2, WHO Archives.

38. "Asociation HIV y Tuberculosis, Guias Tecnicas, Washington D.C., 19–21 de noviembre de 1992," A20/180/16AM.1, WHO Archives.

39. "Guidelines for National Tuberculosis Control Programmes in View of the HIV Epidemic," 1 March 1990, IUATLD Archives. In 1995 two researchers made a definitive causal link between the rise in HIV-related TB in Tanzania

between 1985 and 1989. Maarten R. A. van Cleef and H. J. Chum, "The Proportion of Tuberculosis Cases in Tanzania Attributable to Human Immunodeficiency Virus," *International Journal of Epidemiology* 24, no. 3 (1995): 637–642; on AIDS and TB in Tanzania see also Philip W. Setel, *A Plague of Paradoxes: AIDS, Culture, and Demography in Northern Tanzania* (Chicago: University of Chicago Press, 1999).

40. Tuberculosis Trend, 1980–1988, table appended to Professor C. Chintu, University of Zambia to H. G. ten Dam, Sec. TB/HIV Research, Coordinating Committee, Tuberculosis Programme and Global Programme on AIDS, 18 June 1990, A20–181–244.3; see also Annex 4, "Notifications of Tuberculosis Cases from 1964 till 1993," in Maarten C. J. Bosman, "Report No. 1 of the Visit to the National AIDS/STD/Tuberculosis/Leprosy Control Program of Zambia, 2–16 October 1994," REAP/HTM1/STB/TBS/Zambia, both in WHO Archives.

41. Ministry of Health, Tuberculosis and Leprosy Control Unit, "Annual Report on Tuberculosis and Leprosy in Zambia, 1990," REAP/HTM1/STB/TBS/Zambia/6, WHO Archives.

42. See study protocol for "A Study of the Efficacy of 2EHRZ/6H3E3 for the Treatment of Smear Positive Pulmonary Tuberculosis in HIV-infected Ugandans," 1995, in T9/181/166, WHO Archives.

43. "Progress Report on Research Project 'TB-HIV Infection Trends,'" October 1990–March 1991, A20/181/159.3, WHO Archives.

44. USAID, *HIV/AIDS: The Evolution of the Pandemic, the Evolution of the Response*, 33.

45. W. A. Githui, D. Kwamanga, J. M. Chakaya, F. G. Karimi, and P. G. Waiyaki, "Anti-Tuberculous Initial Drug Resistance of Mycobacterium Tuberculosis in Kenya: A Ten-Year Review," *East African Medical Journal* 70, no. 10 (1993): 609–612, 609.

46. Tuberculosis Programme and the Global Programme on AIDS, "Tuberculosis/HIV Research, Report of a WHO Review and Planning Meeting, Geneva, 24–26 February 1992," WHO/TB/92.167, 12.

47. "Report of Informal Consultation on Chemoprophylaxis to Prevent Tuberculosis among Persons Infected with Human Immunodeficiency Virus."

48. Joint Working Group on HIV Infection and Tuberculosis, "Geneva, 18–19 January 1988, Meeting Report and Recommendations," 17.

49. See, for example: "Interrelations of Tropical Diseases and HIV Infection: Report of an Informal Consultation Held at the Kenya Medical Research

Institute (KEMRI), Co-sponsored by the UNSP/World Bank/WHO Special Programme for Training in Tropical Diseases (TMR) and the Global Programme on AIDS (GPA)," 1–4 December 1987, TDR/GPA/TD-HIV/87.3; "Report of a Technical Advisory Meeting on Research on AIDS and Tuberculosis," Geneva, 2–4 August 1988, WHO/GPA/BMR/89.3; Gary Slutkin to Tom Daniel, 19 September 1988, A20/180/16AF.7, WHO Archives.

50. Project SIDA, Department of Public Health, Kinshasa, Zaire, "Secondary Mycobacterium Tuberculosis in Household Contacts of HIV Seropositive Individuals with Pulmonary Tuberculosis."

51. Memorandum from Arata Kochi to Jonathan Mann, 17 July 1989, Subject: TB/AIDS WORKSHOP, A20/160/16AM.13, WHO Archives.

52. "Proposal for the Study of HIV-1 and HIV-2 Infections in Patients Attending the Centres Antituberculeaux in Abidjan, Cote D-Ivoire," no date but filed with papers from 1989, A20/181/131.25, WHO Archives.

53. "HIV/TB Research Projects (1990/91)," appended to Minutes of the TB/HIV Coordinating Committee, 29 November 1990, A20/181/244.3; TUB/GPA Collaborative Research Programme, "A Summary of Ongoing Research Projects & Budget Information," 6 May 1993, A20/180/16/2.3, WHO Archives.

54. Chaisson to Richard O'Brien, WHO, 21 April 1995, A20-181-227, WHO Archives.

55. Richard Chaisson of Johns Hopkins and Mark Harrington of the Treatment Action Campaign wrote in 2009 that "following the development of short-course chemotherapy in the 1970s and 1980s, research into TB virtually evaporated." R. E. Chaisson and Mark Harrington, "How Research Can Help Control Tuberculosis," *International Journal of Tuberculosis and Lung Disease* 13, no. 5 (2009): 558–568, 558.

56. WHO Press Release, "Vaccination against Tuberculosis, WHO Experts to Meet in Copenhagen," 27 November 1953, Press Release WHO/70, MOH 3/742, Kenya National Archives.

57. D. E. Snider and J. R. La Montagne, "The Neglected Global Tuberculosis Problem: A Report of the 1992 World Congress on Tuberculosis," *Journal of Infectious Diseases* 169, no. 6 (1994): 1189–1196.

58. Laurie Garrett, *The Coming Plague: Newly Emerging Diseases in a World Out of Balance* (New York: Penguin, 1994), 710 footnote 176.

59. WHO, "The HIV/AIDS and Tuberculosis Epidemics: Implications for TB Control," 1994, WHO/TB/CARG(4)/94.4, p. 2, WHO Library.

60. Global Tuberculosis Programme, "Tuberculosis and HIV Research: Working Towards Solutions," Results of a WHO Workshop on the Formulation of a New TB/HIV Research Strategy, Geneva, 29–31 May 1995, WHO/TB/95.193, p. 2, WHO Archives.

61. For the WHO/IUAT group see *Tuberculosis Control: Report of a IUAT/ WHO Study Group*, World Health Organization Technical Report Series, no. 671 (Geneva: WHO, 1982), 21. WHO Library. The decline in interest in TB is well documented. See Jessica Ogden, Gill Walt, and Louisiana Lush, "The Politics of 'Branding' in Policy Transfer: The Case of DOTS for Tuberculosis Control," *Social Science and Medicine* 57 (2003): 179–188; M.C. Raviglione and A. Pio, "Evolution of WHO Policies for Tuberculosis Control, 1948–2001," *Lancet* 359, no. 9308 (2002): 775–780; Chaisson and Harrington, "How Research Can Help Control Tuberculosis"; Christopher Murray, Karel Styblo, and Annick Rouillon, "Tuberculosis," in *Disease Control Priorities in Developing Countries*, edited by Dean T. Jamison, W. Henry Mosley, Anthony R. Measham, and José Bobadilla (Oxford: published for the World Bank by Oxford University Press, 1993), 233–259, 256; Kraig Klaudt, "The Political Causes and Solutions of the Current Tuberculosis Epidemic," in *The Politics of Emerging and Resurgent Infectious Diseases*, edited by Jim Whitman (London: Macmillan, 2000), 86–109; on the neglect of TB and the WHO's diminished presence see also B. R. Bloom, and C. J. Murray, "Tuberculosis: Commentary on a Reemergent Killer," *Science* 257, no. 5073 (1992): 1055–1064, 1061.

62. "Report of Informal Consultation on Chemoprophylaxis to Prevent Tuberculosis among Persons Infected with Human Immunodeficiency Virus."

63. Johannes Holm, "Tuberculosis Control in the Developing World: It's Time for a Change," *World Health Forum* 5 (1984): 107.

64. Karel Styblo, "Major Problems/Opportunities (Political and Operational Issues)," TUB Informal Discussion, Development of Guidelines for TB Control in HIV Epidemic Countries/Areas, Geneva, 2–3 October 1989, IUATLD Archives.

65. "Guidelines for National Tuberculosis Programmes in View of the HIV Epidemic," IUATLD Archives.

66. P. Sudre, G. ten Dam, and A. Kochi, "Tuberculosis: A Global Overview of the Situation Today," *Bulletin of the World Health Organization* 70, no. 2 (1992): 149–159. See also J. Shiffman, T. Beer, and Y. Wu, "The Emergence of Global Disease Control Priorities," *Health Policy and Planning* 17, no. 3

(2002): 225–234; on the global emergency see *TB: A Global Emergency*, WHO/TB/94.177.

67. For the program in Dar es Salaam being on the verge of collapse, and for the emerging threat of HIV/AIDS in general, see "The National Tuberculosis/Leprosy Programme in Tanzania, Summary Report No. 26 on the Visit to Tanzania, July/August 1990"; for more on Tanzania's program being over-stretched in the face of AIDS see, for example, "The National Tuberculosis/Leprosy Programme in Tanzania, Summary Report No.24 on the Visit to Tanzania, August 1990"; see also Report No. 22, August 1989, among others. All in IUATLD Archives; on Tanzania's program see Karel Styblo, "The National Tuberculosis/Leprosy Programme in Tanzania," WHO/TB/88.153, WHO Library.

68. Dr. D. R. Nagpaul, "Why Integrated Tuberculosis Programmes Have Not Succeeded in Many Developing Countries—A Collection of Observations," Joint IUAT/WHO Study Group, Geneva, 14–18 September 1981, WHO/IUAT/JSG/BP/81.4.

69. Consultation on the Application of Tuberculosis Control within Primary Health Care Activities, Geneva, 22–26 September 1986, "Country Experiences in Integration of Specific Programmes into the Primary Health Care System: Kenya," by Dr. W. Koinange Karuga, Director of Medical Services, Ministry of Health, Nairobi, Kenya, TRI/TB.PHC/86.15, REAP/HTMi/STB/TBS/KENYA/LIBERIA, WHO Archives.

70. WHO/IUATLD, "The HIV/AIDS and Tuberculosis Epidemics: Implications for TB Control," WHO/TB/CARG(4)/94.4, 12, 5.

71. On the extremely weak TB program in Zambia see R. Stoneburner, "Trip Report: Protocol Development and Feasibility Assessment of a Study of the Feasibility of Isoniazid Preventive Therapy for Persons Infected with m. TB and HIV, Uganda and Zambia," A20/181/228.4, WHO Archives.

72. For hospital deaths see J. Andersson, Tuberculosis Specialist, Ministry of Health, Lusaka, Zambia, "Job Report," 10 June 1992, REAP/HTMi/STB/TBS/Zambia, WHO Archives; for 40 percent see Dr. N. C. Syabbalo, Lusaka, Zambia, to the Editor, "Pulmonary Tuberculosis and Acquired Immunodeficiency Syndrome," *Chest* 92 (1987): 383–384; for nearly 60 per-cent see O. O. Simooya et al., "HIV Infection in Newly Diagnosed Tuberculosis Patients in Ndola, Zambia," *Central African Journal of Medicine* 37 (1991): 4–7, 6. Data for this study were collected in 1987.

73. Staff Appraisal Report: Zambia, Health Sector Support Project, October 14, 1994, Document of the World Bank, Report No. 13480-ZA, p. 45. http://

www-wds.worldbank.org/external/default/WDSContentServer/
WDSP/IB/1994/10/14/000009265_3961007062816/Rendered/PDF/
multiopage.pdf.

74. J. Andersson, Tuberculosis Specialist, Ministry of Health, Lusaka, Zambia, "Job Report," 10 June 1992, REAP/HTM1/STB/TBS/Zambia, WHO Archives.

75. C. Chintu to J. Narain, WHO, 28 August 1991, A20/181/226; Maarten Bosman, Report no. 1 of the visit to the National AIDS/STD/Tuberculosis/Leprosy control Program of Zambia, 2–16 October 1994, pp. 31–34, REAP/HTM1/STB/TBS/Zambia/4, both in WHO Archives.

76. "HIV and Tuberculosis: Implications for TB Control Strategies and Agenda for Collaboration of AIDS and TB Programmes," WHO/TB/CARG(4)/94.4, IUATLD Archives.

77. J. Andersson, Tuberculosis Specialist, Ministry of Health, Lusaka, Zambia, "Job Report," 10 June 1992, REAP/HTM1/STB/TBS/Zambia, WHO Archives.

78. Stanford, Grange, and Pozniak, "Is Africa Lost?" The meeting they discussed was in 1990, while the article was published in 1991.

79. Corbett et al., "Tuberculosis in Sub-Saharan Africa," 927.

80. Global Programme on AIDS and Tuberculosis Programme, World Health Organization, in collaboration with the International Union Against Tuberculosis and Lung Disease, "Tuberculosis and AIDS: Statement on AIDS and Tuberculosis: Geneva, March 1989," *Bulletin of the International Union Against Tuberculosis and Lung Disease* 64, no. 1 (1989): 8–11, 8.

81. On this point see Kevin De Cock et al., "Tuberculosis and HIV Infection in Sub-Saharan Africa," *Journal of the American Medical Association* 268, no. 12 (23–30 September 1992): 1581–1587.

82. John Iliffe, *The African AIDS Epidemic* (Athens: Ohio State University Press, 2006), 68.

83. See generally ibid. and Greg Behrman, *The Invisible People: How the U.S. Has Slept Through the Global AIDS Pandemic, the Greatest Humanitarian Catastrophe of Our Time* (New York: Free Press, 2004). On Mahler's support of the Global Program see Barton Gellman, "The Belated Global Response to AIDS in Africa, World Shunned Signs of the Coming Plague," *Washington Post*, 5 July 2001, A1; Kevin De Cock, Dorothy Mbori-Ngacha, and Elizabeth Marum, "Shadow on the Continent: Public Health and HIV/AIDS in Africa in the 21st Century," *Lancet* 360, no. 9326 (2002): 67–72.

84. Iliffe, *African AIDS Epidemic*, 68–79.

85. On this period see Theodore M. Brown, Marcos Cueto, and Elizabeth Fee, "The World Health Organization and the Transition from 'International' to 'Global' Public Health," *American Journal of Public Health* 96, no. 1 (2006): 62–72; Nitsan Chorev, *The World Health Organization between North and South* (Ithaca: Cornell University Press, 2012), 124–159.

86. *UNAIDS: The First Ten Years* (Joint United Nations Programme on HIV/AIDS, 2008), UNAIDS/07.20E/JC1262E, p. 7.

87. Paul Taylor, "The United Nations System under Stress: Financial Pressures and Their Consequences," *Review of International Studies* 17, no. 4 (1991): 365–382, 378.

88. Gil Walt, "WHO under Stress: Implications for Health Policy," *Health Policy* 24, no. 2 (1993): 125–144.

89. G. Slutkin, "Global AIDS 1981–1999: The Response," *International Journal of Tuberculosis and Lung Disease* 4, no. 2, suppl. 1 (2000): S24–S33, S30.

90. *UNAIDS: The First Ten Years*, 20.

91. On this point see Behrman, *The Invisible People*, 96.

CHAPTER 11. PREVENTION, CURE, AND THE SEARCH FOR THE CHEAPEST SOLUTION

1. J. F. Murray, "Cursed Duet: HIV Infection and Tuberculosis," *Respiration* 57 (1990): 210–220, 213.

2. See, for example, Randall Packard, "Visions of Postwar Health and Development and Their Impact on Public Health Interventions in the Developing World," in Randall Packard and Frederick Cooper, eds., *International Development and the Social Sciences* (Berkeley: University of California Press, 1997), 93–115; Marcos Cueto, "The Origins of Primary Health Care and Selective Primary Health Care," *American Journal of Public Health* 94, no. 11 (2004): 1864–1874.

3. For this period Nitsan Chorev, *The World Health Organization between North and South* (Ithaca: Cornell University Press, 2012), 124–159, is essential. See also Theodore M. Brown, Marcos, Cueto, and Elizabeth Fee, "The World Health Organization and the Transition from 'International' to 'Global' Public Health," *American Journal of Public Health* 96, no. 1 (2006): 62–72, 68; on the WHO's transition see also G. Walt, "WHO under Stress: Implications for Health Policy," *Health Policy* 24, no. 2 (1993): 125–144; Jennifer Prah Ruger, "The Changing Role of the World Bank in Global Health," *American Journal of Public Health* 95, no. 1 (2005): 60–70.

4. Michael Specter, "What Money Can Buy," *New Yorker*, 24 October 2005, 56–71, 66; for the report's influence at the time, especially in Africa, see Walt, "WHO under Stress," 140.

5. Matthew Basilico, Jonathan Weigel, Anjali Motgi, Jaco Bor, and Salmaan Keshavee, "Health for All? Competing Theories and Geopolitics," in *Reimagining Global Health: An Introduction*, edited by Paul Farmer, Jim Yong Kim, Arthur Kleinman, and Matthew Basilico (Berkeley: University of California Press, 2013), 212–244, esp. 234–242; Howard Stein, *Beyond the World Bank Agenda: An Institutional Approach to Development* (Chicago: University of Chicago Press, 2008), esp. 207–248; for an excellent case study of the ways in which thinking about health care in this way have had an impact on global health, and from where I borrowed the term "infiltrate," see Salmaan Keshavjee, *Blind Spot: How Neoliberalism Infiltrated Global Health* (Berkeley: University of California Press, 2014), esp. 1–17, 85–109.

6. For my discussion of primary health care I have relied heavily on Cueto's essential article "The Origins of Primary Health Care and Selective Primary Health Care." Quote on 1868.

7. Ibid.

8. J. A. Walsh and K. S. Warren, "Selective Primary Health Care: An Interim Strategy for Disease Control in Developing Countries," *New England Journal of Medicine* 301, no. 18 (1979): 967–974, 969; for the conference and Walsh and Warren's influence see Cueto "The Origins of Primary Health Care and Selective Primary Health Care," esp. 1868.

9. Cueto, "The Origins of Primary Health Care and Selective Primary Health Care," 1871.

10. Karel Styblo, "The National Tuberculosis/Leprosy Programme in Tanzania," WHO/TB/88/153, p. 10, WHO Library.

11. C. J. Murray, K. Styblo, and A. Rouillon, "Tuberculosis in Developing Countries: Burden, Intervention and Cost," *Bulletin of the International Union Against Tuberculosis and Lung Disease* 65, no. 1 (1990): 6–24, 20; see also Gill Walt, "The Politics of Tuberculosis: The Role of Process and Power," in *Tuberculosis: An Interdisciplinary Perspective*, edited by John H. Porter and John M. Grange (London: Imperial College Press, 1999), 67–98, 71–72.

12. C. J. Murray, E. DeJonghe, H. J. Chum, D. S. Nyangulu, A. Salomao, and K. Styblo, "Cost Effectiveness of Chemotherapy for Pulmonary Tuberculosis in Three Sub-Saharan African Countries," *Lancet* 338, no. 8778 (1991): 1305–1308. On this work and its influence see Jessica Ogden, Gill Walt, and

Louisiana Lush, "The Politics of 'Branding' in Policy Transfer: The Case of DOTS for Tuberculosis Control," *Social Science and Medicine* 57 (2003): 179–188, 183.

13. *World Development Report, 1993: Investing in Health* (Oxford: published for the World Bank by Oxford University Press, 1993), 27.

14. "Results of Directly Observed Short-course Chemotherapy in 112,842 Chinese Patients with Smear-positive Tuberculosis: China Tuberculosis Control Collaboration," *Lancet* 347, no. 8998 (1996): 358–362.

15. Jai P. Narain, Mario C. Raviglione, and Arata Kochi, "HIV-Associated Tuberculosis in Developing Countries: Epidemiology and Strategies for Prevention," WHO/TB/92.166, WHO Library.

16. Shirley H. Ferebee, Frank W. Mount, and Carroll E. Palmer, "Tuberculosis Prophylaxis Trials in Preview," *Public Health Reports* 72, no. 8 (1957): 703–704; Shirley H. Ferebee, "Human Trials of Tuberculosis Prophylaxis," *Bulletin of the New York Academy of Medicine* 34, no. 11 (1958): 741–746.

17. A. W. Dahlstrom, J. L. Wilson, and B. B. Sedlacek, "The Immediate Effectiveness of Isoniazid Chemoprophylaxis as Determined by the Tuberculin Test: A Five-Year Study Including 5,555 Navajo and Pueblo Children from Birth to 15 Years of Age and the Use of Isonicotinic Acid Hydrazide in the Prevention of Tuberculosis," *Diseases of the Chest* 38 (1960): 599–603.

18. B. A. Dormer, I. Harrison, J. A. Swart, and S. R. Vidor, "Prophylactic Isoniazid: Protection of Infants in a Tuberculosis Hospital," *Lancet* 2, no. 7108 (1959): 902–903; B. A. Dormer and T. F. B. Collins, "The Prevention of Tuberculosis," *Public Health* (December 1963): 15–25, esp. 21.

19. WHO, "Justification and Design for the Undertaking of a Large-Scale BCG Trial in India," WHO/TB/Int./50, 3 December 1963, WHO Library.

20. T. Egsmose, J. O. Ang'awa, and S. J. Poti, "The Use of Isoniazid among Household Contacts of Open Cases of Pulmonary Tuberculosis," *Bulletin of the World Health Organization* 33, no. 3 (1965): 419–433; for the Tunisian study see "Report on Tuberculosis Chemotherapy Pilot Project (Tunisia 9)," by J. Nyboe, A. R. Farah, and O. W. Christensen, WHO/TB/Techn. Information/10, 22 April 1963, WHO Library.

21. P. Smit, "Chemoprophylaxis of Pulmonary Tuberculosis," *Proceedings of the Mine Medical Officers Association* 48 (1968): 19–28, discussion on 27–28.

22. S. H. Ferebee, "Controlled Chemoprophylaxis Trials in Tuberculosis: A General Review," *Advanced Tuberculosis Research* 26 (1970): 28–106, 95.

23. G. W. Comstock, C. Baum, and D. E. Snider, "Isoniazid Prophylaxis among Alaskan Eskimos: A Final Report of the Bethel Isoniazid Studies," *American Review of Respiratory Disease* 119, no. 5 (1979): 827–830.

24. G. W. Comstock and R. N. Philip, "Decline of the Tuberculosis Epidemic in Alaska," *Public Health Reports* 76 (1961): 19–24, 22.

25. M. E. Porter and G. W. Comstock, "Ambulatory Chemotherapy in Alaska," *Public Health Reports* 77 (1962): 1021–1032; for TB in Alaska at this time see generally Robert Fortuine, *"Must We All Die?": Alaska's Enduring Struggle with Tuberculosis* (Fairbanks: University of Alaska Press, 2005), 101–160.

26. G. W. Comstock, "Isoniazid Prophylaxis in an Undeveloped Area," *American Review of Respiratory Disease* 86 (1962): 810–822, 819.

27. M. L. Hanson, G. W. Comstock, and C. E. Haley, "Community Isoniazid Prophylaxis Program in an Underdeveloped Area of Alaska," *Public Health Reports* 82, no. 12 (1967): 1045–1056, 1054.

28. G. J. Kaplan, R. I. Fraser, and G. W. Comstock, "Tuberculosis in Alaska, 1970: The Continued Decline of the Tuberculosis Epidemic," *American Review of Respiratory Disease* 105, no. 6 (1972): 920–926.

29. O. Horwitz, P. G. Payne, and E. Wilbek, "Epidemiological Basis of Tuberculosis Eradication: 4. The Isoniazid Trial in Greenland," *Bulletin of the World Health Organization* 35, no. 4 (1966): 509–526.

30. Guillaume Lachenal, "A Genealogy of Treatment as Prevention (TASP): Prevention, Therapy, and the Tensions of Public Health in African History," in Tamara Giles-Vernick and James L. A. Webb, editors, *Global Health in Africa: Historical Perspectives on Disease Control* (Athens: Ohio University Press, 2013), 70–91, 81.

31. "Report of the WHO/CCTA Tuberculosis Seminar, Nairobi, Kenya 16–22 November 1960," Basutoland-TB, AFP-136, Correspondence, WHO Archives.

32. The WHO recommends against its use in *WHO Expert Committee on Tuberculosis, Eighth Report*, World Health Organization Technical Report Series, no. 290 (Geneva, WHO, 1964), 12; see also "Report of the WHO Inter-Regional Seminar on Tuberculosis Control in Developing Countries," Kuala Lumpur, 5–11 November 1964, WHO/TB/Techn. Information/37.65, p. 8, WHO Library.

33. *WHO Expert Committee on Tuberculosis, Ninth Report*, World Health Organization Technical Report Series, no. 552 (Geneva: WHO, 1974), 22.

34. *Tuberculosis Control: Report of a Joint IUAT/WHO Study Group*, World Health Organization Technical Report Series, no. 671 (Geneva: WHO,

1982), 20; see also "Address by Dr. H. Mahler, Director General of the World Health Organization," *Bulletin of the International Union Against Tuberculosis* 58, no. 1 (1983): 7–10, esp. 8.

35. Global Programme on AIDS, "Report of a Technical Advisory Meeting on Research on AIDS and Tuberculosis," Geneva, 2–4 August 1988, WHO/GPA/BMR/89.3.

36. Jonathan Mann, memo, "Proposed TB/AIDS Workshop," 24 September 1989, A20–180–16.28, WHO Archives.

37. Memo on Proposed TB/AIDS Workshop from Gary Slutkin, GPA, to Arata Kochi, Chief, TUB, 14 July 1989, A20/160/16AM.10, WHO Archives; Global Programme on AIDS and Tuberculosis, "Statement on AIDS and Tuberculosis," Geneva, March 1989, WHO/GPA/INF/89.4.

38. "Africa's Tuberculosis Burden and Chemoprophylaxis," *Lancet* 335, no. 8700 (26 May 1990): 1249–1250.

39. "Report of Informal Consultation on Chemoprophylaxis to Prevent Tuberculosis among Persons Infected with Human Immunodeficiency Virus," Geneva, 6–8 February 1990, A20-180-16.7, WHO Archives.

40. Keith McAdam, principal investigator, "The Prevention of Tuberculosis in HIV Infected Individuals in Zambia," 1 August 1991, Project Proposal Application, A20/181/272.1, WHO Archives.

41. J. P. Narain, M. C. Raviglione, and A. Kochi, "HIV-Associated Tuberculosis in Developing Countries: Epidemiology and Strategies for Prevention," *Tubercle and Lung Disease* 73, no. 6 (1992): 311–321, 318.

42. Facsimile from J. Narain, WHO Medical Officer, to J. Porter, Subject: Prevention of HIV Related TB in Zambia, 16 September 1991, A20/181/272.1, WHO Archives.

43. Jai P. Narain and Mario C. Raviglione, Travel Summary Report, Kampala, Uganda, 28 September 1991–5 October 1991, A20/160/16UG, WHO Archives.

44. P. Godfrey-Faussett, R. Baggaley, A. Mwinga, M. Hosp, J. Porter, N. Luo, M. Kelly, R. Msiska, and K. McAdam, "Recruitment to a Trial of Tuberculosis Preventive Therapy from a Voluntary HIV Testing Centre in Lusaka: Relevance to Implementation" *Transactions of the Royal Society of Tropical Medicine and Hygiene* 89:4 (1995): 354–358, 355.

45. John Porter to Mario Raviglione, 13 November 1992, A20/181/272/1.1, WHO Archives.

46. R. Stoneburner, "Trip Report: Protocol Development and Feasibility Assessment of a Study of the Feasibility of Isoniazid Preventive Therapy

for Persons Infected with m. TB and HIV, Uganda and Zambia," A20/181/228.4, WHO Archives.

47. J. W. Pape, S. S. Jean, J. L. Ho, A. Hafner, and W.D. Johnson, "Effect of Isoniazid Prophylaxis on Incidence of Active Tuberculosis and Progression of HIV Infection," *Lancet* 342, no. 8866 (1993): 268–272.

48. K. De Cock, A. Grant, and J. Porter, "Preventive Therapy for Tuberculosis in HIV-Infected Persons: International Recommendations, Research, and Practice," *Lancet* 345, no. 8953 (1995): 833–836, 835. This article also provides a summary of the work done to date, both published and in abstract form.

49. Ferebee, "Controlled Chemoprophylaxis Trials in Tuberculosis," 97–98.

50. Cooper to Jos Perriens, WHO, 6 September 1994, A20.181.272.2.3, WHO Archives.

51. H. Stott, "Drug Acceptability and Chemoprophylaxis in Under-Developed Countries," 4 March 1959, BY/17/189, KNA.

52. Alwyn Mwinga to Marc Karam, WHO, 18 March 1992, A20.181.272, WHO Archives.

53. Joseph Perriens to David Cooper, 26 January 1994, A20/171/272/2.5; for a detailed breakdown see "The Prevention of HIV-Related Tuberculosis in Zambia," Report on period from 1 December 1993–31 May 1994, A20/171/272/2.4, WHO Archives.

54. Global Tuberculosis Programme, "Tuberculosis and HIV Research: Working Towards Solutions," Results of a WHO Workshop on the Formulation of a New TB/HIV Research Strategy, Geneva, 29–31 May 1995, WHO/TB/95.193, p. 10, WHO Library.

55. "The Prevention of HIV-Related Tuberculosis in Zambia," Report on period from 1 December 1993–31 May 1994.

56. "Feasibility of Isoniazid Preventive Therapy of Tuberculosis among HIV-Infected Persons in Chiang Mai, Thailand," Progress Report, May 1995–April 1996, T9/181/146, WHO Archives.

57. Neil Halsey, project description for "Tuberculosis and Immunodeficiency Virus (HIV) Demonstration Project," 23 June 1989, A20/180/16AM.7, WHO Archives.

58. Thomas Aisu, "Feasibility of TB Preventive Chemotherapy in HIV/TB Infected Individuals," Progress Report, 1 August–31 November 1991, A20/181/228.2, WHO Archives.

59. T. Aisu, M. C. Raviglione, E. van Praag, P. Eriki, J. P. Narain, L. Barugahare, G. Tembo, D. McFarland, and F. A. Engwau, "Preventive

Chemotherapy for HIV-Associated Tuberculosis in Uganda: An Operational Assessment at a Voluntary Counselling and Testing Centre," *AIDS* 9, no. 3 (1995): 267–273.

60. M. C. Bosman, "Health Sector Reform and Tuberculosis Control: The Case of Zambia," *International Journal of Tuberculosis and Lung Disease* 4, no. 7 (2000): 606–614.

61. Global Tuberculosis Programme, "Tuberculosis and HIV Research: Working Towards Solutions," Results of a WHO Workshop on the Formulation of a New TB/HIV Research Strategy, Geneva, 29–31 May 1995, WHO/TB/95.193, p. 9, WHO Library.

CHAPTER 12. PREVENTION VERSUS CURE

1. WHO Tuberculosis Programme, "Framework for Effective Tuberculosis Control," WHO/TB/94.179, p. 3, WHO Library.

2. Ibid., 7.

3. Charles D. Wells, J. Peter Cegielski, Lisa J. Nelson, Kayla F. Laserson, Timothy H. Holtz, Alyssa Finlay, Kenneth G. Castro, and Karin Weyer, "HIV Infection and Multidrug-Resistant Tuberculosis: The Perfect Storm," *Journal of Infectious Diseases* 196, suppl. 1 (2007): S86–S107.

4. On India accepting the loan see J. Shiffman, T. Beer, and Y. Wu, "The Emergence of Global Disease Control Priorities," *Health Policy and Planning* 17, no. 3 (2002): 225–234, 230; on the controversies see J. D. H. Porter and J. A. Ogden, "Public Health, Ethics, and Tuberculosis: Is DOTs a Breakthrough or Inappropriate Strategy in the Indian Context?" *Issues in Medical Ethics* 7, no. 3 (1999): 79–84.

5. *A Deadly Diagnosis: Tuberculosis in the Era of HIV* (WHO: Geneva, 1996), 21.

6. A. Kochi, "Tuberculosis Control—Is DOTS the Health Breakthrough of the 1990s?" *World Health Forum* 18, nos. 3–4 (1997): 225–232; discussion 233–247, quote on 243.

7. On this point see especially J. M. Grange, "DOTS and Beyond: Towards a Holistic Approach to the Conquest of Tuberculosis," *International Journal of Tuberculosis and Lung Disease* 1, no. 4 (1997): 293–296.

8. Jessica Ogden, Gill Walt, and Louisiana Lush, "The Politics of 'Branding' in Policy Transfer: The Case of DOTS for Tuberculosis Control," *Social Science and Medicine* 57, no. 1 (2003): 179–188, 184.

9. Christopher Dye, Catherine J. Watt, Daniel M. Bleed, S. Mehran Hosseini, and Mario C. Raviglione, "Evolution of Tuberculosis Control and Prospects

for Reducing Tuberculosis Incidence, Prevalence, and Deaths Globally," *Journal of the American Medical Association* 293, no. 22 (2005): 2767–2775, 2767; Christopher C. Whalen, "Failure of Directly Observed Treatment for Tuberculosis in Africa: A Call for New Approaches," *Clinical Infectious Diseases* 42, no. 7 (2006): 1048–1050.

10. See generally J. Volmink and P. Garner. "Directly Observed Therapy for Treating Tuberculosis," *Cochrane Database of Systematic Reviews* 4 (2007): 1–31; Christian Lienhardt and Jessica Ann Ogden, "Tuberculosis Control in Resource-Poor Countries: Have We Reached the Limits of the Universal Paradigm?" *Tropical Medicine and International Health* 9, no. 7 (2004): 833–841; R. Bayer, C. Stayton, M. Desvarieux, C. Healton, S. Landesman, and W. Y. Tsai, "Directly Observed Therapy and Treatment Completion for Tuberculosis in the United States: Is Universal Supervised Therapy Necessary?" *American Journal of Public Health* 88, no. 7 (1998): 1052–1058.

11. Christian Lienhardt, Philippe Glaziou, Mukund Uplekar, Knut Lönnroth, Haileyesus Getahun, and Mario Raviglione, "Global Tuberculosis Control: Lessons Learnt and Future Prospects," *Nature Reviews: Microbiology* 10 (2012): 407–416, 409.

12. On being harmful see P. Farmer, J. Bayona, M. Becerra, J. Furin, C. Henry, H. Hiatt, J.Y. Kim, C. Mitnick, E. Nardell, and S. Shin, "The Dilemma of MDR-TB in the Global Era," *International Journal of Tuberculosis and Lung Disease* 2, no. 11 (1998): 869–876, 872; Paul Farmer, "Cruel and Unusual: Drug-Resistant Tuberculosis as Punishment," in Farmer, *Pathologies of Power: Health, Human Rights, and the New War on the Poor* (Berkeley: University of California Press, 2005), 181, 192; Paul Farmer, "DOTS and DOTS-Plus: Not the Only Answer," *Annals of the New York Academy of Sciences* 953 (2001): 165–184.

13. R. Bayer and D. Wilkinson, "Directly Observed Therapy for Tuberculosis: History of an Idea," *Lancet* 345, no. 8964 (1995): 1545–1548; Ogden, Walt, and Lush, "The Politics of 'Branding' in Policy Transfer"; Grange, "DOTS and Beyond"; on Fox paying patients see Niels Brimnes, "Magic Bullets: Chemotherapy," unpublished manuscript in author's possession, 35.

14. C. J. Murray and J. A. Salomon, "Modeling the Impact of Global Tuberculosis Control Strategies," *Proceedings of the National Academy of Sciences* 95, no. 23 (1998): 13881–13886, 13881, 13885.

15. Sarah Bosely, "Profile: Arata Kochi: Shaking up the Malaria World," *Lancet* 367, no. 3267 (2006): 1973.

16. D. B. Young, "New Tools for Tuberculosis Control: Do We Really Need Them?" *International Journal of Tuberculosis and Lung Disease* 1, no. 3 (1997): 193–195, esp. 194.

17. On this point see Jotam G. Pasipanodya and Tawanda Gumbo, "A Meta-Analysis of Self-Administered vs. Directly Observed Therapy Effect on Microbiologic Failure, Relapse, and Acquired Drug Resistance in Tuberculosis Patients," *Clinical Infectious Diseases* 57 (2013): 21–31, 22.

18. Thomas R. Frieden, Paula I. Fujiwara, Rita M. Washko, and Margaret A. Hamburg, "Tuberculosis in New York City—Turning the Tide," *New England Journal of Medicine* 333, no. 4 (1995): 229–233.

19. Salim S. Abdool Karim, Gavin J. Churchyard, Quarraisha Abdool Karim, and Stephen D. Lawn, "HIV Infection and Tuberculosis in South Africa: An Urgent Need to Escalate the Public Health Response," *Lancet* 374, no. 9693 (2009): 921–933, 923; for Africa more generally see E. L. Corbett, B. Marston, G. J. Churchyard, and K. M. De Cock, "Tuberculosis in Sub-Saharan Africa: Opportunities, Challenges, and Change in the Era of Antiretroviral Treatment," *Lancet* 367, no. 514 (2006): 926–937, 928.

20. Stephen D. Lawn, Linda-Gail Bekker, Keren Middelkoop, Landon Myer, and Robin Wood, "Impact of HIV Infection on the Epidemiology of Tuberculosis in a Peri-urban Community in South Africa: The Need for Age-specific Interventions," *Clinical Infectious Diseases* 42, no. 7 (2006): 1040–1047, 1044.

21. See Corbett et al., "Tuberculosis in Sub-Saharan Africa," 928.

22. Dye et al., "Evolution of Tuberculosis Control and Prospects for Reducing Tuberculosis Incidence, Prevalence, and Deaths Globally," 2772.

23. Lixia Wang, Hui Zhang, Yunzhou Ruan, Daniel P. Chin, Yinyin Xia, Shiming Cheng, Mingting Chen, Yanlin Zhao, et al., "Tuberculosis Prevalence in China, 1990–2010: A Longitudinal Analysis of National Survey Data," *Lancet*, published online 18 March 2014, DOI: http://dx.doi.org/10.1016/S0140-6736(13)62639-2.

24. Daiyu Hu, Xiaoyun Liu, Jing Chen, Yang Wang, Tao Wang, Wei Zeng, Helen Smith, and Paul Garner, "Direct Observation and Adherence to Tuberculosis Treatment in Chongqing, China: A Descriptive Study," *Health Policy and Planning* 23, no. 1 (2008): 43–55.

25. On the China program's influence see A. Pio, F. Luelmo, J. Kumaresan, and S. Spinaci, "National Tuberculosis Programme Review: Experience over the Period 1990–95," *Bulletin of the World Health Organization* 75, no. 6 (1997): 569–581, 575; Chen Xianyi, Zhao Fengzeng, Duanmu Hongjin, Wan Liya,

Wang Lixia, Du Xin, and Daniel P. Chin, "The DOTS Strategy in China: Results and Lessons after 10 Years," *Bulletin of the World Health Organization* 80, no. 6 (2002): 430–436.

26. K. Floyd, D. Wilkinson, and C. Gilks, "Comparison of Cost Effectiveness of Directly Observed Treatment (DOT) and Conventionally Delivered Treatment for Tuberculosis: Experience from Rural South Africa," *British Medical Journal* 315, no. 7120 (1997): 1407–1411; D. Wilkinson, G. R. Davies, and C. Connolly, "Directly Observed Therapy for Tuberculosis in Rural South Africa, 1991 Through 1994," *American Journal of Public Health* 86, no. 8 (1996): 1094–1097; D. Wilkinson, "Eight Years of Tuberculosis Research in Hlabisa—What Have We Learned?" *South African Medical Journal* 89, no. 2 (1999): 155–159; D. Wilkinson and G. R. Davies, "Coping with Africa's Increasing Tuberculosis Burden: Are Community Supervisors an Essential Component of the DOT Strategy?" *Tropical Medicine and International Health* 2, no. 7 (1997): 700–704; M. Colvin, L. Gumede, K. Grimwade, D. Maher, and D. Wilkinson, "Contribution of Traditional Healers to a Rural Tuberculosis Control Programme in Hlabisa, South Africa," *International Journal of Tuberculosis and Lung Disease* 7, no. 9, suppl. 1 (2003): S86–S91.

27. D. Wilkinson and K. M. De Cock, "Tuberculosis Control in South Africa—Time for a New Paradigm?" *South African Medical Journal* 86, no. 1 (1996): 33–35, 34.

28. G. R. Davies, C. Connolly, A. W. Sturm, K. P. McAdam, and D. Wilkinson, "Twice-Weekly, Directly Observed Treatment for HIV-Infected and Uninfected Tuberculosis Patients: Cohort Study in Rural South Africa," *AIDS* 13, no. 7 (1999): 811–817.

29. For other flexible programs from India and Nepal not adhering strictly to the WHO model see J. Ogden, S. Rangan, M. Uplekar, J. Porter, R. Brugha, A. Zwi, and D. Nyheim, "Shifting the Paradigm in Tuberculosis Control: Illustrations from India," *International Journal of Tuberculosis and Lung Disease* 3, no. 10 (1999): 855–861, esp. 858; for the problems with DOTS and the private market see Stefan Ecks and Ian Harper, "Public-Private Mixes: The Market for Anti-Tuberculosis Drugs in India," in *When People Come First: Critical Studies in Global Health*, edited by João Biehl and Adriana Petryna (Princeton: Princeton University Press, 2013), 252–275. On the formidable problem of the private sector for TB treatment in India see also Michael Specter, "A Deadly Misdiagnosis," *New Yorker*, 15 November 2010, 48–53.

30. Ricardo Steffen, Dick Menzies, Olivia Oxlade, Marcia Pinto, Analia Zuleika de Castro, Paula Monteiro, and Anete Trajman, "Patients' Costs and Cost-effectiveness of Tuberculosis Treatment in DOTS and Non-DOTS Facilities in Rio De Janeiro, Brazil," *PloS One* 5, no. 11 (2010): e14014.

31. M. A. Khan, J. D. Walley, S. N. Witter, S. K. Shah, and S. Javeed, "Tuberculosis Patient Adherence to Direct Observation: Results of a Social Study in Pakistan," *Health Policy and Planning* 20, no. 6 (2005): 354–365.

32. J. G. Pasipanodya and T. Gumbo, "A Meta-Analysis of Self-Administered vs. Directly Observed Therapy Effect on Microbiologic Failure, Relapse, and Acquired Drug Resistance in Tuberculosis Patients," *Clinical Infectious Diseases* 57, no. 1 (2013): 21–31.

33. Helen S. Cox, Martha Morrow, and Peter W. Deutschmann, "Long Term Efficacy of DOTS Regimens for Tuberculosis: Systematic Review," *British Medical Journal* 336, no. 7642 (2008): doi:10.1136/bmj.39463.640787.BE.

34. E. A. Dosumu, "Compliance in Pulmonary Tuberculosis Patients Using Directly Observed Treatment Short Course," *African Journal of Medicine and Medical Sciences* 30, nos. 1–2 (2001): 111–114, 113.

35. J. C. M. Macq, S. Theobald, J. Dick, and M. Dembele, "An Exploration of the Concept of Directly Observed Treatment (DOT) for Tuberculosis Patients: From a Uniform to a Customised Approach," *International Journal of Tuberculosis and Lung Disease* 7, no. 2 (2003): 103–109.

36. J. Peter Cegielski, "Extensively Drug-Resistant Tuberculosis: 'There Must Be Some Kind of Way Out of Here,'" *Clinical Infectious Diseases* 50, suppl. 3 (2010): S195–S200, S197.

37. Tracy Kidder, *Mountains beyond Mountains: The Quest of Dr. Paul Farmer, a Man Who Would Cure the World* (New York: Random House, 2003), esp. 138–164; Anne Becker, Anjali Motgi, Jonathan Weigel, Giuseppe Raviola, Salmaan Keshavjee, and Arthur Kleinman, "The Unique Challenges of Mental Health and MDRTB: Critical Perspectives on the Metrics of Disease," in *Reimagining Global Health: An Introduction*, edited by Paul Farmer, Jim Yong Kim, Arthur Kleinman, and Matthew Basilico (Berkeley: University of California Press, 2013), 212–244, esp. 234–242.

38. Farmer, "DOTS and DOTS-Plus: Not the Only Answer."

39. WHO, "Tuberculosis Preventive Therapy in HIV-Infected Individuals: A Joint Statement of the WHO Tuberculosis Programme and the Global Programme on AIDS, and the International Union Against Tuberculosis and Lung Disease (IUATLD)," *Weekly Epidemiological Record* 68 (3 December 1993): 361–368, 363.

40. Ibid., 361.

41. J. P. Narain, M. C. Raviglione, and A. Kochi, "HIV-Associated Tuberculosis in Developing Countries: Epidemiology and Strategies for Prevention," *Tubercle and Lung Disease* 73, no. 6 (1992): 311–321, 318.

42. Eric De Jonghe, Christopher J. L. Murray, H. J. Chum, D. S. Nyangulu, A. Salomao, and Karel Styblo, "Cost-Effectiveness of Chemotherapy for Sputum Smear-Positive Pulmonary Tuberculosis in Malawi, Mozambique and Tanzania," *International Journal of Health Planning and Management* 9, no. 2 (1994): 151–181, 152.

43. K. Styblo, "Preventive Chemotherapy for Tuberculosis Control in Developing Countries: The Case Against Preventive Chemotherapy," *Bulletin of the International Union Against Tuberculosis and Lung Disease* 66, suppl. (1990): 27–28; see his earlier comments in K. Styblo, "Recent Advances in Epidemiological Research in Tuberculosis," *Advanced Tuberculosis Research* 20 (1980): 1–63, 46.

44. A similar logic prevailed in the early years of the Roll Back Malaria campaign: when some countries wanted to use residual spraying with DDT they were denied funding based on the fact that bed nets were more cost effective, even though in the places where spraying was sought it was the more effective intervention. Randall M. Packard, *The Making of a Tropical Disease: A Short History of Malaria* (Baltimore: Johns Hopkins University Press, 2007), 227.

45. P. Godfrey-Faussett, R. Baggaley, A. Mwinga, M. Hosp, J. Porter, N. Luo, M. Kelly, R. Msiska, and K. McAdam, "Recruitment to a Trial of Tuberculosis Preventive Therapy from a Voluntary HIV Testing Centre in Lusaka: Relevance to Implementation," *Transactions of the Royal Society of Tropical Medicine and Hygiene* 89, no. 4 (1995): 354–358, 357.

46. Global Tuberculosis Programme, "Tuberculosis and HIV Research: Working Towards Solutions," Results of a WHO Workshop on the Formulation of a New TB/HIV Research Strategy, Geneva, 29–31 May 1995, WHO/TB/95.193, p. 15, WHO Library.

47. S. J. Heymann, "Modelling the Efficacy of Prophylactic and Curative Therapies for Preventing the Spread of Tuberculosis in Africa," *Transactions of the Royal Society of Tropical Medicine and Hygiene* 87, no. 4 (1993): 406–411.

48. WHO and UNAIDS, "Preventive Therapy against Tuberculosis in People Living with HIV: Policy Statement," *Weekly Epidemiological Record* 74 (1999): 385–400, 391, 395.

49. Ibid., 395, 396.

50. Ibid., 396.

51. Ibid., 398.

52. Richard Chaisson, interview with author, 30 April 2013.

53. Jim Yong Kim, Aaron Shakow, Kedar Mate, Chris Vanderwarker, Rajesh Gupta, and Paul Farmer, "Limited Good and Limited Vision: Multidrug-Resistant Tuberculosis and Global Health Policy," *Social Science and Medicine* 61, no. 4 (2005): 847–859, esp. 852.

54. This series of events will sound to some readers like an epistemic community at work, whose members Peter Haas says work at "bringing about their preferred outcomes to the exclusion of others." P. M. Haas, "Introduction: Epistemic Communities and International Policy Coordination," *International Organization* 46, no. 1 (1992): 1–35, 5.

55. Christian Lienhardt, Philippe Glaziou, Mukund Uplekar, Knut Lönnroth, Haileyesus Getahun, and Mario Raviglione, "Global Tuberculosis Control: Lessons Learnt and Future Prospects," *Nature Reviews: Microbiology* 10 (2012): 407–416, 413. For a review of the WHO's repeated recommendations of IPT and still current barriers to its use see Haileyesus Getahuhn, Reuben Granich, Delphine Sculier, Christian Gunnenberg, Leopold Blanc, Paul Nunn, and Mario Raviglione, "Implementation of Isoniazid Preventive Therapy for People Living with HIV Worldwide: Barriers and Solutions," *AIDS* 24, suppl. (2010): S7–S65; for the figure of 2 percent to 2.5 percent see Anthony D. Harries, Rony Zachariah, Elizabeth L. Corbett, Stephan D. Lawn, Ezio T. Santos-Filho, Rhehab Chimzizi, Mark Harrington, Dermot Maher, Brian G. Williams, and Kevin M. De Cock, "The HIV-Associated Tuberculosis Epidemic—When Will We Act?" *Lancet* 375, no. 9729 (2010): 1906–1919, 1909.

56. C. J. Murray and J. A. Salomon., "Modeling the Impact of Global Tuberculosis Control Strategies," *Proceedings of the National Academy of Sciences* 95, no. 23 (1998): 13881–13886, 13881.

57. Ibid., 13884, 13885.

58. The following two meta-analyses cite all the published work to date: D. Wilkinson, S. B. Squire, and P. Garner, "Effect of Preventive Treatment for Tuberculosis in Adults Infected with HIV: Systematic Review of Randomised Placebo Controlled Trials," *British Medical Journal* 317, no. 7159 (1998): 625–629; H. C. Bucher, L. E. Griffith, G. H. Guyatt, P. Sudre, M. Naef, P. Sendi, and M. Battegay, "Isoniazid Prophylaxis for Tuberculosis in HIV Infection: A Meta-analysis of Randomized Controlled Trials," *AIDS* 13, no. 4 (1999): 501–507.

59. S. Foster, P. Godfrey-Faussett, and J. Porter, "Modelling the Economic Benefits of Tuberculosis Preventive Therapy for People with HIV: The Example of Zambia," *AIDS* 11, no. 7 (1997): 919–925; P. Masobe, T. Lee, and M. Price, "Isoniazid Prophylactic Therapy for Tuberculosis in HIV-Seropositive Patients—A Least-Cost Analysis," *South African Medical Journal* 85, no. 2 (1995): 75–81; on Thailand see Chewalit Natrapratan, "Feasibility of Isoniazid Preventive Therapy of Tuberculosis among HIV-Infected Persons in Chiangmai, Thailand," 1994, T9/181/146.2, WHO Archives.

60. J. C. Bell, D. N. Rose, and H. S. Sacks, "Tuberculosis Preventive Therapy for HIV-Infected People in Sub-Saharan Africa Is Cost-Effective," *AIDS* 13, no. 12 (1999): 1549–1556, 1555; see also D. N. Rose, "Short-Course Prophylaxis against Tuberculosis in HIV-Infected Persons: A Decision and Cost-Effectiveness Analysis," *Annals of Internal Medicine* 129, no. 10 (1998): 779–786.

61. On the lack of substantive work on TB/HIV see Haileyesus Getahun, Christian Gunneberg, Reuben Granich, and Paul Nunn, "HIV Infection-Associated Tuberculosis: The Epidemiology and the Response," *Clinical Infectious Diseases* 50, suppl. 3 (2010): S201–S207, S201.

62. Luke Messac and Krishna Prabhu, "Redefining the Possible: The Global AIDS Response," in *Reimagining Global Health: An Introduction*, edited by Paul Farmer, Jim Yong Kim, Arthur Kleinman, and Matthew Basilico (Berkeley: University of California Press, 2013), 111–132, esp. 120–130.

63. See the enlightening article by TAG's director Mark Harrington, "From HIV to Tuberculosis and Back Again: A Tale of Activism in 2 Pandemics," *Clinical Infectious Diseases* 50, suppl. 3 (2010): S260–S266; on this point see especially S263; the Treatment Action Campaign's Zackie Achmat also took on TB. See Z. Achmat, "Science and Social Justice: The Lessons of HIV/AIDS Activism in the Struggle to Eradicate Tuberculosis," *International Journal of Tuberculosis and Lung Disease* 10, no. 12 (2006): 1312–1317.

64. For this claim see Gavin J. Churchyard, Fabio Scano, Alison D. Grant, and Richard E. Chaisson, "Tuberculosis Preventive Therapy in the Era of HIV Infection: Overview and Research Priorities," *Journal of Infectious Diseases* 196, suppl. 1 (2007): S52–S62, S55.

65. Richard Chaisson, interview by author, 30 April 2013.

66. World Health Organization, "Interim Policy on Collaborative TB/HIV Activities," WHO/HTM/TB/2004.330; WHO/HTM/HIV.2004.1, p.2, WHO Library.

67. Erika Check, "Mandela Launches Fight against HIV and TB," published on-line 15 July 2004, *Nature*, doi: 10.1038/news040712–15. On the importance of the Gates grant see Harrington, "From HIV to Tuberculosis and Back Again," S264.

68. WHO, "WHO Three Is Meeting Intensified Case Finding (ICF), Isoniazid Preventive Therapy (IPT), and TB Infection Control (IC) for People Living with HIV," Report of a Joint World Health Organization HIV/AIDS and TB Department Meeting, 2–4 April 2008, Geneva, Switzerland, p. 2; on its cost effectiveness see WHO, "Guidelines for Intensified Tuberculosis Case-Finding and Isoniazid Preventive Therapy for People Living with HIV in Resource-Constrained Settings," Department of HIV/AIDS, Stop TB Department, WHO, Geneva, Switzerland, p. 11. For a recent assessment see S. Gupta, T. Abimbola, A. Date, A. B. Suthar, R. Bennett, N. Sangrujee, and R. Granich, "Cost-Effectiveness of the *Three I's for HIV/TB* and ART to Prevent TB among People Living with HIV," *International Journal of Tuberculosis and Lung Disease* 18, no. 10 (2014): 1159–1165.

69. Reuben Granich, Haileyesus Getahun, Alasdair Reid, Mario Raviglione, and Kevin M. De Cock, "Erring on the Side of Action: Time for HIV Programmes to Implement Isoniazid Preventive Therapy [Editorial]," *International Journal of Tuberculosis and Lung Disease* 13, no. 8 (2009): 925–926.

70. Jonathan E. Golub, Paul Pronyk, Lerato Mohapi, Nkeko Thsabangu, Mosa Moshabela, Helen Struthers, Glenda E. Gray, James A. McIntyre, Richard E. Chaisson, and Neil A. Martinson, "Isoniazid Preventive Therapy, HAART and Tuberculosis Risk in HIV-Infected Adults in South Africa: A Prospective Cohort," *AIDS* 23, no. 5 (2009): 631–636.

71. Haileyesus Getahun, Reuben Granich, Delphine Sculier, Christian Gunneberg, Leopold Blanc, Paul Nunn, and Mario Raviglione, "Implementation of Isoniazid Preventive Therapy for People Living with HIV Worldwide: Barriers and Solutions," *AIDS* 24, suppl. 5 (2010): S57–S65; N. Aït-Khaled, E. Alarcon, K. Bissell, F. Boillot, J. A. Caminero, C.-Y. Chiang, P. Clevenbergh, et al., "Isoniazid Preventive Therapy for People Living with HIV: Public Health Challenges and Implementation Issues," *International Journal of Tuberculosis and Lung Disease* 13, no. 8 (2009): 927–935.

72. Chris Bateman, "Doctor IPT Ignorance Contributing to TB Epidemic—Study," *South African Medical Journal* 101, no. 2 (2011): 88, 90. See also Rebecca Lester, Robin Hamilton, Salome Charalambous, Thobeka

Dwadwa, Clare Chandler, Gavin J. Churchyard, and Alison D. Grant, "Barriers to Implementation of Isoniazid Preventive Therapy in HIV Clinics: A Qualitative Study," *AIDS* 24, suppl. 5 (2010): S45–S48.

73. Katherine L. Fielding, Alison D. Grant, Richard J. Hayes, Richard E. Chaisson, Elizabeth L. Corbett, and Gavin J. Churchyard, "Thibela TB: Design and Methods of a Cluster Randomised Trial of the Effect of Community-wide Isoniazid Preventive Therapy on Tuberculosis amongst Gold Miners in South Africa," *Contemporary Clinical Trials* 32, no. 3 (2011): 382–392, 388. The theoretical possibilities of TB elimination via the prophylactic treatment of latent TB was recently explored and predicted to be successful in P. C. Hill, C. Dye, K. Viney, K. Tabutoa, T. Kienene, K. Bissell, B. G. Williams, R. Zachariah, B. J. Marais, and A. D. Harries, "Mass Treatment to Eliminate Tuberculosis from an Island Population," *International Journal of Tuberculosis and Lung Disease* 18, no. 8 (2014): 899–904.

74. Gavin J. Churchyard, Katherine L. Fielding, James J. Lewis, Leonie Coetzee, Elizabeth L. Corbett, Peter Godfrey-Faussett, Richard J. Hayes, Richard E. Chaisson, Alison D. Grant, and Thibela TB Study Team, "A Trial of Mass Isoniazid Preventive Therapy for Tuberculosis Control," *New England Journal of Medicine* 370, no. 4 (2014): 301–310, 309.

75. For the uncertainty surrounding optimal treatment duration see the following meta-analysis: Christopher Akolo, Ifedayo Adetifa, Sasha Shepperd, and Jimmy Volmink, "Treatment of Latent Tuberculosis Infection in HIV Infected Persons," *Cochrane Database of Systematic Reviews* 1 (2010): 1–82, 8; for the numbers see World Health Organization, *Global Tuberculosis Report, 2012* (Geneva: World Health Organization, 2012), 2.

76. WHO, Department of HIV/AIDS, Stop TB Department, "Guidelines for Intensified Tuberculosis Case Finding and Isoniazid Preventive Therapy for People Living with HIV in Resource Constrained Settings" (Geneva: World Health Organization, 2011). See also C. C. Bristow, E. Larson, A. K. Vilakazi-Nhlapo, M. Wilson, and J. D. Klausner, "Scale-up of Isoniazid Preventive Therapy in PEPFAR-Assisted Clinical Sites in South Africa," *International Journal of Tuberculosis and Lung Disease* 16, no. 8 (2012): 1020–1022.

77. Stephen D. Lawn and Robin Wood, "Short-Course Untargeted Isoniazid Preventive Therapy in South Africa: Time to Rethink Policy?" *International Journal of Tuberculosis and Lung Disease* 16, no. 8 (2012): 995–996, 995.

78. O. Horwitz, P. G. Payne, and E. Wilbek, "Epidemiological Basis of Tuberculosis Eradication: 4. The Isoniazid Trial in Greenland," *Bulletin of the World Health Organization* 35, no. 4 (1966): 509–526.

79. Samandari, Taraz, Tefera B. Agizew, Samba Nyirenda, Zegabriel Tedla, Thabisa Sibanda, Nong Shang, Barudi Mosimaneotsile, et al., "6-month Versus 36-month Isoniazid Preventive Treatment for Tuberculosis in Adults with HIV Infection in Botswana: A Randomised, Double-blind, Placebo-Controlled Trial," *Lancet* 377, no. 9777 (2011): 1588–1598.

80. For a discussion of these issues see Rein M. G. J. Houben, Tom Sumner, Alison D. Grant, and Richard G. White, "Ability of Preventive Therapy to Cure Latent Mycobacterium Tuberculosis Infection in HIV-Infected Individuals in High-Burden Settings," *Proceedings of the National Academy of Sciences* 111, no. 14 (2014): 5325–5330; for drug resistance see Harriet L. Mills, Ted Cohen, and Caroline Colijn, "Community-wide Isoniazid Preventive Therapy Drives Drug-Resistant Tuberculosis: A Model-Based Analysis," *Science Translational Medicine* 5, no. 180 (2013): doi:10.1126/scitranslmed.3005260; Stephen D. Lawn, Robin Wood, Kevin M. De Cock, Katharina Kranzer, James J. Lewis, and Gavin J. Churchyard, "Antiretrovirals and Isoniazid Preventive Therapy in the Prevention of HIV-Associated Tuberculosis in Settings with Limited Health-Care Resources," *Lancet Infectious Diseases* 10: 7 (2010): 489–498.

81. Joel C. Chehab, Amanda K. Vilakazi-Nhlapo, Peter Vranken, Annatjie Peters, and Jeffrey D. Klausner, "Current Integration of Tuberculosis (TB) and HIV Services in South Africa, 2011," *PloS One* 8:3 (2013): 1–6.

82. Salmaan Keshavjee and Paul E. Farmer, "Picking Up the Pace—Scale-up of MDR Tuberculosis Treatment Programs," *New England Journal of Medicine* 363, no. 19 (2010): 1781–84, 1781.

83. For the dismantling of cost effectiveness vis-à-vis MRD-TB see Kim et al., "Limited Good and Limited Vision: Multidrug-Resistant Tuberculosis and Global Health Policy"; see also Paul Farmer and Jim Y. Kim, "Community Based Approaches to the Control of Multidrug Resistant Tuberculosis: Introducing 'DOTS-Plus,'" *British Medical Journal* 317, no. 7159 (1998): 671–674; see generally Salmaan Keshavjee and Paul E. Farmer, "Tuberculosis, Drug Resistance, and the History of Modern Medicine," *New England Journal of Medicine* 367, no. 10 (2012): 931–936.

84. For the shift in thinking see Jim Yong Kim, Joia S. Mukherjee, Michael L. Rich, Kedar Mate, Jaime Bayona, and Mercedes C. Becerra, "From Multidrug-Resistant Tuberculosis to DOTS Expansion and Beyond: Making the Most of a Paradigm Shift," *Tuberculosis* 83, nos. 1–3 (2003): 59–65; for an overview of the era see Victor Roy, "The Politics of Reform in Global Health Policy: The Case of Multi-Drug Resistant Tuberculosis, 1991–2001"

(M.Phil. thesis, University of Cambridge, 2010), esp. pp. 27–67; for the reduction in drug costs see, for example, Rajesh Gupta, Jim Y. Kim, Marcos A. Espinal, Jean-Michel Caudron, Bernard Pecoul, Paul E. Farmer, and Mario C. Raviglione, "Responding to Market Failures in Tuberculosis Control," *Science* 293, no. 5532 (2001): 1049–1051.

85. Salmaan Keshavjee and Paul E. Farmer, "Time to Put Boots on the Ground: Making Universal Access to MDR-TB Treatment a Reality," *International Journal of Tuberculosis and Lung Disease* 14, no. 10 (2010): 1222–1225, 1224.

86. Remarks made during his keynote address at "TB/HIV: Distinct Histories, Entangled Futures: Towards an Epistemology of Co-Infection," 27 and 28 February 2014, Fondation Brocher, Geneva.

CONCLUSION

1. Randall M. Packard and Paul Epstein, "Epidemiologists, Social Scientists, and the Structure of Medical Research on AIDS in Africa," *Social Science and Medicine* 33, no. 7 (1991): 771–783; discussion 783–794.

2. Kurt Toman, "Private and Strictly Confidential, Preliminary Assessment Report, 5 December 1965–16 January 1966," FD 12/556, National Archives of the United Kingdom. In the margin of the report next to the paragraph quoted, suggesting Toman had actually had ample time, someone wrote: "He had five weeks!"

3. Similar questions regarding the past's impact on the present animate an excellent recent collection of essays: Tamara Giles-Vernick and James L. A. Webb, eds., *Global Health in Africa: Historical Perspectives on Disease Control* (Athens: Ohio University Press, 2013); see also Virginia Berridge, "Thinking in Time: Does Health Policy Need History as Evidence?" *Lancet* 375, no. 9717 (2010): 798–799; Berridge, "History Matters? History's Role in Health Policy Making," *Medical History* 52, no. 3 (2008): 311–326, in which she outlines how policy makers might think historically, in the case of vaccines, for instance, when making decisions; see also Vinh-Kim Nguyen, Nathalie Bajos, Françoise Dubois-Arber, Jeffrey O'Malley, and Catherine M. Pirkle, "Remedicalizing an Epidemic: From HIV Treatment as Prevention to HIV Treatment Is Prevention," *AIDS* 25, no. 3 (2011): 291–293, in which the authors warn that "remedicalizing" AIDS, and divorcing it from its social context, is history repeating itself rather than transcending itself.

4. Alison Bashford and Carolyn Strange, "Thinking Historically about Public Health," *Medical Humanities* 33, no. 2 (2007): 87–92.

5. For the example of "treatment as prevention" and the strategic use of history see Guillaume Lachenal, "A Genealogy of Treatment as Prevention (TASP): Prevention, Therapy, and the Tensions of Public Health in African History," in Giles-Vernick and Webb, eds., *Global Health in Africa*, 70–91, 72; on simplifying history to draw lessons from the past see Allan M. Brandt, "From Analysis to Advocacy: Crossing Boundaries as a Historian of Health Policy," in Frank Huisman and John Harley Warner, eds., *Locating Medical History: The Stories and Their Meanings* (Baltimore: Johns Hopkins University Press, 2004), 460–484, esp. 465. Randall M. Packard, *The Making of a Tropical Disease: A Short History of Malaria* (Baltimore: Johns Hopkins Univ. Press, 2007), esp. 113.

6. Available at http://www.historians.org/publications-and-directories/perspectives-on-history/january-2007/what-does-it-mean-to-think-historically. See also Samuel S. Wineburg, *Historical Thinking and Other Unnatural Acts: Charting the Future of Teaching the Past* (Philadelphia: Temple University Press, 2001).

Index